Alternative and Complementary Therapies for Children with Psychiatric Disorders, Part 2

Editors

DEBORAH R. SIMKIN
CHARLES W. POPPER

CHILD AND ADOLESCENT PSYCHIATRIC CLINICS OF NORTH AMERICA

www.childpsych.theclinics.com

Consulting Editor
HARSH K. TRIVEDI

July 2014 • Volume 23 • Number 3

ELSEVIER

1600 John F. Kennedy Boulevard • Suite 1800 • Philadelphia, Pennsylvania, 19103-2899

http://www.theclinics.com

CHILD AND ADOLESCENT PSYCHIATRIC CLINICS OF NORTH AMERICA Volume 23, Number 3
July 2014 ISSN 1056–4993, ISBN-13: 978-0-323-31159-5

Editor: Joanne Husovski
Developmental Editor: Stephanie Carter

Child and Adolescent Psychiatric Clinics of North America (ISSN 1056-4993) is published quarterly by Elsevier Inc., 360 Park Avenue South, New York, NY 10010-1710. Months of issue are January, April, July, and October. Business and Editorial Offices: 1600 John F. Kennedy Boulevard, Suite 1800, Philadelphia, PA 19103-2899. Periodicals postage paid at New York, NY and additional mailing offices. Subscription prices are $310.00 per year (US individuals), $491.00 per year (US institutions), $155.00 per year (US students), $360.00 per year (Canadian individuals), $598.00 per year (Canadian institutions), $200.00 per year (Canadian students), $430.00 per year (international individuals), $598.00 per year (international institutions), and $200.00 per year (international students). International air speed delivery is included in all *Clinics* subscription prices. All prices are subject to change without notice. **POSTMASTER:** Send address changes to *Child and Adolescent Psychiatric Clinics of North America*, Elsevier Health Sciences Division, Subscription Customer Service, 3251 Riverport Lane, Maryland Heights, MO 63043. **Customer Service: 1-800-654-2452 (U.S. and Canada); 314-447-8871 (outside U.S. and Canada). Fax: 314-447-8029. E-mail: JournalsCustomer Service-usa@elsevier.com (for print support) or journalsonlinesupport-usa@elsevier.com (for online support).**

Reprints. For copies of 100 or more of articles in this publication, please contact the Commercial Reprints Department, Elsevier Inc., 360 Park Avenue South, New York, New York 10010-1710 Tel.: 212-633-3874; Fax: 212-633-3820, E-mail: reprints@elsevier.com.

Child and Adolescent Psychiatric Clinics of North America is covered in *MEDLINE/PubMed (Index Medicus), ISI, SSCI, Research Alert, Social Search, Current Contents,* and *EMBASE/Excerpta Medica.*

Contributors

CONSULTING EDITOR

HARSH K. TRIVEDI, MD
Associate Professor of Psychiatry, Vanderbilt University School of Medicine; Executive Medical Director, Chief of Staff, Vanderbilt Psychiatric Hospital, Nashville, Tennessee

CONSULTING EDITOR EMERITUS

ANDRÉS MARTIN, MD, MPH

FOUNDING CONSULTING EDITOR

MELVIN LEWIS, MBBS, FRCPSYCH, DCH

EDITORS

DEBORAH R. SIMKIN, MD, DFAACAP
Member, Committee on Integrative Medicine, American Academy of Child and Adolescent Psychiatry; President, Medical Director, Attention, Memory and Cognition Center, LLC, Destin, Florida; Clinical Assistant Professor, Department of Psychiatry, Emory University School of Medicine, Atlanta, Georgia

CHARLES W. POPPER, MD
Child and Adolescent Psychiatry, McLean Hospital; Harvard Medical School, Belmont, Massachusetts

AUTHORS

L. EUGENE ARNOLD, MD, MEd
Department of Psychiatry, Nisonger Center, The Ohio State University, Columbus, Ohio

NANCY B. BLACK, MD, DFAACAP
Colonel, Medical Corps, U.S. Army; Member, Committee on Integrative Medicine, American Academy of Child and Adolescent Psychiatry; Program and Training Director, National Capital Consortium, Child and Adolescent Psychiatry Fellowship, Walter Reed National Military Medical Center, Bethesda, Maryland

LORI GOODING, PhD, MT-BC
Director of Music Therapy, University of Kentucky School of Music, College of Fine Arts, Lexington, Kentucky

RACHEL V. GOW, PhD
Section of Nutritional Neurosciences, Laboratory of Membrane Biochemistry and Biophysics, National Institute of Alcohol Abuse and Alcoholism, National Institutes of Health, Rockville, Maryland

CAPT JOSEPH R. HIBBELN, MD
Acting Chief, Section of Nutritional Neurosciences, Laboratory of Membrane Biochemistry and Biophysics, National Institute of Alcohol Abuse and Alcoholism, National Institutes of Health, Rockville, Maryland

ELIZABETH HURT, PhD
Postdoctoral Fellow/Instructor, School of Professional Psychology, Wright State University, Dayton, Ohio

NICHOLAS LOFTHOUSE, PhD
School of Professional Psychology, Columbus, Ohio

JOEL LUBAR, PhD
Professor Emeritus, University of Tennessee, Knoxville, Tennessee; Director, Southeastern Neurofeedback Institute, Inc, Pompano Beach, Florida; Past President of International Society for Neurofeedback and Research, McLean, Virginia

CHARLES W. POPPER, MD
Child and Adolescent Psychiatry, McLean Hospital; Harvard Medical School, Belmont, Massachusetts

DEBORAH R. SIMKIN, MD, DFAACAP
Member, Committee on Integrative Medicine, American Academy of Child and Adolescent Psychiatry; President, Medical Director, Attention, Memory and Cognition Center, LLC, Destin, Florida; Clinical Assistant Professor, Department of Psychiatry, Emory University School of Medicine, Atlanta, Georgia

ROBERT W. THATCHER, PhD
Neuroimaging Laboratory, Director, Applied Neuroscience Research Institute, Seminole, Florida

OLIVIA SWEDBERG YINGER, PhD, MT-BC
Assistant Professor of Music Therapy, University of Kentucky School of Music, College of Fine Arts, Lexington, Kentucky

Contents

This article explores the science surrounding neurofeedback. Both surface neurofeedback (using 2–4 electrodes) and newer interventions, such as real-time z-score neurofeedback (electroencephalogram [EEG] biofeedback) and low-resolution electromagnetic tomography neurofeedback, are reviewed. The limited literature on neurofeedback research in children and adolescents is discussed regarding treatment of anxiety, mood, addiction (with comorbid attention-deficit/hyperactivity disorder), and traumatic brain injury. Future potential applications, the use of quantitative EEG for determining which patients will be responsive to medications, the role of randomized controlled studies in neurofeedback research, and sensible clinical guidelines are considered.

Neurofeedback (NF) using surface electroencephalographic signals has been used to treat various child psychiatric disorders by providing patients with video/audio information about their brain's electrical activity in real-time. Research data are reviewed and clinical recommendations are made regarding NF treatment of youth with attention deficit/hyperactivity disorder, autism, learning disorders, and epilepsy. Most NF studies are limited by methodological issues, such as failure to use or test the validity of a full-blind or sham NF. The safety of NF treatment has not been thoroughly investigated in youth or adults, although clinical experience suggests reasonable safety.

This article describes the various forms of meditation and provides an overview of research using these techniques for children, adolescents, and their families. The most researched techniques in children and adolescents are mindfulness-based stress reduction, mindfulness-based cognitive therapy, yoga meditation, transcendental meditation, mind-body techniques (meditation, relaxation), and body-mind techniques (yoga poses, tai chi movements). Current data are suggestive of a possible value of meditation and mindfulness techniques for treating symptomatic anxiety, depression, and pain in youth. Clinicians must be properly trained before using these techniques.

This article summarizes the research on music therapy and music medicine for children and adolescents with diagnoses commonly treated by psychiatrists. Music therapy and music medicine are defined, effects of music on the brain are described, and music therapy research in psychiatric treatment is discussed. Music therapy research with specific child/adolescent populations is summarized, including disorders usually diagnosed in childhood, substance abuse, mood/anxiety disorders, and eating disorders. Clinical implications are listed, including suggestions for health care professionals seeking to use music medicine techniques. Strengths and weaknesses of music therapy treatment are discussed, as well as areas for future research.

Nutritional insufficiencies of omega-3 highly unsaturated fatty acids (HUFAs) may have adverse effects on brain development and neurodevelopmental outcomes. A recent meta-analysis reported a small to modest effect size for the efficacy of omega-3 in youth. Several controlled trials of omega-3 HUFAs combined with micronutrients show sizable reductions in aggressive, antisocial, and violent behavior in youth and young adult prisoners. Studies of HUFAs in youth, however, remain lacking. As the evidence base for omega-3 HUFAs as potential psychiatric treatment develops, dietary adjustments to increase omega-3 and reduce omega-6 HUFA consumption are sensible recommendations based on general health considerations.

Several different vitamins and minerals appear to be effective augmenting agents for mood-modifying drugs, but are not potent monotherapies in themselves for treating psychiatric disorders. In contrast, broad-spectrum micronutrient interventions appear in early trials to be as effective as psychiatric medications with fewer adverse effects for treating mood disorders, ADHD, aggressivity, and misconduct in youth and adults. Broad-spectrum treatments also may improve stress responses, cognition, and sense of well-being in healthy adults, but have been less well studied in youth. Current clinical data justify an extensive expansion of research on micronutrient mechanisms and treatments in psychiatry.

CHILD AND ADOLESCENT PSYCHIATRIC CLINICS

RELATED INTEREST

Medical Clinics of North America, May 2010 (Vol. 94, No. 3)
Insomnia and Its Effective Non-pharmacologic Treatment
Allison T. Siebern and Rachel Manber, *Editors*

AACAP Members: Please go to www.jaacap.org for information on access to the Child and Adolescent Psychiatric Clinics. *Resident* Members of AACAP: Special access information is available at www.childpsych.theclinics.com.

**DOWNLOAD
Free App!**

Review Articles
THE CLINICS

NOW AVAILABLE FOR YOUR iPhone and iPad

Preface

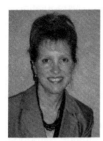
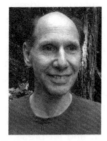

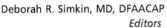

Deborah R. Simkin, MD, DFAACAP   Charles W. Popper, MD
Editors

This is the second of a two-part series on alternative and complementary therapies for psychiatric disorders published in the *Child and Adolescent Psychiatric Clinics of North America*. In Part 1, issued in 2013, the articles were organized to describe the current treatment research on several of the major psychiatric disorders of children and adolescents, including attention deficit hyperactivity disorder (ADHD), mood disorders, autism, and learning disorders. Overviews were also offered regarding the national research effort in complementary and alternative medicine (CAM), translating these treatments into clinical practice, and legal issues regarding CAM treatments that are relevant to child and adolescent psychiatrists.

In Part 2, the emphasis is shifted to specific CAM treatment techniques and the research developments pertaining to their use in treating child and adolescent psychiatric disorders. There are an enormous number of CAM treatments, many that have been proposed for treating psychiatric disorders, and each of these CAM treatments has potential applications for managing a range of psychiatric disorders. Some of the methods are already widely utilized by patients and clinicians, but research on these techniques is limited in psychiatry, especially in child and adolescent psychiatry. The selection of treatments in this issue was based on the availability of systematic research on the treatments specifically in children and adolescents, and also on the general public interest in these approaches. These selected interventions include neurofeedback, mindfulness/meditation, music therapy and music medicine, essential fatty acids, and micronutrients (vitamins and minerals).

Neurofeedback is a relatively new intervention that has been built on modern science and technology. Several neurofeedback techniques have been developed, and the clinical research on youth is described in two articles. One article reports on surface neurofeedback, which is the most commonly studied neurofeedback technique in children and adolescents, particularly for youth with attention deficit disorder, autism, epilepsy, and learning disorders. The second article discusses the few research studies using surface neurofeedback for children and adolescents with depressive disorders, anxiety disorders, comorbid addiction/ADHD disorders, and traumatic brain injury. The second article also explains the science behind the use of quantitative EEG and describes a newer neurofeedback approach that has so far received little

http://dx.doi.org/10.1016/j.chc.2014.04.002
1056-4993/14/$ – see front matter
childpsych.theclinics.com

study in youth: low-resolution electromagnetic tomography (LORETA) neurofeedback. LORETA targets deeper neuronal hubs, modules, and circuits. Clinically, LORETA holds promise as a novel intervention for addressing the central dysregulation associated with psychiatric disorders in youth by normalizing brain function at the level of neuronal circuits and by improving symptom clusters based on connectivity between specialized neuronal populations. This approach of targeting functions that are based on neuronal dysregulation is consistent with the "transdiagnostic" approach exemplified by the Research Domain Criteria of the National Institute of Mental Health. Although the best evidence for the use of neurofeedback concerns ADHD (and to a lesser extent, autism and learning disorders), there remains some degree of controversy regarding the suitability of neurofeedback for general clinical application, due to the time demands, cost, and (at present) lack of insurance reimbursement. Neurofeedback treatment requires referral to a clinician who has received significant training in the appropriate protocols and technologies.

In contrast to neurofeedback, mindfulness and meditation approaches are derived from several ancient traditions that originated centuries ago, and their powers have often been viewed as mystical or mysterious. Modern neuroimaging and EEG technology have helped scientists and clinicians understand the powerful effects that these techniques have on the brain and their benefits for patients with psychiatric disorders. With so many distinct techniques used in mindfulness/meditation, these techniques are presented in five categories: focused attention, open monitoring, transcendental meditation (automatic self-transcending), mind-body techniques, and body-mind techniques. Both mind-body and body-mind techniques often utilize many mindfulness/meditation methods; however, mind-body also includes relaxation components, and body-mind also uses movement techniques (such as Tai Chi) or body postures (such as yoga). Several mindfulness and meditation techniques have been examined for medical indications, but only transcendental medicine has been recognized by the American Heart Association as effective in reducing hypertension in adults. There are few well-conducted randomized controlled trials in children and adolescents for medical and/or psychiatric indications, but the minimal adverse effects make them particularly appealing despite the scarce scientific support. These techniques can be applied in schools and clinics, but the methods should be taught by highly trained personnel. Differences in therapeutic effectiveness among these methods are likely to be uncovered when used as adjunctive treatments for various psychiatric indications, and the effectiveness of the different methods may differ from adults in youth at different ages.

Music has been used as a clinical treatment in medicine for more than three decades, especially with youth and the elderly. In the past, music medicine involved mainly passive listening and did not require trained specialists. More recently, several techniques of actual music therapy have been developed and have been shown to decrease pain and anxiety in adults and youth with cancer. Music therapy has also been used for mental and emotional problems in children and adolescents, with some studies suggesting benefits for intellectual disabilities, emotional and behavioral conditions, and learning disorders. Preliminary data have also examined youth with autism, mood and anxiety disorders, substance abuse, and eating disorders. Music therapy for brain-injured patients became publically prominent when it was employed in the recovery and rehabilitation of former US Congresswoman Representative Gabrielle Gifford. Music therapy has been shown to induce physiological changes in youth and adults as well as hormonal changes in adults, giving credence to the neurobiological legitimacy of this intervention. To acquire clinical sophistication in this field, music therapists receive 2 to 4 years of comprehensive training to become eligible for board certification. Despite the scarcity of substantive data on music therapy as an adjunctive treatment for youth with psychiatric disorders, this promising field deserves clinicians' attention, especially in view of its low risks.

Essential fatty acids are well-established to be critical for proper brain development, and nutritional deficiencies of omega-3 fatty acids appear to have significant effects on neurodevelopmental outcomes. Psychiatric research in youth is not extensive, but available data suggest their value as adjunctive treatments for youth with ADHD, depression, and possibly bipolar disorder. The effect on ADHD appears small but sufficient to justify its use as an adjunctive agent. Some studies of essential fatty acids (when combined with micronutrients) have shown clear-cut and clinically significant benefits for youth (and young adults) with violent, aggressive, and antisocial behaviors associated with conduct disorder in school settings and even in young adult prisoners. It is unclear whether these improvements in conduct disorder are related to symptomatic improvements in ADHD or in mood disorders, and current studies are insufficient to determine what effect essential fatty acid treatments might have in children and adolescents with major depression or bipolar disorder. Further research is needed as well to assess which of the essential fatty acids (and in what relative ratios) may be most relevant for different psychiatric disorders in youth. While treatment outcome data are gathering, the easiest justifications for the clinical use of omega-3 fatty acids are their minimal profile of adverse effects and their broad-ranging (although still debated) benefits to general health.

Micronutrient (vitamin and mineral) supplements have been investigated for their potential for treating psychiatric disorders, especially mood disorders. Certain vitamins, such as folate and perhaps chromium, show significant potential as adjunctive psychiatric treatments in adults. An alternative treatment approach is the use of a broad spectrum of micronutrients, rather than single vitamins or minerals. Although few randomized controlled trials have been conducted, a series of publications on broad-spectrum micronutrient treatments has described clinically significant improvements in youth and adults with mood disorders and ADHD. Based on the preliminary findings in the literature, it appears that broad-spectrum micronutrient approaches may be comparable in clinical effectiveness to psychiatric medications for treating mood disorders, but with much fewer adverse effects than conventional psychiatric medications. Drug-nutrient interactions are surprisingly extensive and complex. Clinicians who wish to employ these treatments will need to become savvy in some aspects of nutritional pharmacology before applying the broad-spectrum treatments, and patients would need to provide well-informed consent in view of the dearth of controlled trials. Broad-spectrum micronutrient treatment appears to have the potential to eventually become a primary monotherapy for bipolar disorder (and probably for non-bipolar major depression as well) and an adjunctive therapy for ADHD, based on currently available studies in youth and adults. The data are limited, but impressive, and justify further research in youth as well as in adults.

In comparing these very different approaches, our authors have employed the US Preventive Service Task Force system to grade the quality of available research supporting the different treatments. This element of continuity will allow clinicians to sense the relative strengths and weaknesses of the evidence base for the different approaches, and it is hoped, will guide researchers toward fruitful areas of investigation.

All of these CAM treatments illustrate the abundance of new directions that are being explored with a new openness and inquisitiveness in medicine. Novel "alternative" treatments of yesterday (eg, cognitive behavior therapy) can become the conventional treatments of today, and a bit ironically, some conventional treatments of today become "alternative" treatments as they are replaced by newer methods. What counts as "alternative" is time-based and culture-based. The current culture of psychiatry is increasingly exhibiting the curiosity and imagination that have been hallmarks of the best of medical research and innovative care. By shedding light on new and promising "CAM" research and the neuroscience underlying these approaches, it is hoped that newer and more diverse interventions will become available to support the health and development of children and adolescents.

We want to again express our gratitude to our series editor, Dr Harsh Trivedi, for granting two issues of the *Child and Adolescent Psychiatric Clinics of North America* to present this unorthodox side of our field, and to Joanne Husovski and Stephanie Carter, our editors at Elsevier, whose devoted work, kindness, prudence, intellect, and grace have been a vital force for us.

Deborah R. Simkin, MD, DFAACAP
American Academy of Child and Adolescent Psychiatry
Attention, Memory and Cognition Center, LLC
4641 Gulfstarr Drive, Suite 106
Destin, FL 32541, USA

Charles W. Popper, MD*
Child and Adolescent Psychiatry
McLean Hospital and Harvard Medical School
Belmont, MA 02478, USA

E-mail addresses:
Deb62288@aol.com (D.R. Simkin)
Charles_Popper@harvard.edu (C.W. Popper)

*385 Concord Avenue, Suite 204
Belmont, MA 02478-3037, USA

Quantitative EEG and Neurofeedback in Children and Adolescents

Anxiety Disorders, Depressive Disorders, Comorbid Addiction and Attention-deficit/Hyperactivity Disorder, and Brain Injury

Deborah R. Simkin, MD, DFAACAP[a,b,]*, Robert W. Thatcher, PhD[c], Joel Lubar, PhD[d,e,f]

KEYWORDS

- Quantitative EEG • Neurofeedback • LORETA • Anxiety disorders • Depression
- Addiction • ADHD • Brain injury in children and adolescents

KEY POINTS

- The waveforms on an electroencephalogram (EEG) result directly from synaptic activity in brain networks, and neurofeedback offers the opportunity for patients to use operant conditioning to alter their waveforms and brain functioning.
- Quantitative EEGs (qEEGs) represent a patient's waveforms compared with normative EEG databases and may be corepresented with functional magnetic resonance imaging (fMRI), single-photon emission computed tomography, positron emission tomography (PET), and magnetic resonance imaging.
- qEEG, modern PET, magnetoencephalography, and fMRI studies concur in showing that the brain is organized by a small set of modules or hubs that represent clusters of neurons characterized by high within-cluster connectivity and sparse long-distance connectivity.
- During child development, functional brain connectivity is substantially reorganized, but several large-scale network properties seem to be preserved over time, suggesting that functional brain networks in children are organized like other complex systems in adults.

Continued

Disclosures: Research support received from Eli Lilly and Company; Pfizer Inc; Novartis Pharmaceutical Corporation.
[a] Committee on Integrative Medicine, American Academy of Child and Adolescent Psychiatry, Attention, Memory and Cognition Center, 4641 Gulfstarr Drive, Suite 106, Destin, FL 32541, USA; [b] Department of Psychiatry, Emory University Medical School, Atlanta, Georgia; [c] Neuroimaging Laboratory, Applied Neuroscience Research Institute, 7985 113th Street, Suite 210, Seminole, FL 33772, USA; [d] University of Tennessee, Knoxville, TN, USA; [e] Southeastern Neurofeedback Institute, Inc, 111 North Pompano Beach Boulevard, Suite 1214, Pompano Beach, FL 33062, USA; [f] International Society for Neurofeedback and Research
* Corresponding author. 4641 Gulfstarr Drive, Suite 106, Destin, FL 32541.
E-mail address: deb62288@aol.com

Child Adolesc Psychiatric Clin N Am 23 (2014) 427–464
http://dx.doi.org/10.1016/j.chc.2014.03.001   childpsych.theclinics.com
1056-4993/14/$ – see front matter © 2014 Elsevier Inc. All rights reserved.

Key Points (*Continued*)

- Circuitry dysconnections (in and between these hubs or networks) have been associated with symptoms of psychiatric illness, and these dysconnections can be targeted using neurofeedback.
- Quantitative EEG provides an opportunity for new evaluation techniques permitting more efficient treatment matching, such as determining which patients will be responsive to certain medications or which areas of the brain should be targeted during neurofeedback treatment.
- Clinicians must be intensively trained in appropriate protocols and technologies in order to provide appropriate clinical neurofeedback treatment and to develop research sound research.
- Although little research has been done using neurofeedback in children and adolescents with anxiety disorders, mood disorders, comorbid addiction and attention-deficit/hyperactivity disorder, and brain injury, the adult literature and more recent advances in neurofeedback interventions (eg, low-resolution electromagnetic tomography) hold particular promise for future research using fewer sessions.

Abbreviations: Quantitative EEG and Neurofeedback	
ADHD	Attention-deficit/hyperactivity disorder
ApoE	Apolipoprotein E
BET	Brain electromagnetic tomography
BRIEF-R	Behavior Rating Inventory of Executive Function-R
DRD2	Dopamine D2 receptor
DSI	Diffuse spectral imaging
EEG	Electroencephalogram
EMG	Electromyography
fMRI	Functional magnetic resonance imaging
GABA	Glutamate and gamma-aminobutyric acid
HD	High dysregulation
IVA-Plus	Integrated Visual and Auditory Continuous Performance Test
JTFA	Joint time-frequency analysis
LD	Low dysregulation
LFP	Local field potentials
LORETA	Low-resolution electromagnetic tomography
LPFC	Lateral prefrontal cortex
LTP	Long-term potentiation
MEG	Magnetoencephalography
NF	Neurofeedback
NIMH	National Institute of Mental Health
PET	Positron emission tomography
PFC	Prefrontal cortex
PTSD	Posttraumatic stress disorder
qEEG	Quantitative electroencephalogram
RDoC	Research domain criteria
rIFG	Right inferior frontal gyrus
ROIs	Subregions of interest
SMR	Sensory motor rhythms
SPECT	Single-photon emission computed tomography
SPM	Statistical parametric mapping
TOVA	Test of variable assessment
USPSTF	United States Preventive Services Task Force
vmPFC	Ventromedial prefrontal cortex
WISC-R	Weschler Intelligence Scale for Children-Revised

INTRODUCTION

Neurofeedback (NF) is a treatment method for altering brain functioning by the use of signals provided to a patient that reflect the moment-to-moment changes in the patient's electroencephalogram (EEG). The method typically uses advanced statistical analysis of quantitative data from the EEG (quantitative EEG [qEEG]) to provide biofeedback to the patient in real time. This approach allows the operant conditioning of the patient's EEG, which, perhaps surprisingly, can have the effect of therapeutically altering cognition, emotions, and behavior.

This article explores the science surrounding NF and reviews the early research on the use of NF technology for treating psychiatric disorders in children and adolescents. Although surface NF (using 2–4 electrodes, which did not use qEEG initially) has long been used, several new NF interventions have been developed. Many of these new interventions, along with surface NF, can now incorporate the use of quantitative electroencephalography to enhance their clinical value.

Three major NF methodologies are real-time z-score surface NF, low-resolution electromagnetic tomography (LORETA), and functional magnetic resonance imaging (fMRI) NF.

Real-time z-score surface NF (EEG biofeedback) uses 2 to 4 or more scalp electrodes to monitor the brain's electrical activity in a particular anatomic location. It uses continuous real-time computerized calculations based on qEEG data comparing the way that the patient's brain is functioning on different variables with an age-matched normative database, using z scores to measure differences from normal EEG activity. The z score is the number of standard deviations of an observation (data on EEG waveform) more than (positive) or less than (negative) the mean. The z scores or standard deviations relative to an age-matched reference population provide a real-time indication of abnormal instabilities in brain networks. These z scores provide a guide to train patients toward quantitatively normal waveforms ($z = 0$) in brain regions associated with particular disorders.

If the surface NF involves the use of 2 or more electrodes, coherence (the measure of the number of connections and communications between groups of neurons) can also be trained during NF training. However, if only 1 electrode is used during NF training, no coherence training can occur. In addition, surface NF involves measuring the amplitude of neurons directly beneath the electrode where 95% of the neurons arise from a distance of 6 cm and all frequencies are mixed together at each electrode. However, LORETA uses three-dimensional source localization applied to human qEEG in which the mixture of frequencies under each scalp electrode are unscrambled and linked to three-dimensional sources in the interior of the brain with accuracies of approximately 1 cm in many situations.

LORETA NF uses a different kind of qEEG NF analysis that provides an estimation of the location of the deep underlying brain generators, called modules or hubs (eg, the anterior cingulate, insula, fusiform gyrus) and networks of the patient's EEG activity within a frequency band. It allows the clinician to translate qEEG data into a three-dimensional figure that corresponds with and looks like the images in fMRI that are associated with disease states. It requires more labor-intensive preparation, because an electrode cap with 19 electrodes must be applied in every session, but it can shorten the length of treatment. Coherence training can include multiple areas.

fMRI NF's advantage is that it can examine functioning at deep subcortical areas of the brain. However, the practical disadvantage of fMRI NF is that it is expensive, with equipment that costs $1 million or more and is not portable.

NF research has been limited in children and adolescents, especially with regard to anxiety, mood, addiction, and traumatic brain injury (TBI). Research has shown that functional hub architecture matures in late childhood and remains stable from adolescence to early adulthood. Thus, LORETA NF, which targets modules and connections between modules, is expected to work the same in patients from 10 years of age to adulthood.

New transdiagnostic approaches, proposed by the National Institute on Mental Health, to defining psychiatric disorders based on dysfunctional connectivity are particularly significant because NF targets dysfunctional connectivity. Clinicians want to familiarize themselves with possible new treatment interventions that target these transdiagnostic symptoms. Other uses of qEEG include determining whether patients will be responsive to medications. In addition, the initial findings on NF research for treating psychiatric symptoms in youth will be covered.

NEUROFEEDBACK BASICS

NF is based on operant conditioning. NF is based on measurements of evoked potentials as measured in electroencephalography. An evoked potential can be negative or positive relative to the average baseline potential. An N100 is a negative evoked potential that is generated by a network of neurons, usually provoked by an unexpected stimulus, in a brain location depending on the sensory modality. P100 is a positive evoked potential in the same region.

Suppose an electrode is recording a P100 evoked potential in a particular area of the brain, and the goal of the NF intervention (to treat a symptom) is to change the P100 positive evoked potential to an N100 negative evoked potential. Following the methods used in operant conditioning, every time an N100 evoked potential begins to occur by chance, a positive reinforcement is provided. The positive reinforcement could be milk delivered into a bowl for a cat. In NF, the patient is provided with a positive reinforcement through the biofeedback presentation of a signal that is linked to the desired alteration in brain wave pattern. The brain would eventually learn to search for this N100 evoked potential in order to receive the positive reinforcement associated with this evoked potential. This example shows how, through operant conditioning, NF can provide a reward for the appearance of a particular electrical event in the brain. The electrical pattern soon begins to appear before the reward, leading to increased frequency of appearance of that electrical pattern. In a similar way in humans, if a dot appears on the screen during an NF session with each occurrence of a particular targeted EEG pattern or rhythm (eg, delta 0–4 Hz, theta 4–8 Hz, alpha 8–12 Hz, beta 12–20 Hz, gamma 20–300 Hz), the rhythm eventually continue to occur in anticipation of the dot appearing.

By knowing the anatomic location of a particular electrical pattern associated with a targeted brain function, NF can be used to change a wide variety of brain functions, including depressed states, anxiety, addiction, injury-induced abnormalities, and attention-deficit/hyperactivity disorder (ADHD). Thus, a precise system for mapping locations in the brain is essential to NF.

To detect specific electrical patterns in the brain, EEG electrodes are placed on the scalp corresponding with anatomic areas associated with particular Brodmann areas, with the aim of targeting certain functions associated with these areas. A targeted rhythm can be pinpointed by an electrode placed on the scalp (for example, corresponding with T3, using the International 10–20 System illustrated in **Fig. 1**, which corresponds with a particular area of the brain). For example, T3 is associated with Brodmann areas 22/42 on the superior temporal gyrus. Affective prosody is

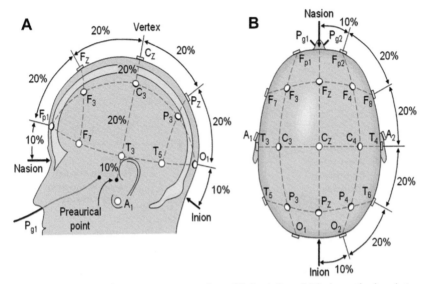

Fig. 1. The International 10–20 System seen from (*A*) the left and (*B*) above the head. A, ear lobe; C, central; F, frontal; F_p, frontal polar; O, occipital; P, parietal; P_g, nasopharyngeal. (*From* Ferreira A, Celeste WC, Cheein FA, et al. Human-machine interfaces based on EMG and EEG applied to robotic systems. J Neuroeng Rehabil 2008;5:10.)

associated with this Brodmann area on the right and language processing on the left. Abnormal evoked potentials (representing abnormal brain wavelengths) in this region may be identified on an EEG. Using NF to target specific Brodmann areas that have abnormal evoked potentials that are found in an individual to be associated with symptoms or specific disorders may change that area of the brain back to a normal pattern and, it is hoped, decrease the symptoms of the disorder.[1]

NF is based on the clinician's ability to link a patient's symptoms and complaints to dysregulation or deviation from normal in EEG patterns in particular brain regions known to be related to specific functions. **Fig. 2** shows the various anatomic regions of the brain, originally delineated by Brodmann[2] in 1909 based on their microarchitecture and their links to particular functions, as based on the findings of various techniques across many patients. Brodmann areas are macroscopic brain regions of common functional cytoarchitecture ranging in size from about 1 cm to 6 cm, and a qEEG can give a precise delineation of these Brodmann areas for each individual. Following qEEG assessment of abnormal brain rhythms in precisely defined brain regions in an individual, NF treatment aims to modify dysregulated subsystems and global linkages toward the normal range of function. Periodic qEEG assessments during treatment can be used to monitor treatment efficacy. The assessment is similar to the use of a blood test to identify deviant constituents of the blood (eg, increased liver enzymes) that can be linked to the patient's symptoms and aid in making treatment decisions and monitoring treatment efficacy.[3]

HOW NEUROFEEDBACK CHANGES ACTION POTENTIALS

The science and techniques involved in NF are described in more detail in the *Handbook on Quantitative Electroencephalography and EEG Biofeedback* by Thatcher.[1]

The registration of wavelengths on a raw EEG results directly from synaptic electrical action potentials produced by chemical synapses in neuronal networks. There are

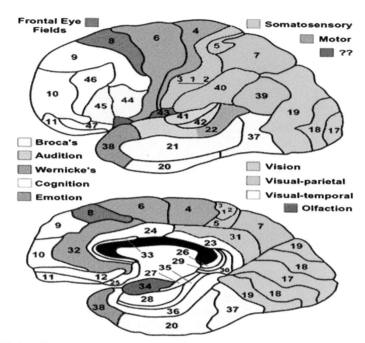

Fig. 2. Various functions associated with particular Brodmann areas based on fMRI, PET, EEG/magnetoencephalography (MEG), and lesion/tumor studies. (*Data from* Refs.[1-5]; and *Courtesy of* M. Dubin, PhD, Boulder, CO.)

2 types of chemical synapses that produce the EEG wavelengths. First, fast synapses involve the neurotransmitters glutamate and gamma-aminobutyric acid (GABA), which are associated with fast gated ion channels (which occur from 0–80 milliseconds). Second, slow synapses involve dopamine, serotonin, acetycholine, and norepinephrine, which are associated with slow voltage gated ion channels (which occur from 100 milliseconds to 1 second). These excitatory and inhibitory postsynaptic potentials give rise to local field potentials (LFPs). LFPs influence the firing of action potentials in pyramidal neurons near the surface of the brain.[1,6] These wavelengths can be changed by operant conditioning that targets these networks. Operant conditioning of the EEG involves changes in synapses caused by what is referred to as a phase reset. Operant conditioning begins by reinforcing a frequency (eg, 5 Hz) associated with a particular wavelength (eg, theta) detected by EEG electrodes near the surface of the brain. When a desired wavelength occurs, there is a burst of action potentials that impinges on the dendrites and cell bodies of pyramidal neurons. The time it takes for this wavelength shift to occur is referred to as phase shift duration and it can be seen on an EEG when the same wavelengths are not in sync (**Fig. 3**). When a phase lock occurs, the desired wavelengths will be synchronized (see **Fig. 3**).

To describe a phase shift or wavelength shift, Thatcher[1] gave the following example. Imagine a family is at a Thanksgiving dinner, and an unexpected relative suddenly arrives whom no one has seen in years. The family shifts from focusing on the dinner to focusing on the relative at the door. Over time, as more and more of the family members recognize the unexpected relative, more family members shift their attention and move toward the door. If more time is given (phase shift duration), more family members move to the door. This analogy also applies for phase shifts in the brain. The

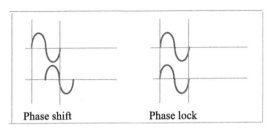

Phase shift   Phase lock

Fig. 3. Phase lock.

longer the duration of the phase shift, the greater the number of neurons that are recruited.[1] When this burst of neuronal activity synchronously occurs in millions of neurons, then a detectable change in the EEG frequencies occurs, (eg, from theta 4–8 Hz to alpha 8–12 Hz).[7]

When all the family members arrive at the door, a phase lock occurs (when all of the EEG frequencies are the same for a particular rhythm). During operant conditioning, a wavelength rhythm is reinforced when the duration of phase lock is increased and the frequency of phase shift is decreased. Likewise, a rhythm is inhibited when the duration of phase lock is decreased and the frequency of phase shift is increased.[1] During NF, a change in an individual's EEG activity can be reinforced by a visual and/or auditory stimulus. As NF continues, the reinforcement is more difficult to obtain because the length of time the individual has to sustain the preferred wavelength is increased. As the individual masters the level of difficulty in sustaining the preferred wavelength, the clinician increases the level of difficulty in order to continually challenge the brain by increasing the length of time the individual must hold the preferred wavelength.

Fast excitatory chemical synapses dominate long-distance corticocortical loops and fast inhibitory synapses dominate short-distance loops. However, long-duration neurotransmitters shape and mold the mechanisms of long-term potentiation (LTP).[1,8] Synapse modifications occur during the phase lock. Neurotransmitters, such as dopamine, are released in anticipation of these rewarding experiences that occur when particular wavelength patterns are elicited during phase lock. Neurotransmitters released during phase lock can influence structural plasticity within the brain. Phase lock produces a long-lasting enhancement in signal transmission between 2 neurons that results from their synchronous firing, which is associated with increased dendrite formation and increase neurotransmitter delivery into the cleft. This process of synapse modification is called LTP, and it requires synapse growth and the development of new synapses during learning. Kandel[9] received the Nobel Prize in 2000 for his work linking LTP to DNA, RNA, and protein production associated with learning and memory formation. Phase lock results in LTP or neuronal learning at the molecular level that moves the patient having NF treatment toward normal functioning.

In effect, EEG NF uses operant conditioning to (1) reinforce particular brain rhythms by reinforcing phase lock and decreasing phase shift, or (2) inhibiting rhythms by decreasing the frequency of phase lock and increasing the frequency of phase. The phase shifts and phase locks reinforced by NF are associated with long-term synaptic modifications characterized by changes in neurotransmitter release and neuronal functioning. For example, if the symptoms of ADHD are known to be associated with an abnormal wavelength in a particular area of the brain, then NF can change the wavelength to those found in normal individuals. By using NF, clinicians may be able to effectively treat the symptoms of ADHD by selectively enhancing dopamine transmission in the relevant parts of the brain.

In addition to frequency changes and phase shifts, NF can be used to modify synaptic and network functioning by operating on EEG data reflecting brain coherence. Coherence is a measure of coupling between groups of neurons, or more precisely a measure of the number of connections and communications (or frequency of activity) between groups of neurons with a constant phase relationship. Coherence is proportional to phase lock and inversely proportional to phase shift; when coherence is working well in desired networks, several areas of the brain are in phase lock.

IS ALL BRAIN BIOFEEDBACK ALIKE?

NF is a subtype of EEG biofeedback in which EEG data, or signals based on EEG data, are used as the feedback to the patient. Other types of biofeedback include electromyography (EMG) biofeedback and thermal (or temperature) biofeedback. EMG biofeedback measures electrical activity associated with muscle contractions, and it is often used for relaxation training, stress management, peak performance training, and pain management. Thermal biofeedback uses a temperature sensor (electronic, computerized, liquid crystal, or a glass thermometer) to detect temperature changes in the extremities (usually fingertips or toes). Stress and nervous system excitation/arousal causes blood vessels in the extremities to constrict, and the reduced blood flow leads to cooling. Thermal biofeedback is used to train people to quiet the nervous system arousal mechanisms that produce hand or foot cooling, and this is often used for relaxation training, stress management, and pain management.[10]

In contrast, NF specifically uses data based on brain functioning, specifically EEG data. Surface NF, involving 2 to 4 electrodes, started before the advent of qEEG, but modern surface NF often uses qEEG data for assessment before NF treatment is begun. LORETA, which involves many more electrodes and can capture EEG data from deeper structures, is a newer approach that makes integral use of qEEG data. Other forms of NF are discussed by Hurt and colleagues elsewhere in this issue.

QUANTITATIVE ELECTROENCEPHALOGRAPHY AND ITS ROLE IN NEUROFEEDBACK

Quantitative electroencephalography involves computerized data analysis to precisely quantify the electrical potentials or frequency bands from 0 Hz to transform the EEG to a format that elucidates relevant information, such as highlighting specific waveforms components.[11] The mathematical technique used to decompose and transform the mixture of waves in the human EEG is Fourier transform or, given the periodic nature of EEG data, the Fourier series coefficients. Joint time-frequency analysis (JTFA) is another mathematical procedure developed in the late 1980s that gave rise to precise time-frequency measures and quantification of phase locks and phase shifts.[12]

For technically informed readers, some features of qEEG that can be used as the basis for NF include absolute power (the average amount of power uV2 in each frequency band or wavelength and in the total frequency spectrum recorded from each electrode site), relative power (the percentage of total power contributed by each frequency band or wavelength in the spectrum from each electrode site), coherence (the amount of synchronization of electrical events in corresponding brain regions, separately for each frequency band and for the entire frequency spectrum), and symmetry (the ratio of power in each band between a symmetric pair of electrodes).

A qEEG can only be validly interpreted after artifacts are removed from the digital record. If a clinician does not have the training to interpret EEGs, then a skilled and trained professional consultant should be involved. The artifact-free information is then compared with normative databases to identify brain regions whose EEG data are deviant by 2 or more standard deviations more than or less than the mean. These brain regions are targeted for NF training if the z scores (the number of standard deviations off the mean) are thought to be relevant to the patient's symptoms and if these symptoms are associated with the area of the brain that is typically responsible for the patient's malfunctioning.

The uses of normative databases have been validated in the scientific literature. The normative databases contain the raw EEG records and features derived from analysis of data from individuals aged 6 months to about 90 years. The number of subjects required for reliability at each age point were statistically determined and increased until consistent split-half replications were obtained. The sampling requirement was interesting because each age required different numbers of participants. For example, in the ages from 6 months to 13 years, when brain maturation changes are rapid, higher numbers of subjects were needed. This use of age-regression normative equations and z scores, good test-retest reliability, and lack of ethnic bias allows the use of qEEG that is not only noninvasive but highly sensitive to abnormalities in brain function found in psychiatric populations.[13–15] Replications of normative databases have been extended to cover the range from 1 to 95 years of age for each of the electrode positions in the standardized International 10–20 System, and they have been broadened to include measures of absolute power, relative power, mean frequency, coherence, and symmetry.[14–20]

Distinctive patterns of qEEG abnormalities have been described in diverse psychiatric disorders in adults and youth. These distinctive diagnostic patterns allow differentiation of these disorders from normal and from each other.[8,13] A large body of peer-reviewed published data from independent laboratories reports the sensitivity of neurometrics in varied clinical populations, including head injury,[13,14,21] schizophrenia,[22] depression,[23] marijuana abuse,[24] and ADHD.[25,26]

VALIDATION OF QUANTITATIVE ELECTROENCEPHALOGRAPHY BY USE OF NEUROIMAGING AND OTHER TECHNIQUES

In the early 1990s, efforts were made to identify the three-dimensional location of deep sources in the interior of the brain of the surface (scalp) EEG data, and then to correlate these deep sources with MRI tomographic data.[27] This coregistration of deep EEG sources to MRI slices is known as EEG tomography (tEEG), electrical neuroimaging,[28] or brain electromagnetic tomography.[15] These efforts were expanded to coregister all imaging modalities, including, positron emission tomography (PET), single-photon emission computed tomography (SPECT), and fMRI, and to create a common anatomic atlas. Based on neurosurgical identification of areas pertinent to function, the Talaraich atlas and later the Montreal Neurological Atlas were subsequently used to incorporate EEG data into the Human Brain Mapping Project.[27,29–32] It was used to visualize Brodmann areas as they were defined for the Talairach brain[33] and to compare Brodmann areas across subjects.

tEEG is based on the ability to measure the location of three-dimensional sources of the scalp surface EEG in the interior of the brain and then register the sources to MRI tomographic slices. The advent of tEEG is important because it provides coregistration of 2 imaging modalities that have similar spatial localization characteristics, in which fMRI measures blood flow and the qEEG adds a high temporal resolution of changes in the electrical sources in the brain that are associated with changes in blood flow.[1]

In 1994, Robert Marqui-Pascual[4] devised accurate estimates of the deep (lower) brain sources of the EEG patterns in small regional voxels (approximately 4 mm to

1 cm cubic voxels) coregistered to MRI slices. He transformed these raw EEG signals into three-dimensional images that were then coregistered on the Talairach MRI atlas. This new method was called LORETA. The Web site to obtain additional information on LORETA is http://uzh.ch/keyinst/loreta.htm. LORETA provides better temporal resolution than can be achieved with either PET or fMRI. This high temporal resolution is important for studies using event potentials (ie, time-locked events) and also for investigating brain changes proposed to be associated with psychological states, such as depression.[34] Using LORETA allows a clinician to translate qEEG data into a three-dimensional figure that corresponds with and looks like the images in fMRI that are associated with the same disease state. Furthermore, during NF treatment, as waveforms are adjusted toward normal, the three-dimensional images generated by LORETA also become more consistent with a normal fMRI.

A statistical normalization was later applied to LORETA and was called sLORETA.[35,36] The first normative tEEG databases, using z scores and Gaussian or normal distributions similar to fMRI, are referred to as statistical parametric mapping (SPM) and were introduced by Valdez in 2001[32] and followed by Thatcher and colleagues[37,38] in 2005.

Modern PET, qEEG, magnetoencephalography (MEG), and fMRI studies all agree that electrical activity in the brain is organized by a small set of modules or hubs that represent clusters of neurons with high within-cluster connectivity and sparse long-distance connectivity (**Fig. 4**).[29,39–41]

Quantitative electroencephalography and MEG are the only 2 imaging methods that have sufficient spatial and temporal resolution to measure the millisecond dynamics of

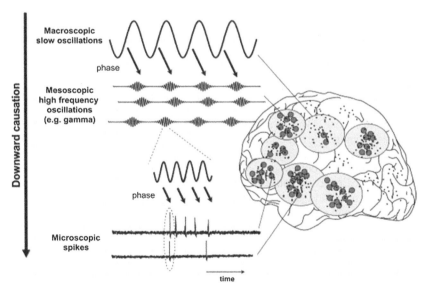

Fig. 4. Quantitative EEG measures short-distance and long-distance coherence, phase delays, phase locking, and phase shifting of different frequencies. The qEEG reflects top-down causality at the macro level (scalp surface EEG) coordinating the meso and micro levels of neural organization. The dysregulation of groups of neurons at the micro and meso levels, which simultaneously mediate specialized functions, can be measured at the macro level using quantitative EEG. (*From* Le Van Quyen M. The brainweb of cross-scale interactions. New Ideas Psychol 2010;29:57–63; with permission.)

hubs and modules. Both use z scores to estimate dysregulation in these brain areas, and these z scores can be linked to a patient's symptoms. However, quantitative electroencephalography can better detect deeper cortical sources and is much less expensive than MEG. For that matter, a qEEG is less expensive than fMRI and PET scans.[29]

COREGISTRATION OF QUANTITATIVE ELECTROENCEPHALOGRAPHY WITH DIFFUSE SPECTRAL IMAGING AND OTHER NEUROIMAGING METHODS

The human cortex has been arranged in 6 basic cluster modules that have been measured using diffuse spectral imaging (DSI) (**Fig. 5**). Coregistration of quantitative electroencephalography to these 6 modules based on DSI can be used to determine phase dynamics and fine temporal coherence within and between these modules.[38]

Hagmann and colleagues[39] developed these 6 modules. They used DSI to trace cortical white matter connections of the human cerebral cortex between 66 cortical regions, using clear anatomic landmarks, based on Brodmann areas.[42] From the 66 cortical regions, 998 subregions of interest (ROIs) were calculated using a connection matrix of inter-regional cortical connectivity. Network spectral analyses of nodes and edges of the 998 ROIs were grouped into 6 anatomic modules.[38] These 6 anatomic modules include, but are not exclusive to, the posterior cingulate, the bilateral precuneus, the bilateral paracentral lobule, the unilateral cuneus,

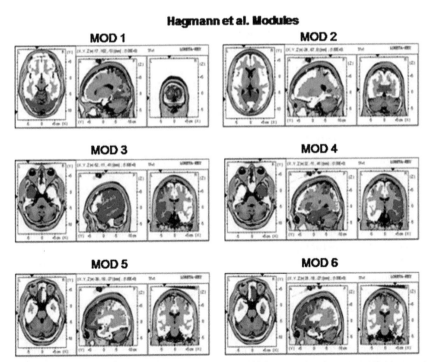

Hagmann et al. Modules

MOD 1   MOD 2

MOD 3   MOD 4

MOD 5   MOD 6

Fig. 5. The locations of the 6 Hagmann modules (MOD1–6). These modules represent the Hagmann DSI-based modules coregistered to quantitative electroencephalography. (*From* Thatcher W, North DM, Biver CJ. Diffusion spectral imaging modules correlate with EEG LORETA neuroimaging modules. Hum Brain Mapp 2011;33:1062–75; with permission.)

the bilateral isthmus of the cingulate gyrus, and the bilateral superior temporal sulcus. A replication of the 6 modules described by Hagmann and colleagues[39,43] using DSI and coregistered to quantitative electroencephalography is shown in **Fig. 5**.

In summary, z scores (based on qEEGs) allow clinicians to determine the location and extent of dysregulation with respect to a group of age-matched controls. A tEEG normative database of Brodmann areas and hub and modules when linked to a patient's symptoms aids a clinician in making a diagnosis. The goal is to target weak systems and avoid compensatory systems. The z scores or standard deviations with respect to an age-matched reference population provides a real-time guide to train patients toward z = 0 in brain regions associated with particular disorders.[1,44–46] The clinical use of qEEG in neuropsychiatry involves 3 distinct steps: (1) a clinical interview and evaluation of the patient's symptoms and complaints, (2) linking the patient's symptoms to functional specialization in the brain based on the scientific literature (qEEG/MEG; fMRI; PET; SPECT, and so forth) and, (3) real-time z-score surface or LORETA to modify deviant or deregulated brain regions associated with the patient's symptoms and complaints.[1,29]

Z scores derived from a normative qEEG database can be used as an aid to diagnosis, but they cannot be used as a stand-alone approach to diagnosis (just as PET scans can help but not make a diagnosis). However, qEEG normative database z scores, like PET scans or fMRI, can be used to monitor the course of treatment (eg, of transcranial magnetic stimulation, NF training, or psychopharmacologic interventions) or evaluate the comparative efficacy of treatments.

QUANTITATIVE ELECTROENCEPHALOGRAPHY AND NF FOR PSYCHIATRIC CONDITIONS
Role of the EEG Power Spectrum, Neuromodulators, and Psychiatric Disorders

As discussed earlier, the changes in wavelengths produced during phase lock can cause the release of neuromodulators, which in turn can cause synaptic modifications. However, these neuromodulators also have a role in specific systems or circuits in the brain that influence the expression of clinical psychiatric symptoms.

How Complex Homeostatic Systems Regulate the EEG Power Spectrum

Hughes and John[47] provide a more detailed explanation of the brief summary given here. Large neuronal populations in the brainstem, thalamus, and the cortical areas mediate EEG power spectrums.[47] The thalamus is part of the brainstem through which all sensory information (except olfactory information) flows. This sensory-driven information is sent to the cortex, and the cortex relays information back to the thalamus (the thalamic-cortical-thalamic pathway); the thalamus then sends the information to the other parts of the brain.

Changes in the EEG frequency in the thalamus can increase or decrease the flow of information by way of large pacemaker neurons that are distributed throughout the thalamus. Inhibition of information flow in the thalamic-cortical-thalamic pathway occurs when the rhythm increases from a theta (4–8 Hz) and low alpha (8–10 Hz) range to the faster rhythms in the high alpha (11–12 Hz) range and still faster beta (12.5–2.0 Hz) range. These faster activity ranges are thought to be involved in corticocortical and corticothalamic interactions during information processing.[47] When phase shift and phase lock are functioning efficiently (eg, in a patient without ADHD), neuromodulators influence rhythms that are responsible for selectively inhibiting cortical regions during cognitive processing. Deficiencies or excesses of neurotransmitters or modulators can therefore affect the efficiency of the relay of information, and thereby the homeostasis of the brain (and potentially play a role in psychiatric disorders). Thus, NF, by changing theta waves to high alpha and beta waves, may correct these deficiencies and bring the brain back to a more normative and efficient way of processing.

Comparison with normative databases shows that raw EEG power spectrums (conventional EEG) of alpha, beta, theta, and delta frequency bands for each electrode in the standardized International 10–20 System have links to psychiatric disorders. Normal distributions of power in these frequency bands in normal, healthy individuals also show high test-retest reliability. However, although the conventional EEG can be used in the diagnostic work-up of such things as acute confusional states; first presentation of schizophrenia; major mood or mania; and refractory behavioral problems such as obsessions, panic, or violence, qEEG is particularly well suited to identify subtle changes in the topographic distributions of background activity. qEEG may aid in identifying difficult differential diagnosis, such as: distinguishing between mood disorders and schizophrenia; assessing cognitive, attentional, or developmental disorders; distinguishing between environmentally induced and endogenously induced mediated behavioral disorders; evaluating alcohol and substance abuse; and evaluating postconcussion syndrome.[47] More research using NF in children and adolescents is needed to determine whether NF may be able to change these disease states as well.

How May This Occur in the Case of ADHD?

ADHD provides an example of how changes in the flow between these pathways can influence psychiatric symptoms. The major qEEG frequency abnormalities seen in ADHD involve an excess of theta and, in some cases, low alpha.[48–50] Furthermore, an excess of theta and low alpha waves might result from low dopamine levels that may be caused by a hypofunctioning prefrontal cortex (PFC) and/or the nigrostriatal system, via low dopaminergic firing. These qEEG findings are in agreement with the dopaminergic theory of ADHD expressed by Levy,[51] which conceptualizes ADHD of the polysynaptic dopaminergic circuits between prefrontal and striatal centers of activity. These findings are also compatible with the neurophysiologic model of ADHD proposed by Niedermeyer and Naidu,[52] which emphasizes prefrontal, frontal and striatal, and thalamic interconnections. The Levy[51] model is also supported by MRI and PET imaging studies and by behavioral, pharmacologic, and neuroanatomic studies on the nature of cortical and subcortical disturbances in function that characterizes children with attention and learning problems.[16]

In summary, the dysregulation of the thalamic-cortical-striatal system in ADHD is still not completely understood. However, the high levels of theta and low alpha wavelengths registered on qEEG, which are associated with ADHD in specific regions of the brain, are thought to be changed by NF through operational conditioning, changing the theta waves (inattentive state) to high alpha and beta waves (attentive state). However, the effects of NF training are not limited to ADHD alone.

Psychiatry as Related to Circuitry: Moving from Categorical Disorders to Transdiagnostic Symptoms

As psychiatry prepares to better understand psychiatric disorders from a neurobiological perspective, clinicians are developing a new way of describing psychiatric symptoms. Core connectivity circuits may be disrupted in the brain, which leads to the expression of these symptoms. Buckholtz and Myer-Lindenberg[53] expanded on this idea. Populations of neurons are segregated to perform specialized functions (ie, language processing in the left inferior frontal gyrus). Simple execution of these functions requires that specialized output of each of these segregated neuron populations be integrated or connected. The notion that schizophrenia is a disorder of dysconnectivity has a long history. Connectivity analysis (using fMRI research) in healthy individuals has uncovered specific networks associated with cognition, affect, motivation, and social function.

These networks have been identified as part of an initiative at the National Institute of Mental Health (NIMH). The Research Domain Criteria (RDoC) at NIMH[54] have organized symptom domains that correspond with neuropsychological junctions based on connectivity between specialized neuronal populations. There are 4 domains: the corticolimbic, the corticocortical, the frontoparietal, and the default mode network (**Fig. 6**). These circuits underpin core executive, affective, motivational, and social domains. Heritable variation in the function of these circuits produces deficits in circuit-specific cognitive domains that manifest as psychiatric symptoms. Using these domains, these symptoms are seen to be common to multiple disorders rather than specific to unique categorical disorders.

Buckholtz and Meyer-Lindenberg[53] summarized these circuits and their function as follows (see **Fig. 6**):

1. The amygdala, medial prefrontal cortex (ventromedial and medial orbital aspects along with the perigenual cingulated cortex), and lateral prefrontal cortex (LPFC)

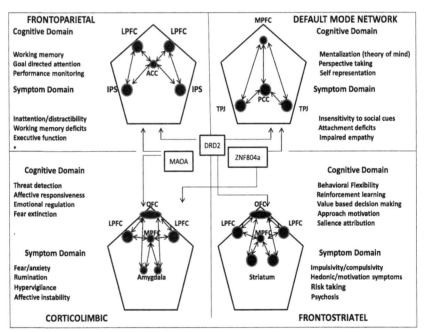

Fig. 6. Genetic variation affects risk for mental disorder by disrupting cognition-specific brain circuits. dACC, dorsal anterior cingulate; DRD2, dopamine D2 receptor (associated with substance abuse, ADHD, schizophrenia, and antisocial personality disorder); LPFC, lateral prefrontal cortex; MAOA, monoamine oxidase A (associated with serotonin and mood disorder and antisocial personality disorder); MPFC, ventromedial prefrontal cortex (ventromedial and medial orbital cortex, and perigenual cingulate cortex); OFC, orbital frontal cortex; PCC, posterior cingulate cortex; TPJ, temporal parietal junction; ZNF804a, a series of genome-wide association with schizotypal and decreased social cognition. (*Adapted from* Buckholtz JW, Meyer-Lindenberg A. Psychopathology and the human connection: toward a transdiagnostic model of risk for mental illness. Neuron 2012;74(6):990–1004. http://dx.doi.org/10.1016/j.neuron.2012:06.002; with permission.)

make up the corticolimbic circuit and is associated with affective symptoms, such as anger, anxiety, rumination, and hypervigilance. This circuitry in healthy individuals is engaged during negative emotional arousal and requires regulation of these negative emotions. The dysregulation of these affective symptoms is associated with mood, anxiety, schizophrenia, conduct, substance abuse, and personality disorders.

2. The default mode network is thought to be more commonly engaged when people think about the thoughts, beliefs, emotions, and intentions of others. It involves the temporoparietal junction, posterior cingulate, and ventromedial prefrontal cortex (vmPFC). Dysfunction of this circuitry is associated with poor social cognition and is associated with psychosis, personality disorders, mood disorders, and ADHD.

3. The frontostriatal network is made up of the vmPFC, LPFC, orbital frontal cortex, and the striatum. Dysconnectivity can lead to impairment of motivational and hedonic responses, cognitive flexibility, value-based learning, and decision making. Such impairments cut across many mental disorders, including anhedonia in schizophrenia and mood disorders; impulsivity in ADHD, substance abuse, schizophrenia, and personality disorders; and compulsivity in obsessive-compulsive disorder and substance abuse.

4. In addition, the frontoparietal network involves the dorsal LPFC, dorsal cingulate, and parietal cortex, which are critical to executive function. Executive function involves tasks that use working memory, goal-directed attention, conflict detection, and performance monitoring. Deficits in executive function span several disorders, including schizophrenia, ADHD, major depression, and substance abuse.

These pathways are influenced by multiple small effect risk alleles, like the DRD2 allele, which can affect different circuitry in these 4 networks as shown in **Fig. 6**. Therefore, a genetic variant of DRD2 affecting, for instance, the frontoparietal network can cause a deficit in executive function. This deficit increases susceptibility to multiple disorders because the resulting deficits are not disorder specific. For instance, the dopamine DRD2 receptor shows significant effects associated with schizophrenia, ADHD, substance abuse, and antisocial behavior. The reader is referred to the article by Buckholtz and Meyer-Lindenberg[53] for further explanation of how genetic variations of particular genes in **Fig. 6**, as well as other variants of genes, can disrupt circuitry in these networks.

Hence, certain genes can influence connectivity in networks linked to symptom domains, which implies that connectivity changes seen in mental illness reflect the cause of the illness and are not consequences of the illness.

These pathways can also be influenced by environmental risk factors, as well as epigenetics. Nonetheless, this hypothesis could lead to a new way to organize psychiatric disorders. Instead of discrete categorical disorders, the influence of genes and environment can disrupt system-level circuits for several dimensions of cognition, producing instead transdiagnostic symptoms or symptoms that overlap several disorders, which may why comorbidity among diagnoses is so frequently observed. Correcting dysfunction in circuits in these 4 networks can explain how interventions using transmagnetic stimulation, qEEG, and (for deeper structures) LORETA NF may work to relieve symptoms associated with broad domains of mental disorder. For instance, LORETA can target every brain area listed in all 4 networks with the exception of the striatum.

Research that gives credibility to targeting these circuits has already begun. For instance, the Longitudinal Assessment of Mania Study[55] was designed to identify distinct developmental trajectories of behavioral and emotional dysregulation in youth with bipolar disorder and high dysregulation (HD) and youth without bipolar who had low dysregulation (LD). Youth with LD had greater activity in the dorsolateral prefrontal cortex and greater functional connectivity among the amygdala, dorsolateral and ventrolateral prefrontal cortex, and anterior cingulate. Therefore, a possible use of LORETA NF in youth with HD with bipolar disorder is to target the dorsolateral prefrontal cortex and, perhaps, improve coherence in the less functional circuits (ventral LPFC to amygdala).

Targeting specific networks in youths who are already ill is not the only way LORETA NF may be used. Research using MRI is now beginning to identify dysfunctional areas of the brain that may predict the risk of developing a particular disease. For instance, in a study by Hajek,[56] youths who had a risk of developing bipolar disorder (identified by having 1 or 2 parents with a diagnosis of bipolar disorder) were compared with unaffected youths who did not have one or more parents with a diagnosis for bipolar disorder. Of those who were unaffected (and who had a risk of developing bipolar disorder), 8 of 21 had an abnormally large right inferior frontal gyrus (rIFG) compared with controls. The individuals were followed 4.5 years after the scanning. Of the 8 who had a larger rIFG, 4 converted to a psychiatric disease, 3 developed a major depression, 1 an anxiety disorder, and 1 a personality disorder (all requiring medication). Of the unaffected with a risk for developing a bipolar disorder who had rIFGs that were comparable with controls, only 2 converted to an axis I disorder (1 who developed an adjustment disorder following a motor vehicle accident and 1 who had a milder depressive disorder). Therefore, it can be postulated from this study that the development of more severe forms of psychiatric disorders can be better associated with certain abnormal circuits before the diseases develop. Also, the identified circuits at risk can develop into a variety of disorders, congruent with the idea behind transdiagnostic symptoms. Therefore, future studies of these networks may help to predict who may be at risk and interventions to correct these abnormalities may help prevent the development of psychiatric disorders. More research is needed.

In summary, targeting networks in individuals with known symptoms associated with one or several psychiatric diseases and cross-correlating the research with qEEG may provide an avenue to target these areas using LORETA NF. It is speculated that, by using LORETA NF, the symptoms of these diseases may be relieved or decreased in severity. The new trend to consider psychiatric illnesses as transdiagnostic entities may be an avenue for many new interventions, not limited to LORETA NF, such as repetitive Transcranial Magnetic Stimulation (rTMS) or cognitive training programs.

NEUROFEEDBACK TREATMENT IN CHILDREN AND ADOLESCENTS

Two types of NF have been described in case reports in adults and youth. Z-score surface NF training, using 2 to 4 or more scalp electrodes, uses continuous real-time computerized calculations comparing the way that the patient's brain is functioning with a normative database on different variables (eg, power, asymmetries, phase-lag, and coherence). LORETA uses a different kind of qEEG NF analysis that provides an estimation of the location of the underlying brain generators (eg, the anterior cingulate, insula, fusiform gyrus) and networks of the patient's EEG activity within a frequency band. There is no current published research on the use of LORETA NF in youths. It requires more labor-intensive preparation, because an entire electrode cap with 19 electrodes must be applied in every session, but it can shorten the length of treatment. fMRI NF's advantage is that it can examine functioning at deep subcortical areas of the brain. However, the practical disadvantage of fMRI NF is that it is very expensive, with equipment that costs $1 million or more and is not portable.

Unless specifically stated, the following research has been done in adults.

Neurofeedback Treatment of Depression

qEEG research in adults with depression has focused on the structures involved in processing emotions, which are found in the left and right hemispheres, including the amygdala, orbitofrontal cortex, basal ganglia, and the hippocampus. Most of the research has been done in adults and involves surface NF. The left hemisphere is involved in processing positive emotions and the right is involved in processing negative emotions.[57] Depression is associated with hypometabolism in the cingulate and occasionally in the orbitofrontal cortex, insula, anterior temporal cortices, amygdala, basal ganglia, and thalamus.

The details of the associations between brain wavelength rhythms and behavioral states are complex and do not need to be understood in order to understand NF; however, some of these details are mentioned here. Delta (0–4 Hz) and theta (4–8 Hz) rhythms are associated with hypoactive states, and alpha (8–12 Hz) is associated with activated states. However, higher alpha in the right frontal cortex and lower alpha in the left frontal cortex are associated with positive mood. Beta rhythms (12–30 Hz) are usually associated with activated states, but can be subdivided: beta 1 (12–15 Hz) on the right is associated with a calm and observant state, beta 2 (15–18 Hz) on the left is associated with a fully attentive and less depressed state, and beta 3 (19–30 Hz) on the left and right is associated with the anxious and irritable state. These known associations between behavioral states and wavelengths can provide targets for NF treatment of depression.[58–62]

Quantitative EEG has been used to distinguish between unipolar depression and bipolar disorder in adults.[59] Increases in alpha power in the left hemisphere and decreases in left parietal-occipital beta and hypercoherence in the right anterior region were found in adults with unipolar depression, whereas decreased alpha on the left and increased left parietal-occipital beta were found in adults with bipolar disorder.[16,59–61]

The hypercoherence in depression can be related to networks being oversaturated in order to attempt to overcompensate for the inefficiency in the networks and therefore being unable to process emotional information appropriately. Higher theta and alpha coherence is found primarily in longer-distance connections between the frontopolar prefrontal cortex (Brodmann area 10, **Fig. 2**) and the temporal or parieto-occipital regions. Higher beta coherence is primarily found in connections within and between electrodes overlying the dorsolateral prefrontal cortex or the temporal regions.[60,61]

Adults with depression show alpha asymmetry on qEEG, and this alpha asymmetry has been used as a primary target in the treatment of depression in adults and also as a target in some reports in youth: in alpha asymmetry, the frontal lobes show higher alpha on the left and lower alpha on the right; in contrast, posterior (parietal-temporal) regions show lower alpha on the left and higher alpha on the right.[59,60] Individuals showing the frontal alpha asymmetry mentioned earlier typically are prone to experiencing negative withdrawal states. Those who experience increased alpha activity on the right relative to the left tend to experience more positive affective states.[61]

In female adolescents with depression, one study showed that the right posterior lobe had findings typically found in adult depression.[62] However, the same study showed that, in those female adolescents with depression and anxiety disorders, the posterior asymmetry was reduced. These findings highlight the importance of looking for comorbid conditions that may offset the effects of depression and account for inconsistencies found in posterior asymmetry in adolescents with depression. In the same study, female adolescents with depression alone did not show the same anterior alpha asymmetry found in adults with depression. These findings may be caused by adolescent frontal regions developing later in life and the findings therefore not correlating with findings is seen in adults with depression. These facts may indicate that, in female adolescents, posterior alpha asymmetry may be a more predictive way of detecting depression than anterior asymmetry. This study highlights the importance of using qEEG findings that match the symptoms of individual patients based on their developmental age, especially when attempting to use alpha asymmetry as a target of NF treatment in adolescents.

qEEG may also be used to estimate the risk for developing a mood disorder.[63] Baseline electroencephalographic activity was recorded from adolescents from 12 to 14 years old whose mothers had a history of depression (high-risk group) and whose mothers were lifetime free of axis I mental disorder (low-risk group). High-risk adolescents showed the hypothesized pattern of relative left frontal hypoactivity on alpha-band measures. These findings may indicate that individuals with left frontal hypoactivation should be followed closely for the development of depression.

Another potentially useful qEEG parameter is cordance, which combines absolute power (the amount of power in a frequency band or wavelength at a given electrode) and relative power (the percentage of power contained in a frequency band relative to the total spectrum) normalized across electrode sites and frequency bands. Cordance has a stronger association with regional cerebral blood flow than other EEG measures. Hunter and colleagues[64] showed that cordance can be used to predict antidepressant treatment response or remission with 70% or greater accuracy. Changes in prefrontal theta-band cordance within the first week of medication treatment predicted 8-week treatment outcome in 27 adult subjects. Early change in theta-band cordance in those treated with either serotonin selective reuptake inhibitors or mixed serotonin-norepinephrine agents predicted a good response to medication.[64] Similar findings have been reported for the treatment of bipolar depression in adults.[65] There are no qEEG studies predicting antidepressant treatment effectiveness in children or adolescents.

Although many studies in adults have effectively treated depression in adults by targeting alpha asymmetry, only 1 published study has been conducted using the alpha asymmetry model in a depressed adolescent. The adolescent had nonbipolar major depression and had not responded to psychotherapy. Surface EEG biofeedback was used until the alpha asymmetry changes occurred, which appeared normal for a nondepressed individual. This treatment required 67 sessions and the patient did not require medication.[66] More research is needed.

This is the first and, at present, only reported case of NF treatment of depression in an adolescent, and there are no reported cases in children. There are no case reports in youth regarding the qEEG prediction of response to treatment with psychiatric medications. However, based on findings on the treatment of adults with depression and of adults with bipolar disorder, this area needs further development in youth.

Neurofeedback Treatment of Anxiety Disorders

Available qEEG studies suggest a high incidence of abnormalities in adults with anxiety, panic, and obsessive-compulsive disorder (OCD).[16,67–70]

Two subtypes of (OCD) in adults have been described. One subgroup had excess alpha throughout most of the brain along with excess beta in the frontal, central, and midtemporal regions. The other group had a theta excess mostly in the frontal areas and at posterior temporal electrodes.[71]

Youth (aged 10–14 years) with anxiety who responded to 19 channel surface NF based on EEG characteristics had significant increases in the ratio of amplitudes of alpha and theta rhythms, sensorimotor and theta rhythms, as well as the modal frequency of alpha rhythm.[72] The study was small (n = 7 in experimental group and n = 10 in control group). The groups were divided into those with high levels of anxiety versus low levels of anxiety based on the Prikhojan questionnaire, the Spielberger-Khanin test, and the House-Tree-Person projective test. Between 10 and 12 NF sessions were performed. Feedback was used with acoustic sounds when eyes were closed and with visual stimuli when eyes were opened. Different feedback protocols were used. When patients tried to control the loudness of white noise (with eyes closed) or the intensity of colors in pictures (with eyes opened), the NF sessions were more effective. In the experimental group, estimates of the level of anxiety decreased in all scales of the psychological tests but were not significant. Significant decreases in the experimental group were observed in the scales of feelings of inferiority and frustration. In both groups, before and after reports by parents indicated decreases in emotional instability. Also, in the control group, significant decreases on the scale of feelings of inferiority were observed. The study is small and more research is needed.

In OCD, adults whose qEEG showed increased alpha relative power responded positively to serotonergic antidepressants (82% response rate), whereas 80% of adults with increased theta relative power (especially in the frontal area) failed to improve. Responders to placebo showed increased prefrontal cordance and medication responders showed decreased cordance within 48 hours of treatment.[73,74] No studies of response to antidepressant medication using qEEG have been done on children and adolescents with OCD or depression.

In summary, qEEGs may help to predict response to medication treatment in depression and OCD, but none of these studies have been done in children and adolescents. One study using NF in adolescents with anxiety has been published with fair to good results. Quantitative EEG in adolescents with depression and anxiety may indicate that those with anxiety may be protective against developing more severe symptoms of depression.

Neurofeedback Treatment of Substance Abuse

The effects of drug abuse on a qEEG vary depending on the substance and the duration, acute versus chronic, use or abuse. There seems to be a consensus that chronic cannabis and cocaine use are associated with an increase in alpha brainwave activity[75] and that chronic alcohol abuse is associated with an increase in beta brainwave activity.[76] In addition, several research studies show that, in both alcoholics and cocaine addicts, the best predictor of relapse is the excessive amount of fast beta brainwave activity.[75,76] EEG investigations of the children of alcoholics have documented that they also have an excess of fast beta activity, and this predicts a risk of developing alcohol abuse in adulthood. Alcoholics and their children frequently have lower levels of alpha and theta brainwaves, which similarly predict a risk for developing alcohol abuse. Following the intake of alcohol, alcoholics and/or their children feel more relaxed and show an increase in the levels of alpha and theta brainwaves, suggesting self-medication of symptoms.[10,75,76]

NF has been used to train adult alcoholics to promote stress reduction and achieve profoundly relaxed states by increasing alpha and theta brainwaves and decreasing fast beta brainwaves[77] when the patients' eyes were closed. Increasing theta brainwaves with eyes closed was felt to produce a relaxed state, which is not to be confused with theta brainwaves that are produced in the eyes-opened state (indicating the inattention state) as is seen in ADHD. This same study showed promising potential as an adjunct to alcoholism treatment. In a 4-year follow-up in which only 20% of the traditionally treated group of alcoholics remained sober, 80% of the subjects who had received NF training showed sustained reductions in alcohol use. Furthermore, these subjects showed improvement in psychological adjustment on 13 scales of the Millon Clinical Multiaxial Inventory, compared with the traditionally treated alcoholics who improved on only 2 scales and became worse on 1 scale.[10,77] This single study suggests that NF may have some potential to improve treatment effectiveness in adults with chronic alcohol use. There have been no studies using alpha/theta training in adolescents with a history of substance abuse, but, speculatively, NF might in the future have a role in preventing or treating alcohol abuse in youth.

Neurofeedback Treatment of Substance Use Disorders in the Context of Comorbid ADHD

Although there have not been any studies using NF for the treatment of substance abuse disorders in adolescents, qEEG research has discovered a difference in individuals who started using cocaine chronically before age 20 years as opposed to those who became chronic users after age 20 years.[78] For example, there was significantly more theta excess in adolescents who began abusing cocaine before age 20 years compared with those whose abuse began after age 20 years. A significantly larger proportion of early cocaine users had ADHD. It has been known for some time that many youth with ADHD have increased theta.[79,80] Therefore, ADHD may be a risk factor for the development of cocaine abuse during adolescents and using NF to suppress theta in these youth may decrease the risk of developing chronic cocaine abuse.

This example shows how treating ADHD by suppressing theta may be helpful in reducing the risk of developing cocaine abuse in youth. However, some protocols used to treat ADHD and a comorbid substance abuse may increase the risk of using specific substances of abuse. To understand why the risk may be increased, a brief summary of surface NF protocols is needed. Lubar and colleagues[79,80] were the first to introduce these protocols. In individuals with combined type ADHD, either increasing sensory motor rhythms (SMR) and suppressing theta (at electrodes C3 and C4 and linked earlobes) or increasing SMR and suppressing beta 2 (C4 and linked earlobes followed by the first protocol) has led to positive results. SMR involves strengthening sensory motor inhibition in the cortex. For the inattentive type of ADHD, Clarke and colleagues[81] described a protocol involving theta suppression and beta 1 enhancement, which was done at electrode Cz with linked ears, at FCz-PCz with single ear reference or at Cz-Pz with single ear reference.[82]

If an adolescent has alcohol abuse (decreased theta and alpha and increased beta) and ADHD combined type, increasing theta (although helpful in some alcoholics) may cause the ADHD to worsen. In this case, if the adolescent has increased beta at baseline, the first half of the Lubar protocol (suppressing theta and increasing SMR) may be of more benefit because decreasing beta may help reduce alcohol abuse and the symptoms of ADHD. Suppressing theta and increasing SMR may also be advantageous in ADHD youth who are abusing cocaine because both of these conditions increase theta.

It has also been shown that individuals who abuse both cocaine and marijuana have excess alpha activity.[75,83] In this case, any protocol in youth with comorbid ADHD and marijuana and cocaine abuse that increases alpha activity may not be preferred. Instead, decreasing theta, which reduces ADHD symptoms and decreases the abuse of cocaine, may be preferred.

Because increases in beta activity seem to predict the risk of developing alcohol abuse in children of alcoholics[75,76] and can increase the risk of relapse in cocaine and alcohol abusers, any protocol used in youth engaged in alcohol and cocaine abuse with comorbid ADHD that increases beta activity (as suggested in Clarke and colleagues[81] NF protocol) should be used with caution. The previously mentioned limitations to surface NF in youth with comorbid substance abuse and ADHD are speculative and baseline and subsequent qEEGs performed during NF along with correlation to clinical symptoms and outcomes should guide the clinician in treatment protocols used in youth with comorbid ADHD and substance abuse. These suggested protocols are summarized in **Table 1**.

Table 1 Proposed surface NF treatment of comorbid ADHD and substance abuse using qEEG findings		
Findings in Chosen Substance of Abuse	**ADHD Protocol**	**ADD Protocol**
Alcoholics: decreased theta and alpha and increased beta	Decrease beta 2 and increase SMR and increase alpha	Decrease beta 1 and increase alpha
Cocaine users in whom increased theta is found and the predictor of cocaine relapse may be caused by increased beta and increased theta in those who started using before age 20 y	Decrease beta 2, increase SMR and decrease theta, or increase SMR	Decrease beta 1 and decrease theta
Cocaine and marijuana users with increased alpha	Avoid increasing alpha and decrease beta 2	Avoid increasing alpha and decrease beta 1
Children of alcoholics with increased beta and decreased theta and alpha	Decrease beta 2 and increase SMR	Decrease beta 1 and increase SMR

Abbreviation: ADD, attention deficit disorder.

Surface Neurofeedback Treatment of Posttraumatic Stress Disorder

The first study of posttraumatic stress disorder (PTSD) in adults examined surface NF as an adjunct to conventional treatment of Vietnam combat veterans in a Veterans Administration hospital.[84] To target PTSD symptoms, a sequence of thirty 30-minute sessions of alpha-theta NF training was provided to 15 veterans, and a contrast group of 14 veterans received treatment as usual. No attempt was made to provide a sham or alternative adjunctive treatment of the contrast group. At the end of the study, among the patients receiving traditional treatment and medication (n = 14), only 1 patient decreased medication needs, 2 reported no change, and 10 required an increase in psychiatric medications. On the Minnesota Multiphasic Personality Inventory, patients receiving NF training improved significantly on all 10 clinical scales, whereas the traditionally treated patients showed no significant improvements on any of the scales. At follow-up 30 months after treatment, all 14 patients in traditional treatment had relapsed and were rehospitalized, whereas only 3 of 15 patients having NF treatment had relapsed. All 14 of the patients having NF treatment receiving medication were able to be managed on less psychiatric medication at follow-up.

The only surface NF study of PTSD symptoms in youth examined 26 adopted children, aged 6 to 15 years, with histories of abuse and/or neglect.[85] Most of the subjects showed symptoms of reactive attachment disorder and were taking a variety of psychiatric medications before and during the NF trial. All of the children had increased theta waves in at least one frontal site, and most had decreased delta waves in frontal regions. NF training consisted of thirty 30-minute sessions involving auditory and visual feedback, with feedback initially contingent on reduction of delta/theta activity. Before-and-after Child Behavior Checklists were completed by the adoptive parents. Before-and-after Test of Variable Assessment (TOVA) evaluation was also done. All but 3 subjects completed a posttreatment TOVA evaluation. Total syndrome scale scores decreased an average of 23.05 points (standard deviation = 21.44) with a 95% CI of 12.73 to 33.39, and were significant at $t(18) = 4.69$, $P<.001$. Six of the 8 CBCL syndrome scale scores significantly improved (medium effect sizes [ESs] $d>0.55$), although only nonsignificant improvements were observed in somatic complaints and withdrawn scale scores. The TOVA scores showed significant improvements on omission errors, commission errors, and total variability ($d>0.60$). Limitations of the study include the small and nonrandomized sample, lack of control group, and failure to control for potential effects of medications and other concurrent therapies. This single study provides encouragement for further NF studies in abused or neglected children with PTSD.

NEUROFEEDBACK TREATMENT OF INTRAUTERINE BRAIN DAMAGE, MILD HEAD INJURY, CONCUSSION, AND TBI

Numerous qEEG studies of severe (Glasgow Coma Scale 4–8) and moderate head injury (Glasgow Coma Scale 9–12) on patients aged 14 years and older have shown that such injuries produce persistent qEEG abnormalities. These qEEG abnormalities may include increased theta and decreased alpha power, decreased coherence, and increased asymmetry.[16,86]

Regarding treatment of TBI, a recent research review by Thornton and Carmody[87] suggests that qEEG-guided NF is superior to both neurocognitive rehabilitation strategies and medication treatment in the rehabilitation of TBI in adults, especially for auditory memory. There have been no studies of this type published with regard to children and adolescents.

Only 1 study in children was conducted that examined EEG NF versus physical/occupational therapy in 12 children (aged 7 months to 14 years) who had had a stroke before birth. The mothers had no history of drug use, hypertension, or viral infection. All children were evaluated for baseline range of motion, and the older children provided self-descriptions of mood and completed a short-term memory test (how these tests were administered was not available for this publication). Six children were selected randomly for EEG NF, for 30 minutes a week, whereas 6 children received physical or occupational therapy once a week. The EEG NF targeted brain regions T4, C4, T3, and C3 to inhibit theta waves (4–7 Hz) and reduce their voltage, and to produce beta waves (15–18 Hz) for 0.5 seconds at 1 μV. After 3 months of treatment, children receiving EEG NF had improved range of motion, improvement in concentration (or, in young children, eye tracking), improved short-term memory, and fewer mood swings. The control group showed only improved range of motion, but no improvement in cognitive or emotional status.[88] This lone report suggests that NF might be useful for treating a variety of effects of intrauterine stroke, although further studies are needed.

With regard to EEG indicators of postconcussion syndrome in adults, there is also a broad consensus that common EEG indicators include increased focal or diffuse theta, decreased alpha, decreased coherence, and increased asymmetry, similar to the changes observed in TBIs in general. Multiple reports suggest that these qEEG variables also successfully separate patients with a history of mild to moderate head injury, even years after apparent clinical recovery, from normal individuals.[21] Compared with postconcussion syndrome, TBI seems to show increases in slow frequencies (delta, theta, slow alpha 8–10 Hz), and decreases in fast frequency alpha (10.5–13.5 Hz), and increases in beta levels.[89]

A study of patients (aged 18–65 years) with TBI (and who had a Glasgow Coma Scale of 9 or higher) examined qEEG 1 to 3 days after the TBI. Subjects were screened to determine whether they were carriers of the apolipoprotein E (ApoE), whose E4 allele is thought to decrease blood cerebral blood flow. ApoE4 carriers had fewer alpha and beta waves and more delta and theta waves compared with noncarriers and controls. This finding suggests that ApoE carriers may show more abnormal qEEG effects in the early stages of TBI, which supports the Buckholtz and Meyer-Lindenberg[53] theories that different alleles of certain genes are more likely to be associated with connectivity dysfunction.[90] These findings may open opportunities for research to determine whether using NF to target these abnormalities (in ApoE carriers after TBI) would be a complementary treatment of those who regain consciousness.

Many cognitive functions are affected by TBI, and studies indicate that some of these same cognitive functions are impaired in ADHD.[91] MRI and qEEG studies suggest that the same brain regions are dysfunctional in both conditions.[92] Gerring and colleagues[93] found that children who had thalamic injuries had a 3.6 times higher risk for developing ADHD. The same logistic regression models used in Gerring and colleagues'[93] analysis also showed a 3.15 times higher risk for developing ADHD if injuries occurred in the basal ganglia. Using variable-resolution electromagnetic tomography qEEG data of children with ADHD, the same study found that excess theta seemed to be generated from the septal-hippocampal pathway of the basal ganglia, whereas excess alpha derived from the thalamus.[94] These studies emphasized the possible correlation between TBI-acquired ADHD and the underlying mechanisms found in ADHD. It may be that some of the NF protocols used in the treatment of ADHD are similar to protocols used to improve cognitive function in children with TBI.

Although Down syndrome is not classified as a brain injury disorder, some of the cognitive functions found in TBI and ADHD are also found in these children. In a study of 8 medication-free children (aged 6–14 years) with Down syndrome, qEEGs generally showed excess delta and theta EEG patterns. All children displayed limited vocabulary (5–10 words), poor attention and concentration, weak memory, impulsivity, and behavior problems. All 7 children who completed 60 sessions of surface NF training showed significant ($P<.02$) improvement in all areas, as evaluated by questionnaire and parent interviewing, and beneficial changes were found in qEEGs.[95]

The overlap of qEEG findings in ADHD, TBI, and mental retardation was further explored in 23 subjects (7–16 years old) with mild to moderate mental retardation. Most subjects showed increased theta, increased alpha, and coherence abnormalities, and a few showed increased delta over the cortex. Of 23 patients who received NF training, 22 showed clinical improvement according to the Developmental Behavior Checklist-Parent scores, and patients showed significant improvement on the Weschler Intelligence Scale for Children-Revised (WISC-R) and the TOVA. The WISCV-R was repeated at 6 months' follow-up after the completion of NF treatment. The mean verbal intelligence quotient (IQ) score was 49.6 before treatment and 53.05 after treatment ($P<.0295$). Performance IQ scores were 55.45 before treatment and 63.20 after treatment ($P<.0007$). Full scale mean was 49.0 before treatment and 54.6 after treatment ($P<.0003$). The mean and standard deviation of the number of sessions were 134.78 and 7.874 respectively. The range of the sessions was from 80 to 200. There were significant TOVA improvements and significant decreases in impulsivity, temper tantrums, problems with sleep, telling lies, attention, and distractibility. All improvements in behavior and attention that had been observed during the treatment remained stable in the 2 years of follow-up according to parents' reports.[96] This study indicates that the use of qEEG may have some indication for increasing IQ and targeting disruptive behaviors.

These studies suggest that there are similarities in some clinical features and qEEG findings in TBI, postconcussive symptoms, ADHD, Down syndrome, and other forms of mental retardation. There is some promising evidence that NF may be helpful in treating these various conditions using generally similar NF protocols. However, the research is limited, the qEEG for each individual needs to be carefully evaluated for potential NF targets, and treatment needs to be matched with the symptoms in order to develop appropriate qEEG protocols.[96]

Looking to the future, the United States Army is implementing LORETA z-score biofeedback as a clinical treatment of active duty military personnel involved in an extensive rehabilitation program for treating PTSD/TBI at the Fort Campbell Warrior Resiliency and Recovery Center, headed by Dr Marc Zola in collaboration with Drs Joel Lubar and Robert Thatcher. The areas targeted include symptoms associated with concussion, posttraumatic stress, depression, chronic pain, headache and substance abuse disorder. A qEEG assessment is used to rank order the most deviant nodes and hubs of the networks most commonly associated with these symptoms and periodic follow-up qEEG analyses are used to assess the progress of treatment. The US Army program is just getting started and is scheduled to continue for the next 5 years, during which extensive pretreatment versus posttreatment assessments and statistical analyses will be conducted. Most of the patients will be between 18 and 25 years of age, and preliminary findings suggest promising results in as little as 12 sessions.

Neurofeedback in Reducing Performance Anxiety

Alpha/theta NF training was used in 2 studies involving musical performance. The effects of alpha/theta training were the same in both studies. In both studies, NF training occurred over 10 sessions and involved alpha/theta training with eyes closed and auditory feedback intended to increase theta more than alpha waves. In a replication study, students were randomized to one of 6 interventions, including 3 different NF techniques and 3 other techniques: alpha/theta NF training, beta training (intended to reduce fast waves at the beta frequencies), or SMR NF (which involved strengthening sensorimotor inhibition in the cortex and inhibiting alpha frequencies), and mental skills performance, aerobic fitness, and the Alexander technique (postural retraining and somatic stress reduction). The results provided confirmation of the beneficial effects of alpha/theta NF, which was the only intervention that improved music performance (overall quality, musical understanding, stylistic quality, and interpretive imagination). All 6 interventions were successful in reducing preperformance anxiety, so the performance enhancement by alpha-theta training could not be attributed to anxiety reduction alone.[97]

Alpha/theta training has been used with university dancers who compete in ballroom dancing. Twenty-four male/female pairs were randomly assigned to either alpha/theta training, heart rate coherence (HRC) training (involving heart rate variability training), or a nonintervention control group before and after performance was judged by 2 dance experts who were blinded to which groups got the intervention. Both the HRC and alpha/theta training groups improved on the overall rating of execution more than the control group. Subscale ratings revealed that HRC improved technique, but alpha/theta training improved timing.

As noted by the investigators, theta oscillations are speculated to affect meditative concentration, and reduce anxiety and sympathetic autonomic activation. Theta oscillations may also affect virtual spatial navigation, focused and sustained attention, and working and recognition memory.

In summary, it is thought that alpha-theta training targets optimal performance and enhancement of technical, communication, and artistic domains of performance in the arts.

Does Neurofeedback Technique Have to be Modified for Developmental Age?

Recent research[98,99] has shown that the major brain networks develop early in life and are essentially the same in adolescents and adults. One study[99] used measures of network topology to investigate the development of functional hubs in 99 normal subjects, aged 10 to 20 years. Hub architecture was evident in late childhood (age 10 years) and was stable from adolescence to early adulthood, but the strength of connectivity changed with development. From childhood to adolescence, the strength of connections increased between frontal hubs and frontal, parietal, temporal, and cerebellar spoke regions, whereas connections decreased in the posterior part of the brain. It was hypothesized that this pattern reflects the gradual maturation of the ability of the frontal lobe to coordinate distributed cortical functions for goal-directed behaviors. The subsequent developmental increases in hub-spoke connectivity between adolescence and adulthood were fewer and tended to be more posterior, involving connections between subcortical hubs (the putamen and cerebellum) and frontal, occipital, and temporal spoke regions. These findings suggest that developmentally stable functional hub architecture provides the foundation of information flow in the brain, whereas connections between hubs and spokes continue to develop, presumably supporting the maturation of cognitive functions. Based on these findings, it is expected that NF would work in a manner that is identical from age 10 years to adulthood.

Controversies

Although there is extensive scientific evidence to validate the use of qEEG, there has been limited acceptance in the United States. There are several reasons for this. First, psychiatrists do not often follow the EEG literature and are unaware of developments in the field. Second, because of the evolving understanding about technology and appropriate protocols, some falsely negative findings have been reported[16,100,101] and adopted by some expert panels[102] but rejected by others.[103] More recent studies provide substantial additional support for the validity and clinical use of qEEG in several areas of psychiatry.[16,104] The American Academy of Pediatrics has recently listed EEG biofeedback as a level 1, best-support (a valid first-line) intervention for ADHD (www.aap.org/en-us/advocacy.../aap.../CRPsychosocialInterventions.pdf).

Questions continue to be raised concerning the available normative databases, but current methodological adjustments and mathematical techniques allow cross-validation among different normative databases that have high intradatabase similarity.[12] Confidence in normative databases is based on widespread independent replications,[16] test-retest reliability confirmed in short-term and long-term follow-up large samples,[105,106] and small gender differences.

Some critics have argued that NF should not be an accepted intervention until double-blind placebo-controlled studies using sham controls have been conducted. There has been considerable debate and controversy in the NF literature about the pitfalls of attempted sham-NF controls, what technical innovations can be introduced to provide better controls, the validity of proceeding with randomized controls in the absence of an acceptable sham procedure, and the use of altered qEEG patterns in an individual as corroboration of the validity of the intervention (eg, as is often used with other interventions).

This issue of whether a sham is as effective, more effective, or less effective than contingent reinforcement may involve a serious misconception. Both experimental and sham groups are operating under the contingencies of classical and operant conditioning. Imagine a child with ADHD who already spends a lot of time playing computer games and is now placed in front of a display that purportedly is going to help but he is in the sham group. The child becomes engaged by the display, tries to make it occur more frequently, and in the process is releasing dopamine in both the dorsal and ventral attention networks and from dopamine-producing regions within the brain such as the nucleus accumbens and related areas. The display elicits an unconditioned response of increasing EEG activation in many areas including the one in which the sensor has been placed, such as FZ or CZ, resulting in more beta and less theta. Sometimes when a burst of beta activity associated with decreased theta activity occurs at the location where the sensor is placed, reinforcement is delivered. Now the child is experiencing partial noncontingent reinforcement on a variable ratio schedule. This same type of reinforcement, used in the gambling industry, is the most powerful reason why casinos make billions of dollars. As a result, the child in the sham conditioning group often has an activated EEG, tries hard to get the noncontingent reinforcement, which is sometimes contingent, and shows improvements in several ADHD indices such as rating scales and perhaps even academic performance.

So what is the answer? It has been repeatedly stated that, because an operant conditioning of a particular EEG pattern reinforcement is usually delivered after 0.5 to 1 second of the production of that pattern, the EEG recording can be marked every time reinforcement is delivered in both the experimental and sham control group. In the sham group, a simple correlation can be run between the percentage time that the reinforcement was contingent and the degree to which the measured EEG parameters changed in the desired direction along with all of the appropriate before and after measures. It would not be surprising that, even if there was a 20% contingency in the sham group, powerful learning effects might occur. As a result it is impossible to develop a sham in which reinforcement never coincides with the EEG pattern that is being trained in the experimental group.

Until a generally agreed on placebo can be developed, continuing active randomized controlled studies should be encouraged.

Furthermore, the lack of understanding of NF has led to several other problems regarding research. For instance, some studies that have questioned the effectiveness of NF have been poorly done for many reasons.

First, some studies have been done that have little to support the role of a feasible sham. One reason has to do with the use of different NF protocols that are not recognized as proven and the use of technology that has little proven effectiveness. In a study that was done to show the effectiveness of a double-blind, sham-controlled, randomized pilot feasibility trial in patients with ADHD, there were no significant differences between the NF group and the sham group. However, the investigators appropriately admitted that they did not use NF technology that is considered effective.[107] The equipment used was Smart Brain by Cybert Learning Technology (www.smarttech.com). This technology allows altering the reinforcement threshold from minute to minute, adopting the threshold to just completed performance, and not requiring focus on the NF training. This technique is referred to as autothresholding. If a patient is not paying attention, the thresholding may be adjusted to a nonlearning event and the reinforcement may not produce the desired effect.

Second, some studies were done without evaluating pre-qEEG data. When participants are selected based on their pre-qEEG data, the protocol used would be better matched to the participant and the use of this protocol would more likely produce a larger ES (an ES is considered large when it is 0.8 or greater). An ES of 0.8 means that the mean of the treated group is at the 79th percentile of the untreated group. As noted in an article by Sherlin and colleagues,[108] when pre-qEEG data are evaluated in, for instance, a study involving preselection of participants based on abnormal theta/beta ratios for ADHD, the ES for inattention was 2.22 and for hyperactivity was 1.2.[109] These ESs are substantially larger than the ES calculated from a meta-analysis of NF by Arns and colleagues,[110] in which the ES was 0.81 for inattention and 0.4/0.69 for impulsivity/hyperactivity. This later meta-analysis had similar ES discussed in an article by Faraone and Buitelaar,[111] which was comparable with medication for inattention (0.84) but not for the ES for medication for impulsivity/hyperactivity (1.01). Therefore, NF must be based on pre-qEEG data and, in this case, may improve therapeutic outcomes. If children are very hyperactive and unable to be still during NF and a pre-qEEG analysis has occurred, it is suggested that they may require medication (if they are good responders to stimulant medication) initially in order to have good control of their disorder. This can be gradually tapered as the NF proceeds. If the hyperactivity does not subside, but the attention improves, they may still require medication. More research is needed.

Third, meta-analysis of NF studies have concluded that the ES of NF was small because studies were included that did not included standard NF protocols, which again points to the lack of knowledge surrounding NF. In a meta-analysis of non-pharmacologic interventions for ADHD by Sonuga-Barker and colleagues[112] Arns and Strehl[113] pointed out that, when statistics were recalculated using only studies with standard NF protocols, parent ratings obtained a significant standardized difference of 0.58 (95% CI = 0.12–0.94; z = 3.52; P = .0004) and for teacher ratings a significant standardized mean difference was found of 0.39 (95% CI = 0.07; z = 2.39; P = .02). The inclusion of nonstandardized protocols in a meta-analysis points to a problem in NF: the lack of the standardized protocols that are critical to future research. In addition, for every disorder, best-practice approaches should be individualized and the same before and after instruments should be uniformly used. These instruments should not be limited to rating scales from multiple sources and may include neuropsychological instruments, such as the TOVA (http://www.tovatest.com/), Integrated Visual and Auditory Continuous Performance Test (IVA-Plus) (http://www.braintrain.com/ivaplus/), and the Behavior Rating Inventory of Executive Function-R (BRIEF-R) (http://www4.parinc.com/Products/Product.aspx?ProductID=BRIEF#).

Fourth, with regard to lack of knowledge about standardized protocols, some studies, although well intentioned, do not use well-known facts about learning curves and operant conditioning. For instance, in randomized placebo-controlled trial of NF for children with ADHD done by van Dongen-Boomsma and colleagues,[114] the percentage of reward used was too high (80%) for operant conditioning to occur. If the reward is too easy (rewards are delivered every time) no learning occurs.

However, some users of NF are not trained professionals. Given the evolution of NF, only clinicians who are well trained in neurophysiology, neuroanatomy, and neuroendocrine and metabolic processes should be allowed to do NF. Given the need to remove artifact appropriately in order to use qEEG, only clinicians who are trained to do so should be allowed to extract the artifacts, or a requirement that an untrained clinician must be supervised by someone who is proficient in reading EEGs may be necessary. NF is most appropriately used as an adjunct to a multimodal biological, psychological, and social treatment approach. These points may indicate that the accreditation used in NF may need to be reconsidered.

New mathematical techniques for qEEG analysis are developing rapidly, and new technology will promote this development. The advent of LORETA and z-score NF allows clinicians to selectively target data that are substantial deviations above or below the normative population means, enabling more accurate matching of those deviations to symptoms and to the relevant brain regions. LORETA (19 electrodes) allows targeting of deeper structures than can be reached with surface NF (2–4 electrodes), will likely reduce the number of sessions and costs required to get effective results, and seems to have long-lasting effects after treatment is stopped.

Summary of Tables

In evaluating this limited literature on NF treatment in children and adolescents, the system developed by United States Preventive Services Task Force (USPSTF) can be used.

Table 2 provides a summary of the quality of evidence that is currently available in the published literature as well as a summary of the strength of recommendations that can be offered to clinicians concerning the value of the treatment. **Table 3** is similar, except that the right-hand column provides the authors' clinical expert opinions rather than being based purely on publications.

Table 2
Evaluation of surface NF in youth: the evidence base

Indications	NF Method	Quality of Research	Strength of Recommendation	Evidence Base
Depression	Alpha asymmetry	Fair	Recommend	1 case study[66]
Anxiety	Increase alpha/theta ratio or SMR/theta ratio	Fair	Recommend	1 RCT[72]
Performance anxiety	Alpha/theta training	Good	Recommend	1 RCT and 1 open trial[97,115]
Mental retardation	NF based on individual qEEG	Good	Recommend	2 clinical trials
TBI	Decrease theta/increase beta	Fair	Recommend	1 RCT comparing physical therapy with NF
PTSD	Decrease delta/theta activity	Fair	Recommend	Non–randomized controlled study
Alcohol abuse	Alpha/theta training	ND	ND	ND
Substance abuse	Alpha/theta training	ND	ND	ND

USPSTF quality of evidence grade is a qualitative ranking of the strength of the published evidence in the medical literature. Limited, indirect evidence; good, consistent benefit in well-conducted studies in different populations; fair, data show positive effects, but weak, limited, or indirect evidence; poor, cannot show benefit because of data weakness.

USPSTF strength of recommendations: A, recommend strongly (good evidence of benefit and safety); B, recommend (fair evidence of benefit and of safety); C, neutral (fair evidence for, but seems risky); D, recommend against (fair evidence of ineffectiveness or harm); I, insufficient data.

Abbreviations: ND, no data on youth; RCT, randomized controlled trial.

Table 3			
Evaluation of surface NF in youth: authors' recommendations and personal comments			
Indications	Strength of Recommendations Based on Published Data	Authors' Clinical Recommendations	Authors' Other Comments
Depression	Recommend	Possible benefit	Requires further study given the variance between findings in frontal lobes in alpha asymmetry adolescents vs adults. qEEG should always be used before and during treatment with regard to clinical symptoms. Studies needed using LORETA NF
Anxiety	Recommend	Shows promise and improvement trends	May have greater effect if based on qEEG. Studies needed using LORETA NF
Performance anxiety	Recommend	Shows promise and improvement trends	Promising for decreasing performance anxiety and performance skill. Studies needed using LORETA NF
Mental retardation	Recommend	Shows promise and possible benefit based on pretreatment and ongoing treatment on qEEGs	Promising for possible increase in IQ and decreasing disruptive behaviors and improving attention. May help to reduce medications used to treat these behaviors. Studies needed using LORETA NF
TBI	Recommend	Shows promise	May help to increase range of motion and memory in persons who have had a stroke. Need to use qEEG and watch to see whether increasing beta will make symptoms worse. Studies needed using LORETA NF
PTSD	Recommend	Recommend	Helpful in decreasing PTSD symptoms and improving attention in abused children. Studies needed using LORETA NF
Alcohol and substance abuse	Neutral with comorbid ADHD	See **Table 1** for recommendations	Studies needed using LORETA NF

USPSTF strength of recommendations: A, recommend strongly (good evidence of benefit and safety); B, recommend (fair evidence of benefit and of safety); C, neutral (fair evidence for, but seems risky); D, recommend against (fair evidence of ineffectiveness or harm); I, insufficient data.

SUMMARY

Although most NF research has targeted ADHD, there are some limited studies in children and adolescents suggesting possible applications for treatment of anxiety, depressive disorder, addiction (with or without ADHD), brain injury (including TBI, mild head injury, concussion, and intrauterine brain damage), Down syndrome, and perhaps some other forms of mental retardation in children and adolescents. There are additional data suggesting that NF might also be useful for treating certain intractable seizure disorders in youth,[47,116,117] but a neurologist should be involved in managing those cases. Although some of the data remain controversial, the American Academy of Pediatrics has recently endorsed NF as a valid and possibly first-line treatment of ADHD in youth, and the United States Army is implementing an innovative program to examine the role of NF in treating TBI in veterans. As the technology and statistical analytical methods advance, many of the remaining uncertainties can be expected to be addressed.

Research has documented that many of the same areas targeted in the NF treatment of ADHD (right ventrolateral prefrontal cortex, right dorsal anterior cingulate, left thalamus, left caudate nucleus, and left substantia nigra) are involved in mediating selective attention and response inhibition in children with ADHD, and similar NF treatment is helpful for improving attention in a variety of other psychiatric disorders.[118] The targeting of such transdiagnostic symptoms holds particular promise for the future of NF treatment.

A small study has suggested that NF and methylphenidate similarly improve several behavioral and cognitive functions in children with ADHD.[119] This raises the question of whether nondrug treatment might be able to eventually augment or, conceivably, supplant some of the established current psychopharmacologic interventions. For many families, NF might be a more acceptable option than psychostimulants for treating ADHD. Furthermore, NF might be a particularly valid option for treating ADHD with comorbid substance abuse, especially because NF may be beneficial for both conditions, without the risks associated with using abusable medications in this population.

The use of qEEG to characterize and localize brain dysfunction creates new opportunities. Current data suggest that qEEG might eventually be useful for predicting medication responders and nonresponders,[120] for identifying patients at risk for developing antidepressant-induced treatment-emergent suicidal ideation,[121] and for identifying patients at particularly high risk for relapse (depression, cocaine addiction, nicotine craving).[122] In addition to identifying patients at risk by qEEG monitoring, NF can be used to target the dysfunctional circuitry in relevant brain regions and could conceivably act proactively to reduce the risks.

The newer technologies may eventually be found to be particularly suitable for providing a more penetrating picture of dysfunctional circuitry and for yielding more effective treatments with fewer NF sessions and lower costs. There was a recent presentation of a patient with multiple diagnosis starting in adolescence (including major depression, ADHDF, bipolar I, social phobia, TBI, OCD, and PTSD), and multiple medications (including sertraline, dextroamphetamine mixed salts, Synthroid, lithium carbonate, hydroxyzine, alprazolam, and lorazepam), who had not adequately responded to surface NF and therapy over a 2-year period. He had made 3 previous suicide attempts. Once LORETA NF was used (for 33 sessions over a 6-month period), the patient was off all medications and functioning well.[123] His Global Assessment of Functioning (GAF) score improved from 15 to 90. A single case cannot be the guide for clinicians to use LORETA NF in every person with multiple disorders, but this case presentation highlights the need to do more research using this intervention, especially in patients who are not responding to conventional interventions and therapy.

Although LORETA seems to offer some promise for advances compared with the older surface NF methods, the two approaches can currently be viewed as complementary. Some children are not able to tolerate the many electrodes required for LORETA and may be better candidates for the more user-friendly surface NF methods using 2 to 4 electrodes.

At present, NF can be considered when patients or parents prefer not to use psychopharmacologic treatments or when medication treatments are not well tolerated or adequately effective.

Child and adolescent psychiatrists are well aware of the importance of well-trained clinicians who are skilled in doing biopsychosocial evaluation and treatment. NF should never be used as a single intervention in child and adolescent psychiatry, just as medications should never be the only intervention for depression. NF is properly used when integrated into a multimodal series of interventions for the child and family that precedes and continues after the time period of active NF treatment. Although this may be obvious to child psychiatrists, clinicians should be advised that an increasing number of lay persons are inappropriately obtaining NF equipment and offering to put electrodes on someone's head and to alter the brain functioning of individuals with serious medical and psychological conditions. In less drastic cases, some inadequately trained clinicians have assumed that a patient with ADHD can benefit from a predetermined protocol to increase alpha or beta activity, without having conducted proper individualized assessments. The risk, for example, in a patient who already has excess beta and cortical irritability is the induction of tics, anxiety, or seizure activity.[124]

Psychiatrists who are collaborating with NF specialists are strongly encouraged to use licensed clinicians with certification in NF (eg, from the Biofeedback Certification Institute of America) and or clinicians supervised by clinicians with certification and/or certification in qEEG (eg, from the EEG and Clinical Neuroscience Society, the Quantitative Electroencephalography Certification Board, or the Society for the Advancement of Brain Analysis).

In regards to the effectiveness of neurofeedback, the reader is referred to a recent review by Arns and colleagues[125] which addresses this issue with a concise summary of previous studies. Although double blind placebo controlled studies are clearly the preferred type of research in regards to proving the effectiveness of treatment regimens, until a convincing sham is found, randomized controlled studies based on appropriate protocols and methods should continue. Meanwhile, a collaborative group has been formed to address the issue of a credible sham.[126]

REFERENCES

1. Thatcher RW. Introduction. In: Robert Thatcher, editor. Handbook on quantitative electroencephalography and EEG biofeedback. St Petersburg (FL): Anipublishing; 2012. p. 10–145.
2. Brodmann K. Vergleichende Lokalisationslehre der Grosshirnrinde in ihren Prinzipien dargestellt auf Grund des Zellenbaues. Leipzig (Germany): Johann Ambrosius Barth Verlag; 1909.
3. Nunez P. Neocortical dynamics and human EEG rhythms. New York: Oxford University Press; 1994.
4. Pascual-Marqui RD, Michel CM, Lehmann D. Low resolution electromagnetic tomography: a new method for localizing electrical activity in the brain. Int J Psychophysiol 1994;18:49–65.

5. Pascual-Marqui RD, Lehmann D, Koenig T, et al. Low resolution brain electromagnetic tomography (LORETA) functional imaging in acute, neuroleptic-naive, first-episode, productive schizophrenia. Psychiatry Res 1999;90:169–79.

6. Hughes SW, Crunelli V. Just a phase they are going through: the complex interaction of intrinsic high-thresholding bursting and gap junctions in the generation of thalamic α and 0 rhythms. Int J Psychophysiol 2007;64:3–17.

7. Tiesinga PH, Sejnowski TJ. Mechanisms for phase shifting in cortical networks and their role in communication through coherence. Front Hum Neurosci 2010;4:196.

8. John ER. From synchronous neural discharges to subjective awareness. Prog Brain Res 2005;150:143–71.

9. Kandel ER. The molecular biology of memory storage: a dialogue between genes and synapses [review]. Science 2001;294(5544):1030–8.

10. Hammond DC. What is neurofeedback: an update. J Neurotherapy 2011;15: 305–36.

11. Buzsaki G. Rhythms of the brain. New York: Oxford University Press; 2006.

12. Thatcher RW, Lubar JF. History of scientific standards of qEEG normative bases. In: Budzinsky T, Budzinsky J, Evans J, et al, editors. Introduction to qEEG and neurofeedback: advanced theory and applications. San Diego (CA): Academic Press; 2008.

13. Prichep LS. Use of normative databases and statistical methods in demonstrating clinical utility of qEEG: importance and cautions. Clin EEG Neurosci 2005;36(2):82–127.

14. Thatcher RW, Walker RA, Biver C, et al. Quantitative normative databases: validation and clinical correlation. J Neurotherapy 2003;7:87–122.

15. Valdes-Sosa P, Valdes -Sosa M, Carballo J, et al. qEEG in a public health system. Brain Topogr 1992;4(4):259–66.

16. Chabot RJ, di Michel F, Prichep L. The role of quantitative EEG in child and adolescent psychiatric disorders. Child Adolesc Psychiatr Clin N Am 2005;14: 21–5.

17. John ER, Prichep LS, Ahn H, et al. Neurometric evaluation of cognitive dysfunctions and neurological disorders in children. Prog Neurobiol 1983;21: 239–90.

18. John ER, Prichep LS, Friedman J, et al. Neurometrics: computer assisted differential diagnosis of brain dysfunctions. Science 1988;293:162–9.

19. John ER, Prichep LS. Principles of neurometrics and neurometric analysis of EEG and evoked potentials. In: Niedermeyer E, Lopes Da Silva F, editors. EEG: basic principles, clinical applications and related fields. Baltimore (MD): Williams & Wilkins; 1993. p. 989–1003.

20. Prichep LS, John ER. qEEG profiles of psychiatric disorders. Brain Topogr 1992; 4(4):249–57.

21. Thatcher RW, Walker RA, Gerson I, et al. EEG discriminant analyses of mild head trauma. Electroencephalogr Clin Neurophysiol 1989;73:94–106.

22. Czobor P, Volavka J. Pretreatment EEG predicts short-term response to haloperidol treatment. Biol Psychiatry 1991;30:927–42.

23. Roemer RA, Shagass C, Dubin W, et al. Relationship between pretreatment EEG coherence measures and subsequent response to ECT. Neuropsychobiology 1991;24:121–4.

24. Struve FA, Straumanis JJ, Patrick G. Persistent topographic quantitative EEG sequelae of chronic marijuana use: a replication study and initial discriminant function analysis. Clin Electroencephalogr 1994;25(2):63–75.

25. Chabot RJ, Merkin H, Wood LM, et al. Sensitivity and specificity of qEEG in children with attention deficit or specific developmental learning disorders. Clin Electroencephalogr 1996;27(1):26–34.
26. Suffin SC, Emory WH. Neurometric subgroups in attentional and affective disorders and their association with pharmacotherapeutic outcome. Clin Electroencephalogr 1995;26(2):76–83.
27. Lancaster JL, Woldorff MG, Parsons LM, et al. Automatic Talairach atlas labels for functional brain mapping. Hum Brain Mapp 2000;10:120–31.
28. Michel CM, Koenig T, Brandeis D, et al. Electrical neuroimaging. New York: Cambridge University Press; 2009.
29. Thatcher RW. Neuropsychiatry and quantitative EEG in the 21st century. Neuropsychiatry 2011;1(5):495–514.
30. Thatcher R, Wang B, Toro C, et al. Human neural network dynamics using multimodal registration of EEG, PET and MRI. In: Thatcher R, Hallett M, Zeffiro T, et al, editors. Functional neuroimaging: technical foundations. New York: Academic Press; 1994. p. 269–78.
31. Wang B, Toro C, Zeffiro T, et al. Integrating electrophysiological data with brain images: I- Sources of event related potentials, PET and MRI. In: Thatcher R, Hallett M, Zeffiro T, et al, editors. Functional neuroimaging: technical foundations. New York: Academic Press; 1994. p. 251–6.
32. Thatcher RW, Lyon GR, Rumsey J, et al, editors. Developmental neuroimaging: mapping the development of brain and behavior. London, UK: Academic Press, Limited; 1996.
33. Talairach JT. Co-planar stereotaxic atlas of the brain: 3 dimensional proportional system: an approach to cerebral imaging. New York: Thieme Medical Publishers; 1998.
34. Cannon RL. Introduction to LORETA. In: Cannon RL, editor. Low resolution brain electromagnetic tomography (LORETA) basic concepts and clinical applications. Corpus Christi (TX): BMED Press; 2012. p. 3–6.
35. Pascual-Marqui R. Standardized low-resolution brain electromagnetic tomography (sLORETA): technical details. Methods and Find in Exp. Clin Pharmacol 2002;24(Suppl D):5–12.
36. Bosch-Bayard J, Valdes-Sosa P, Virues-Alba T, et al. 3D statistical parametric mapping of EEG source spectra by means of variable resolution electromagnetic tomography (VARETA). Clin Electroencephalogr 2006;32(2):47–61.
37. Thatcher R, North D, Biver C. EEG inverse solutions and parametric vs. nonparametric statistics of low resolution electromagnetic tomography (LORETA). Clin EEG Neurosci 2005;36(1):1–9.
38. Thatcher RW, North D, Biver C. Evaluation and validity of a LORETA normative EEG database. Clin EEG Neurosci 2005;36(2):116–22.
39. Hagmann P, Cammou L, Gigandet X, et al. Mapping the structural core of human cerebral cortex. PLoS Biol 2008;6:e159.
40. Chen ZJ, He Y, Rosa-Neto P, et al. Revealing modular architecture of human brain structural networks by using cortical thickness from MRI. Cereb Cortex 2008;18:2374–81.
41. He Y, Wang J, Wang L, et al. Uncovering intrinsic modular organization of spontaneous brain activity in humans. PLoS One 2009;4(4):e5226. http://dx.doi.org/10.1371/journal.pone.0005226.
42. Brodmann VK. Localization in the cerebral cortex: the principles of comparative localization in the cerebral cortex based on cytoarchitectonics. London, UK: Springer; 1909. Translated by L. J. Garey, 1994.

43. Thatcher W, North DM, Biver CJ. Diffusion spectral imaging modules correlate with EEG LORETA neuroimaging modules. Hum Brain Mapp 2011;33: 1062–75.

44. Collura TF, Thatcher RW, Smith M, et al. EEG biofeedback training using live Z-scores and a normative database. In: Budzinsky T, Budzinsky H, Evans J, et al, editors. Introduction to qEEG and neurofeedback: advanced theory and applications. San Diego (CA): Academic Press; 2008. p. 123–33.

45. Thatcher RW. EEG operant conditioning (biofeedback) and traumatic brain injury. Clin EEG Neurosci 2000;31(1):38–44.

46. Collura TF, Guan J, Tarrant J, et al. EEG biofeedback case studies using live Z-score training and a normative database. J Neurotherapy 2010;14:22–46.

47. Hughes JR, John ER. Conventional and quantitative electroencephalography in psychiatry. J Neuropsychiatry Clin Neurosci 1999;11(2):190–206.

48. DeBoer P, Abercrombie E. Physiological release of striatal acetylcholine in vivo: modulation of D1 and D2 dopamine receptor subtypes. J Pharmacol Exp Ther 1996;277:775–83.

49. Icarashi Y, Takahashi H, Aral T, et al. Suppression of cholinergic activity via the dopamine D2 receptor in the rat stratum. Neurochem Int 1997;30:191–7.

50. Russel V, de Villiers A, Sagvolden T, et al. Altered dopaminergic function in the prefrontal cortex, nucleus accumbens and caudate-putamen of an animal model of attention deficit hyperactivity disorder. Brain Res 1995;676: 343–51.

51. Levy F. The dopamine theory of attention deficit hyperactivity disorder. Aust N Z J Psychiatry 1991;25:277–83.

52. Niedermeyer E, Naidu SB. Attention deficit disorder and frontal motor cortex disconnection. Clin Electroencephalogr 1998;28:130–6.

53. Buckholtz JW, Meyer-Lindenberg A. Psychopathology and the human connection: toward a transdiagnostic model of risk for mental illness. Neuron 2012; 74(6):990–1004. http://dx.doi.org/10.1016/j.neuron.2012:06.002.

54. Insel T, Cuthbert B, Garvey M, et al. Research domain criteria (RDoC): toward a new classification framework for research on mental disorders. Am J Psychiatry 2010;167:748–51.

55. Phillips ML. More severe developmental trajectory of behavioral and emotional dysregulation in youth is associated with reduced functional integrity prefrontal cortical-amygdala circuitry during emotional regulation. Presented at the American Academy of Child and Adolescent Psychiatry Meeting. Orlando (FL), October 25, 2013.

56. Hajek T. Right inferior frontal gyrus volume and future conversion to psychiatric disorders: Prospective study of subjects at genetic risk for bipolar. Presented at the American Academy of Child and Adolescent Psychiatry meeting in Orlando (FL), October 25, 2013.

57. Adolphs RJ, Tranel D. Emotion. In: Rizzo M, Eslinger PJ, editors. Principles and practice of behavioral neurology and neuropsychology. Philadelphia: Saunders; 2004. p. 451–74.

58. Walke J, Lawson R, Kozlowski G, et al. Current status of qEEG and neurofeedback in the treatment of depression. In: Evans JR, editor. Handbook of neurofeedback. Binghampton (NY): Haworth Medical Press; 2007. p. 341–51.

59. Prichep LS, John ER, Alper K, et al. Quantitative EEG in depressive disorders. In: Shagass C, Josiassen RC, Roemer RA, editors. Brain electrical potentials and psychopathology. Amsterdam: Elsevier; 1986. p. 223–44.

60. Leuchter AF, Coo IA, Hunter AM, et al. Resting state quantitative electroencephalography reveals neurophysiologic connectivity in depression. PLoS One 2012; 7(2):e3250.
61. Wheeler RE, Davidson RJ, Tomarken AJ. Frontal brain asymmetry and emotional reactivity: a biological substrate of affective style. Psychophysiology 1993;30(1): 82–9.
62. Kentgen LM, Tenke CE, Pine DS, et al. Electroencephalographic asymmetries in adolescents with major depression: influence of comorbidity with anxiety disorders. J Abnorm Psychol 2000;109:797–802.
63. Tomarken AJ, Dichter GS, Garber J, et al. Resting frontal brain activity: linkages to maternal depression and socioeconomic status among adolescents. Biol Psychol 2004;67:77–102.
64. Hunter AM, Cook IA, Leuchter AF. The promise of the quantitative electroencephalogram as a predictor of antidepressant treatment outcomes in major depressive disorder. Psychiatr Clin North Am 2007;30:105–24.
65. Bares M, Nova T, Brunovsky M, et al. The change in qEEG prefrontal cordance as a predictor to antidepressant intervention in bipolar depression. A pilot study. J Psychiatr Res 2012;46(2):219–25.
66. Earnest C. Single case study of EEG asymmetry biofeedback for depression and independent replication in an adolescent. J Neurotherapy 1999;3: 28–35.
67. Small JG. Psychiatric disorders and EEG. In: Niedermeyer E, Lopes Da Silva F, editors. Electroencephalography: basic principles, clinical applications, and related fields. Baltimore (MD): Wilkins and Wilkins; 1993. p. 581–96.
68. Jenike MA, Brotman AW. The EEG in obsessive-compulsive disorder. J Clin Psychiatry 1984;45:122–4.
69. Abraham HD. Stimulants, panic, and BEAM EEG abnormalities. Am J Psychiatry 1989;146(7):947–8.
70. Buchsbaum MS, Hazlett E, Sicotte N, et al. Topographic EEG changes with benzodiazepine administration in generalized anxiety disorder. Biol Psychiatry 1985;20:832–42.
71. Prichep LS, Mas F, Hollander E, et al. Quantitative electroencephalographic (qEEG) subtyping of obsessive compulsive disorder. Psychiatry Res 1993; 50(1):25–32.
72. Eismont EV, Lutsyu NV, Pavlenko VB. Moderation of increased anxiety in children and teenagers with the use of neurotherapy: estimation of the efficacy. Neurophysiology 2011;43(1):53–61.
73. Cook IA, Leuchter AF, Morgan M, et al. Early changes in prefrontal activity characterize clinical responders to antidepressants. Neuropsychopharmacology 2002;27(1):120–31.
74. Hanse ES, Prichep LS, Bolwig TG, et al. Quantitative electroencephalography in OCD patients treated with paroxetine. Clin Electroencephalogr 2003;34(2): 70–4.
75. Prichep L, Alper KR, Kowalik SC, et al. qEEG subtypes in crack cocaine dependence and treatment outcome. In: Harris LS, editor. Problems of drug dependence, 1995: proceedings of 57th Annual Scientific Meeting, The College on Problems of Drug Dependence, Inc. Rockville (MD): National Institute on Drug Abuse; 1996. p. 142. Research Monograph. No. 162.
76. Baue LO. Predicting relapse to alcohol and drug abuse via quantitative electroencephalography. Neuropsychopharmacology 2001;25:332–40.

77. Peniston EG, Kulkosky PJ. Alcoholic personality and alpha-theta brainwave training. Medical Psychotherapy 1991;2:37–55.
78. Prichep LS, Alper KR, Sverdlov L, et al. Outcome related electrophysiological subtypes of cocaine dependence. Clin Electroencephalogr 2002;33(1): 8–20.
79. Lubar JO, Lubar JF. Electroencephalographic biofeedback of SMR and beta for treatment of attention deficit disorders in a clinical setting. Biofeedback Self Regul 1994;9:1–23.
80. Lubar JF, Swartwood MO, Swartwood JN, et al. Evaluation of the effectiveness of EEG neurofeedback training for ADHD in a clinical setting as measured by changes in T. O. V. A. scores, behavioral ratings, and WISC-R performance. Biofeedback Self Regul 1995;20:83–99.
81. Clarke AR, Barry RJ, McCarthy R, et al. Excess beta activity in children with attention-deficit hyperactivity disorder: an atypical electrophysiological group. Psychiatry Res 2001;103:205–18.
82. Monastra VJ. Electroencephalographic biofeedback (neurotherapy) as a treatment for attention deficit hyperactivity disorder: rationale and empirical foundation. Child Adolesc Psychiatr Clin N Am 2005;14:55–82.
83. Struve FA, Patrick G, Straumanis JJ, et al. Possible EEG sequelae of very long duration marijuana use: pilot findings from topographic quantitative EEG analyses of subjects with 15 to 24 years of cumulative daily exposure to THC. Clin Electroencephalogr 1998;29(1):31–6.
84. Peniston EG, Kulkosky PJ. Alpha-theta brainwave neuro-feedback therapy for Vietnam veterans with combat related post-traumatic stress disorder. Medical Psychotherapy 1991;4:47–60.
85. Huang-Storms L, Bodenhamer-Davis E, Davis R, et al. qEEG-guided neurofeedback for children with histories of abuse and neglect: neurodevelopmental rationale and pilot study. J Neurotherapy 2006;10(4):3–16.
86. Rimel RW, Giordani B, Barth JT, et al. Moderate head injury: completing the clinical spectrum of trauma. Neurosurgery 1982;11:344–51.
87. Thorton KE, Carmody DP. Efficacy of traumatic brain injury rehabilitation: interventions of qEEG-guided biofeedback, computers, strategies, and medications. Appl Psychophysiol Biofeedback 2008;33(2):101–24.
88. Ayers ME. A controlled study of EEG neurofeedback and physical therapy with pediatric stroke, age seven months to age fifteen, occurring prior to birth. Biofeedback & Self-Regulation 1995;20(3):318.
89. Thorton KE, Carmody DP. Traumatic brain injury rehabilitation: qEEG biofeedback treatment protocols. Appl Psychophysiol Biofeedback 2009; 34:59–68.
90. Jian L, Yin X, Cheng Y, et al. Different quantitative EEG alterations induced by TBI among patients with different APOE genotypes. Neurosci Lett 2011;505: 160–4.
91. Duf J. The usefulness of quantitative EEG and neurotherapy in the assessment and treatment of post- concussion syndrome. Clin EEG Neurosci 2004;35(4): 198–209.
92. Gerring JP, Brady KD, Chen A, et al. Premorbid prevalence of ADHD and development of secondary ADHD after closed head injury. J Am Acad Child Adolesc Psychiatry 1998;37(6):647–54.
93. Gerring J, Brady K, Chen A, et al. Neuroimaging variables related to development of secondary attention deficit hyperactivity disorder after closed head injury in children and adolescents. Brain Inj 2000;14(3):205–18.

94. Chabot RJ, di Michele F, Prichep L, et al. The clinical role of computerized EEG in the evaluation and treatment of learning and attention disorders in children and adolescents. J Neuropsychiatry Clin Neurosci 2001;13(2): 171–86.
95. Sunrmeli T, Ertem A. EEG neurofeedback treatment of patients with Down syndrome. J Neurotherapy 2007;11(1):63–8.
96. Surmeli T, Ertem A. Post WISC-R and TOVA improvement with qEEG guided neurofeedback training in mentally retarded: a clinical case series of behavioral problems. Clin EEG Neurosci 2010;1:32–41.
97. Egner T, Gruzelier JH. Ecological validity of neurofeedback: modulation of slow wave EEG enhances musical performance. NeuroReport 2003;14:1221–4. http://dx.doi.org/10.1097/00001756-200307010-00006.
98. Power JD, Fair DA, Schlaggar BL, et al. The development of human functional brain networks. Neuron 2010;67:736–48.
99. Hwang K, Hallquist MN, Luna B. The development of hub architecture in the Human Functional Brain Network cerebral cortex. Cerebral Cortex 2012. http://dx. doi.org/10.1093/cercor/bhs227. Available at: http://cercor.oxfordjournals.org/content/early/2012/08/28/cercor.bhs227.long.
100. Coutin-Churchman P, Anez Y, Uzctegui M, et al. Quantitative spectral analysis of EEG in psychiatry revisited: drawing signs out of numbers in a clinical setting. Clin Neurophysiol 2003;114:2294–306.
101. Nuwer M. Clinical use of qEEG. Clin Neurophysiol 2003;114:2225.
102. Nuwer M. Assessment of digital EEG, quantitative EEG and brain mapping: mapping: report of the American Academy of Neurology and the American Clinical Neurophysiology Society. Neurology 1997;49:277–92.
103. Duffy FH, Hughes JR, Miranda F, et al. Status of quantitative EEG (qEEG) in clinical practice, 1994. Clin Electroencephalogr 1994;25:6–22.
104. Monastra VJ, Lynn S, Linden M, et al. Electroencephalographic biofeedback in the treatment of attention-deficit hyperactivity disorder. Appl Psychophysiol Biofeedback 2005;30:95–114.
105. Kondacs A, Szabo M. Long-term intra-individual variability of the background EEG in normals. Clin Neurophysiol 1999;110:1708–16.
106. Levesque J, Beauregard M, Mensour B. Effect of neurofeedback training on the neural substrates of selective attention in children with attention-deficit/hyperactivity disorder: a functional magnetic resonance imaging study. Neurosci Lett 2006;394:216–21.
107. Arnold LE, Lofthous N, Hersch S, et al. EEG neurofeedback for ADHD: double blind sham controlled randomised pilot feasibility trial. J Atten Disord 2012; 17(5):1–10.
108. Sherlin L, Arns M, Lubar J, et al. A position paper on neurofeedback for the treatment of ADHD. J Neurotherapy 2010;14(2):66–78.
109. Monastra VJ, Monastr DM, George S. The effects of stimulant therapy, EEG biofeedback, and parenting style on the primary symptoms of attention-deficit-hyperactivity disorder. Appl Psychophysiol Biofeedback 2002;27: 231–49.
110. Arns M, de Ridde S, Strehl U, et al. Efficacy of neurofeedback treatment in ADHD: the effects on inattention, impulsivity and hyperactivity: a meta-analysis. Clin EEG Neurosci 2009;40:180–9.
111. Faraone SV, Buitelaar J. Comparing the efficacy of stimulants for ADHD in children and. adolescents using meta-analysis. Eur Child Adolesc Psychiatry 2009; 14(1):353–64.

112. Sonuga-Barker J, Brandeis D, Cortese S, et al, European ADHD Guidelines Group. Nonpharmacological interventions for ADHD: systematic review and meta-analyses of randomized controlled trials of dietary and psychological treatments. Am J Psychiatry 2013;170:275–89.

113. Arns M, Strehl U. Evidence for efficacy of neurofeedback in ADHD? Am J Psychiatry 2013;170:799–800.

114. van Dongen-Boomsma M, Vollebregt MA, Slaats-Willemse D, et al. A randomized placebo-controlled trial of electroencephalographic (EEG) neurofeedback in children with attention-deficit/hyperactivity disorder. Focus on Childhood and Adolescent Mental Health. J Clin Psychiatry 2013;74(8):821–7.

115. Raymond J, Varney C, Gruzelier JH. The effects of alpha/theta neurofeedback on personality and mood. Cogn Br Res 2005;23:287–92. http://dx.doi.org/10.1016/j.cogbrainres.2004.10.023.

116. Walker JE, Kozlowski GP. Neurofeedback treatment of epilepsy. Child Adolesc Psychiatr Clin N Am 2005;14:163–76.

117. Lubar JF, Shahsin HS, Natelson SE, et al. EEG operant conditioning in intractable epileptics. Arch Neurol 1981;38(11):699–704.

118. Beauregard M, Lévesque JL. Functional magnetic resonance imaging investigation of the effects of neurofeedback training on the neural bases of selective attention and response inhibition in children with attention-deficit/hyperactivity disorder. Appl Psychophysiol Biofeedback 2006;31(1). http://dx.doi.org/10.1007/s10484-006-9001-y.

119. Nazari MA, Querne L, DeBroca AD, et al. Effectiveness of EEG biofeedback as compared with methylphenidate in the treatment of attention-deficit/hyperactivity disorder: a clinical outcome study. Neurosci Med 2011;2:78–86. http://dx.doi.org/10.4236/nm.2011.22012. Available at: http://www.SciRP.org/journal/nm Copyright © 2011 SciRes. NM.

120. Arns M, Drinkenburg W, Kenemans JL. The effects of qEEG-informed neurofeedback in ADHD: an open-label pilot study. Appl Psychophysiol Biofeedback 2012;37:171–80. http://dx.doi.org/10.1007/s10484-012-9191-4.

121. Hunte AM, Leuchter AF, Cook IA, et al. Brain functional changes (qEEG cordance) and worsening suicidal ideation and mood symptoms during antidepressant treatment. Acta Psychiatr Scand 2010;122(6):461–9.

122. Canterberry M, Hanlon C, Hartwell K, et al. Real time neurofeedback: exploring the role of severity of dependence. Nicotine Tob Res 2013;15:1–5. http://dx.doi.org/10.1093/ntr/ntt122.

123. Foster D, Center W, Butler B. Integral neurofeedback is superior to conventional medication in a case of bipolar. Presented at the International Society of Neurofeedback and Research Conference. Dallas, Texas, September 18–22, 2013.

124. Hammond DC, First KL. Do no harm: adverse effects and the need for practice standards in neurofeedback. J Neurotherapy 2008;12(1):79–88.

125. Arns M, Heinrich H, Strehle U. Evaluation of neurofeedback in ADHD: The long and winding road. Biological Psychology 2014;95:108–15.

126. Arnold LE, Arns M, Conners K, et al. The Collaborative Neurofeedback Group, A proposed multisite double-blind randomized clinical trial of neurofeedback for ADHD: Need, rationale, and strategy. Journal of Attention Disorders 2013. http://dx.doi.org/10.1177/1087054713482580.

Quantitative EEG Neurofeedback for the Treatment of Pediatric Attention-Deficit/Hyperactivity Disorder, Autism Spectrum Disorders, Learning Disorders, and Epilepsy

CrossMark

Elizabeth Hurt, PhD[a],*, L. Eugene Arnold, MD, MEd[b],
Nicholas Lofthouse, PhD[c]

KEYWORDS

- Neurofeedback • Neurotherapy • EEG biofeedback • Quantitative EEG • ADHD
- Autism spectrum disorders • Learning disorders • Epilepsy

KEY POINTS

- Quantitative electroencephalogram neurofeedback (qEEG NF) aims to improve brain functioning by targeting brain-wave correlates of functional deficits, based on the quantitative evaluation of the individual's EEG rather than on traditional diagnostic categories or observable symptoms.
- qEEG NF for attention deficit/hyperactivity disorder, based on 12 randomized controlled trials (RCTs) with medium effect sizes ($d = 0.57$–0.72), is recommended with reservations, and only as an adjunctive intervention after families have tried or at least considered conventional treatments.
- For autism, in 4 small RCTs, NF showed improvements in sustained attention, sensory/cognitive awareness, communication, sociability, set shifting/flexibility skills, and some long-term maintenance of treatment gains. NF may be recommended, again with reservations.

Continued

Disclosures: Dr L.E. Arnold has had research funding from CureMark, Lilly, and Shire, been on advisory boards for AstraZeneca, Biomarin, Novartis, Noven, Seaside Therapeutics, and Shire, and had travel support from Noven. Dr E. Hurt has had research funding from Bristol-Meyer-Squibb. Dr N. Lofthouse has no financial disclosures.
[a] School of Professional Psychology, Wright State University, 053 Student Union, Dayton, OH 45435, USA; [b] Department of Psychiatry, Nisonger Center, The Ohio State University, 1581 Dodd Drive, Columbus, OH 43210, USA; [c] School of Professional Psychology, 130 Northwood's Boulevard, Suite B, Columbus, OH 43235, USA
* Corresponding author.
E-mail address: Beth.Hurt@wright.edu

Continued

- For learning disorders, with 2 flawed studies, results of NF treatment suggest improvements in global and performance IQ, spelling, attention/impulsivity, and repeal of learning disorder diagnosis. Treatment gains were maintained over a period of 2 years of follow-up, but limited data do not support treatment recommendations.
- Pediatric epilepsy has no controlled studies, and preliminary data are not promising, but it might be considered for uncontrolled seizures unresponsive to anticonvulsants.
- qEEG NF treatment seems sensible and safe, but not easy or inexpensive (30–40 half-hour treatments, 2–3 times weekly).
- NF should be conducted by a well-trained professional with expertise in brain function beyond simply an ability to operate equipment, to enhance safety and optimize effectiveness.

Abbreviations	
ADHD	Attention Deficit/Hyperactivity Disorder
APA	American Psychological Association
ATEC	Autism Treatment Evaluation Checklist
CNV	Contingent Negative Variation
EEG	Electroencephalogram
ERPs	Event-Related Potentials
ES	Effect Size
FD-VARETA	Frequency Domain Variable Resolution Electromagnetic Tomography
fMRI	Functional Magnetic Resonance Imaging
HEG	Hemoencephalograpic Neurofeedback
Hz	Hertz
ISNR	International Society for Neurofeedback and Research
LD	Learning Disorders
LENS	Low Energy Neurofeedback System
LORETA	Low Resolution Electromagnetic Tomography
MTA	Multimodal Treatment Study of ADHD
NF	Neurofeedback
PDD	Pervasive Developmental Disorder
qEEG	Quantitative Electroencephalography
qEEG NF	Quantitative EEG Neurofeedback
RCTs	Randomized Controlled Trials
SCP-NF	Slow Cortical Potential Neurofeedback
SCPs	Slow Cortical Potentials
USPSTF	US Preventive Services Task Force

This article provides a definition of neurofeedback (NF), theories of its mechanisms of change, types of NF, a brief history of the research, and efforts to measure the specific effects of NF as distinguished from nonspecific treatment effects. The focus is on NF treatment of attention deficit/hyperactivity disorder (ADHD), autism spectrum disorders (from here on referred to as autism), learning disorders (LD), and epilepsy in children and adolescents, using signal from surface electrodes. For each disorder, it is initially noted how this treatment might be beneficial, the results of empirical studies, their strengths and limitations, and directions for future research. The article concludes with clinical recommendations for the use of NF treatment for these disorders.

WHAT IS NEUROFEEDBACK?

Neurofeedback (also called neurotherapy or electroencephalogram [EEG] biofeed-back) is a type of biofeedback that uses operant conditioning to train people to improve regulation of their brain-wave patterns by providing them with real-time video/audio information about their brain's electrical activity measured from scalp electrodes. In effect, the conditioning is based on feedback given to the patient that is contingent on the patient's EEG pattern (see article by Simkin and colleagues in this issue for more technical details).

First described qualitatively as "brain waves" on the EEG by Hans Berger in 1924, the electrical activity of the brain was thought to reflect changes in the brain's functional state while awake or asleep, or to denote brain diseases such as epilepsy.[1] EEG activity, characterized in terms of rhythmic activity measured in hertz (Hz, the number of waves per second), is divided into specifically named frequency bands, corresponding to functional activity and arousal state: the δ band corresponds to slow-wave sleep state (up to 4 Hz), θ to a drowsy/inattentive state (4–8 Hz), α to a relaxed/wakeful/alert state (8–12 Hz), and β to an active/attentive state (12–30 Hz). Most of the brain electrical activity occurs in the 1- to 20-Hz range.

Within each band, there are recognizable functionally significant rhythms. For example, a specific type of low β activity (12–15 Hz) observed in the sensorimotor cortex is called the sensorimotor rhythm. The amplitude of the sensorimotor rhythm is higher when the sensory-motor areas are inactive (eg, during immobile states) and decreases when those areas are activated (eg, during motor tasks). Therefore, the amplitude of the sensorimotor rhythm is a measure of sensory-motor inhibition; that is, higher amplitude when the "brake is on" and lower when the "brake is off." A mathematical approach to analyzing EEG data, called quantitative electroencephalography (qEEG), can be used to develop a visual map of the type and location of brain waves or rhythms. Other more specific wave patterns, such as event-related potentials, can also be seen in the EEG. Event-related potentials are electrical representations associated with sensory and cognitive processing occurring in response to a stimulus or event.[2] Slow cortical potentials (SCPs) are one specific group of event-related potentials. They are slow event-related direct-current shifts of the EEG that correspond to the excitation threshold of large cortical cell assemblies.[3,4] Shifts in the positive direction indicate an increase of the excitation threshold and a corresponding inhibition of activation, whereas shifts in the negative direction, called the contingent negative variation, reflect a reduction of the excitation threshold and represent cognitive preparation and increased cortical activation of a network.[3,5]

The classical conditioning of human EEG was first shown in the mid-1930s, when researchers trained human subjects to block α waves.[6,7] Operant conditioning, in which EEG-derived information is used as instant feedback to the patient in real-time, was first used to alter the human EEG in the 1960s[8,9] (see also Ref.[10] for a historical review). Since the 1960s, mainly using operant conditioning, there has been a significant increase in the clinical application of NF to several neuropsychiatric conditions, including ADHD, LD, developmental disabilities, cognitive/memory enhancement, epilepsy, traumatic brain injury, stroke, alcoholism, substance abuse, antisocial personality, autism, anxiety, depression, insomnia, and migraines.[11] There has also been a significant increase, especially in the 21st century, in the number of published research and dissertation studies (eg, *PsychINFO/Medline* journal searches for title terms neurofeedback, electroencephalographic/EEG biofeedback, or neurotherapy: pre-1970 = 11 studies, 1970–1979 = 212 studies, 1980–1989 = 145 studies, 1990–1999 = 226 studies, 2000–2012 = 1279 studies). The International Society for

Neurofeedback and Research (ISNR; www.isnr.org) and *Journal of Neurotherapy* were established in 1995, with annual ISNR conferences since 1993. More recently, NF was introduced to the general public by Jim Robbins' book, *A Symphony in the Brain: The Evolution of the New Brain Wave Biofeedback*.[12]

TYPES OF NEUROFEEDBACK

Hammond[11] defines 7 types of NF and their use for various disorders:

1. The traditional and most frequently used is *Frequency/Power NF*, and it is the NF method usually meant by the general term "neurofeedback." This technique typically entails the use of 2 to 4 surface electrodes and is sometimes called "surface neurofeedback." Developed in the 1960s to change the amplitude or speed of specific brain waves in particular brain locations, it is used to treat ADHD, anxiety, insomnia, and LD.
2. *Slow Cortical Potential Neurofeedback* (SCP-NF) modifies the direction (positive or negative) of slow cortical potentials and has been used to treat epilepsy, migraines, and ADHD.
3. *Low-Energy Neurofeedback System* (LENS), developed in 1992, is a passive type of NF involving delivery of a very weak electromagnetic signal to change a patient's brain waves while the patient is motionless and has their eyes closed; it has been used to treat traumatic brain injury, fibromyalgia, anger, restless legs syndrome, ADHD, anxiety, depression, and insomnia.
4. *Hemoencephalographic* (HEG) Neurofeedback, developed in 1994, provides feedback about cerebral blood flow to treat migraine.
5. *Live Z-score* Neurofeedback, developed in 1998, involves the continuous comparison of multiple variables of brain electrical activity (eg, power, asymmetries, phase-lag, coherence) to a normative database to give moment-to-moment feedback; it has been used to treat insomnia.
6. *Low-Resolution Electromagnetic Tomography* (LORETA) was developed in 1994 to treat depression, addictions, and obsessive-compulsive disorder. LORETA involves the use of 19 electrodes that are used to monitor phase, power, and coherence (see article by Simkin and colleagues in this issue).
7. The most recent type of NF, developed in 2003, is *functional magnetic resonance imaging* (fMRI) NF, which allows patients to regulate their brain activity based on feedback of activity from deep subcortical areas of the brain.

Although Hammond's article can be found on the web site of the ISNR and is published in their journal, the *Journal of Neurotherapy*, not everyone agrees with these definitions. Martijn Arns, PhD, an NF expert at Research Institute Brainclinics in the Netherlands, noted that "...the simple lack of published controlled efficacy studies does not justify including all them as NF. Furthermore, HEG has not been demonstrated to penetrate the skull, so that should be considered biofeedback, not NF. Also, LENS does not provide any feedback, since LENS consists of measuring a single-channel EEG, having the computer apply a specific algorithm, with no physical or yet measurable form of feedback." (Martijn Arns, PhD, personal communication, 2013). Only one randomized placebo controlled study has been conducted using LENS and found no difference between sham and active-LENS.[13] Unfortunately, the lack of a standard definition of NF, standard protocols of applying different forms of NF to different disorders, and an agreed-on certification process of its professionals has limited the progress of the NF field from its inception.

CONTROLS FOR NEUROFEEDBACK RESEARCH

A methodological topic that is currently being debated in NF is the necessity for double-blind, placebo-controlled randomized trials. The disagreement involves whether NF should be evaluated as an unblindable psychological treatment (like cognitive-behavioral therapy), using American Psychological Association guidelines,[14–16] or as a blindable treatment similar to new medications, using double-blind sham-controlled studies.[17–20]

Randomization is essential for any treatment study,[17–20] conventional or otherwise. Although psychiatrists are well aware of the need for randomized double-blind, placebo-controlled studies, one can forget the full range of advantages that these procedures can provide. Without randomization, it would not be known whether reported results were caused by a specific treatment effect (eg, an actual treatment-induced change in EEG brain waves) or because of nonspecific treatment effects, such as self-selection of treatment, expectations of parents and participants (eg, from choosing their preferred treatment), family motivation and resources to manage the time and cost of NF, nonrandom participant experiences (ie, participant history), practice with assessment measures, maturation, and regression to the mean; or interactions among these factors. Other nonspecific treatment effects can threaten the internal validity of treatment outcome research, including the expectations regarding study outcome of the research staff and raters (ie, parents, teachers, and clinicians), provider qualities, staff attention to the patient, practice paying attention/sitting still/inhibiting responses, treatment structures and apparatus, participants' motivation for improvement and/or therapeutic alliance.[21]

Most of the nonspecific treatment effects of a procedure like NF can be controlled by randomizing part of the sample to a "fake" ("sham") NF condition, akin to a placebo, or to some other treatment comparable to NF except lacking the specific active treatment component, that is, the feedback to the patient that is contingent on the person's EEG. The expectations of subjects, experimenters, trainers, and raters in NF research can all be controlled by blinding them to the treatment condition to which they have been randomly assigned. For effective blinding, the treatment and control groups need to be matched in duration, intensity, and apparatus.

The use of sham controls in NF research to obtain valid double-blinding has been questioned on both ethical and practical levels.[20] On ethical grounds, based on the Declaration of Helsinki,[22] some NF researchers[23] have argued against using a placebo in the form of sham NF, claiming that it would "withhold or deny 'the best proven diagnostic and therapeutic' treatment to any participant" (p. 23); instead they recommend an active-control condition with known clinical efficacy. However, it seems presumptuous and even antiscientific to assert that NF is so obviously effective that there is no need for placebo-controlled studies. Others have disagreed with this recommendation to omit placebo-controlled studies for several reasons and have addressed it by suggesting ethical ways to use a sham-NF condition.[17,20] The practicality of using a sham-NF in research involves 3 sequential questions[20]: (1) Is it possible to develop a truly inert sham NF condition, in accordance with principles of learning theory and conditioning principles,[24] that does not lead to learning via unintentional feedback? (2) If question 1 is answered, can this sham-NF condition then be effectively blinded to participants, informants, and experimenters? (3) Finally, if questions 1 and 2 are both answered, can a sample be recruited and retained throughout the lengthy pretreatment and posttreatment assessments and a full NF treatment schedule (eg, 40 sessions for ADHD) using a truly inert sham treatment that remains validly blind to all? By fulfilling these conditions, the use of a sham-NF control in NF research would be presumably both practical and ethical.

Recently, a collaborative group of researchers from NF and traditional treatment outcome research has, for the first time, proposed, and is seeking funding for, a design that meets these ethical and practical concerns by (1) reinforcing the sham subject based on a pre-recorded EEG from another patient, (2) superimposing the sham subject's real-time artifacts on the stored EEG to keep the technician/trainer/therapist blinded, and (3) time-stamping the reinforcement events on the sham subject's real EEG, to determine post-hoc if there were any contingencies that were inadvertently providing unintended systematic feedback[20] (eg, randomly reinforcing at the same time they were paying attention).

TREATMENT OUTCOMES IN NEUROFEEDBACK RESEARCH

The following sections describe the research on NF for ADHD, autism, LD, and epilepsy based on a PsycINFO/Medline search in September 2012 using the title words: neurofeedback, EEG biofeedback, or neurotherapy crossed with (1) ADHD or attention-deficit; (2) autism, Aspergers, or pervasive developmental disorder (PDD); (3) seizure, epilepsy, epileptic, grand mal, or petite mal; and (4) learning, reading, dyslexia, dyslexic, math, mathematics, dyscalculia, spelling, writing, written, dysgraphia, and dysgraphic.

NEUROFEEDBACK FOR ADHD

NF has been suggested for the treatment of ADHD because research indicates that many patients with ADHD have more slow-wave (especially θ, 3.5–8 Hz) power and less β (12–20 Hz) power, especially in the central and frontal regions, as well as reduced cortical negativity (ie, a deviance in contingent negative variation) during cognitive preparation.[2] These brain-wave patterns probably reflect underarousal of the central nervous system associated with the core ADHD symptoms of inattention, hyperactivity, and impulsivity. The goal of this treatment is to reverse these functional characteristics of abnormal CNS physiology by countering the physiological underarousal associated with ADHD.

To quantify treatment effects in the clinical trials discussed in this article, the effect size (ES) is described using the Cohen's d statistic,[25] based on posttreatment means and standard deviations, with the assumption that randomization controlled for any pretreatment differences between groups. Cohen's d values between 0.2 and 0.4 are considered small ESs; values between 0.5 and 0.8 are considered medium, and values greater than 0.8 are considered large. For comparison with other empirically validated treatments for ADHD, stimulant medications have ESs of 0.8 to 1.2, atomoxetine 0.4 to 1.0, and behavior modification 0.5 to 1.0.

Since the first report of an RCT on NF for ADHD in 1996,[26] 12 RCTs and 2 meta-analyses[14,27] on youth have been published, with 11 RCTs since 2006; most of these RCTs used either traditional NF targeting the θ-β ratio or slow-cortical-potential NF. Summing across the 9 RCTs that provided ESs or the means and standard deviations to calculate them, the mean ES for measures of inattention was 0.72; the mean ES for measures of hyperactivity/impulsivity was 0.70; the mean ES for measures of all ADHD symptoms was 0.62; and the mean ES for measures of all problems (ADHD or otherwise) was 0.57. Four of these studies also showed neurophysiologic changes that were specifically associated with NF treatment (EEG,[28,29] fMRI,[30] and N2-amplitude[31]). One study[32] reported continued improvements for NF at 6 months following the end of treatment, but that study had serious methodological limitations.[18]

However, the reported benefits of NF have only been replicated in one[28] of the 4[19,33,34] double-blinded RCTs conducted, but those studies had methodological flaws, including small samples.

Of the 12 RCTs, only 4 studies used a sham-NF design, and none of them examined the validity of the sham's inertness. Therefore, it is not known whether any of these were truly comparing EEG-contingent feedback to noncontingent feedback rather than, in some manner, giving unintentional contingent feedback in the control condition. Similarly, only 2 of these 4 sham-controlled studies[19,33] tested the accuracy of their blinded testing and found them to be valid, so it is not known whether the other 2 studies were correctly blinded. Another criticism of these 4 studies is that they used unconventional NF protocols that are not typically used in the field, such as the use of automatic (auto-thresholding) rather than manual modulation of training thresholds by the NF clinicians who continuously monitor the subject's qEEG.[35] Recalculating the aforementioned ESs, without these 4 sham-controlled studies, leads to slightly higher values (previous ESs in parentheses): Inattention 0.81 (vs 0.72), hyperactivity/impulsivity 0.73 (vs 0.70), all ADHD problems 0.71 (vs 0.62), and any problems (ADHD or otherwise) 0.68 (vs 0.57). However, these ES are now based on studies that do not include a full-validated blinded control comparator.

A recent open-label clinic-based study examined the effects of qEEG-guided NF for ADHD using a pretreatment qEEG to develop personalized NF protocols for 7 children and 14 adults with ADHD.[35] The use of qEEG indicates that a patient's EEG is compared with a normal database. If the brain-wave pattern of the patient is 2 or more standard deviations above or below the mean, and these abnormal brain-wave patterns are in a part of the brain corresponding with the symptoms, then these brain-wave patterns will be the target of the NF sessions. Pre-post treatment comparisons indicated significant improvements for the entire sample on self-reported ratings of attention ($P = .000$, within-subject ES = 1.78), hyperactivity/impulsivity ($P = .001$, within-subject ES = 1.22), and depression ($P = .003$). The study authors noted these ESs were much larger than those calculated in the meta-analysis of 16 studies (6 RCTs) of NF with pediatric ADHD (inattention = 0.81, impulsivity = 0.69, hyperactivity = .40) and similar to an open-label clinic study that preselected children with deviant θ/β ratio (attention ES = 1.8).[36] Open-label studies, with no double-blind or sham-placebo controls, often show stronger effects than rigorously designed studies and are unable to separate the specific from the nonspecific effects of treatment. However, the personalized approach to NF based on pretreatment qEEG seems sensible and worth pursuing in controlled research. In this open-label study, although results were not reported separately for children and adults, no significant differences were found between children and adults on pre-post measures of attention and impulsivity, suggesting that, in this study, the effects of NF on ADHD in youth and adults were comparable.

The meta-analysis by Arns and colleagues[14] of 15 studies (6 with randomization) on NF for children and adolescents reported ESs of $d = 0.81$ for inattention, $d = 0.69$ for impulsivity, and $d = 0.40$ for hyperactivity, and it concluded that "Neurofeedback treatment for ADHD can be considered 'Efficacious and Specific' Level 5 (p. 180)." However, because of the inclusion of nonrandomized studies and the lack of studies with blinding and sham-NF controls, the authors disagree and instead conclude that NF has not been shown superior to a credible placebo or to established treatment for ADHD in youth.[18]

Readers may also be interested in a paper-commentary-reply series of articles based on the position paper by Sherlin and colleagues[15] on NF for ADHD[15–17] and the authors' recent reviews of published or conference-presented RCTs on this topic.[18,37] **Fig. 1** compares the pre-post improvement in parent-rated inattentive

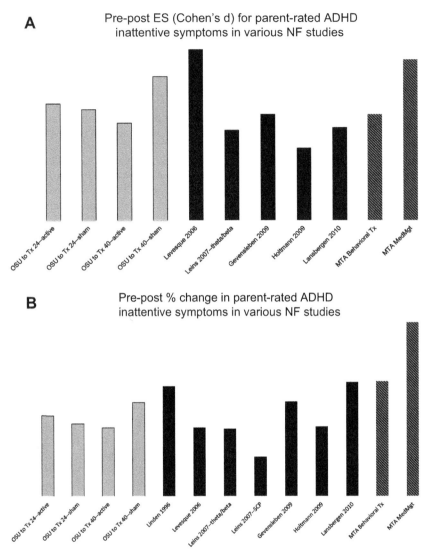

Fig. 1. Comparison of parent-rated pre-post inattention symptoms in controlled randomized studies of NF. Gray columns show improvement with active and sham placebo NF treatment in the Ohio State University (OSU) trial (Arnold and colleagues, 2013[19]) at mid treatment (24 sessions) and end of treatment (40 sessions). Black columns show improvement with active NF treatment in other studies, with varied treatment durations. Striped columns show, for comparison, improvements with 2 standard treatments (carefully monitored medication and multicomponent behavioral treatment) after 14 months in the Multimodal Treatment Study of ADHD (MTA, MTA Cooperative Group, 1999[38]). This figure illustrates the difficulty of assessing efficacy in the absence of a double-blind control group. Parent-rated inattention was the most common measure across studies, presenting the opportunity for comparison. A different outcome measure may have shown a different picture. (A) pre-post ESs; (B) percentage change in ratings.

symptoms across available controlled studies for active treatment and sham placebo treatment in the Ohio State University study. The pre-post improvement in 2 of the 14-month evidence-based treatments in the Multimodal Treatment Study of ADHD[38] is also shown for comparison. Parent-rated inattention was selected for comparison because it was the most common of reported outcomes; other outcomes may show a different picture.

The American Academy of Pediatrics (AAP) recently declared "biofeedback" to be an evidence-based child and adolescent psychosocial intervention with "level 1, best support".[39] "Biofeedback" was used to refer to feedback interventions to train either the brain (ie, NF) or the body (traditionally referred to as biofeedback). This rating was based on recommendations derived from the PracticeWise Evidence-Based Services Database (www.practicewise.com), which attributes "Level 1, Best Support" for treatments with at least 2 RCTs, each involving at least 30 subjects, showing that the treatment approach was better than another active treatment or placebo. Practice-Wise cited Gevensleben and colleagues[32] and Bakhshayesh and colleagues[40] for NF, and for biofeedback, Rivera and Omizo[41] and Omizo and Michael.[42] Although it is true that all of these studies were RCTs with more than 30 subjects and demonstrated that the treatment was more effective than another active treatment, neither PracticeWise nor AAP considered or explained the possible contribution to these results of nonspecific treatment factors and did not alert the public to these potential confounds.

In general, the quality of research on NF for ADHD is mixed but improving. On the positive side, many available studies incorporate randomization, standardized diagnostic assessments, Diagnostic and Statistical Manual of Mental Disorders (DSM) diagnoses, control of concomitant medication, measurement of comorbidity, multidomain assessment, standard treatment outcome measures, some type of blind (typically single) in a few studies, and a sham or control treatment condition in 4 studies. Current limitations in most studies, and so areas to be addressed in future studies, include recruitment of participants with abnormal EEGs, standardization of NF protocols, triple-blinding (of subjects, NF trainers, and raters, such as parents, teachers, and clinicians), testing validity of blinding, testing inertness of sham, reporting of adverse effects, and controlling for concurrent treatments (such as medications, psychotherapy, special education), increased sample size, monitoring of long-term follow-up, and examining for potential age-related (youth vs adult) differences in response.

In summary, applying the US Preventive Services Task Force (USPSTF) Level of Certainty of Research Evidence and Recommendation Grade,[43] which rates the quality of data-based evidence as poor, fair, or good, the authors rate the quality of evidence for the NF treatment of ADHD as fair to good. This rating fits the USPSTF criteria of "recommend," defined as fair evidence of benefit and safety (**Tables 1** and **2**). However, despite the endorsement of this treatment by the AAP, and despite the "recommend" language of the USPSTF criteria, the authors would nonetheless hesitate to place NF for ADHD into a simple "recommend" category, because of the failure of current studies to sufficiently rule out nonspecific effects contributing to the apparent outcome. The authors are concerned that the current data might overestimate the clinical value of NF for ADHD. Nonetheless, for families who have tried or at least considered conventional treatments for ADHD, and who have the time and money to invest in NF, an empirical trial could be considered in conformity with the clinical recommendations at the end of this article. Based on the current standard NF protocols examined in the 12 available RCTs, a typical treatment course for ADHD would involve about 30 to 40 sessions, lasting 30 minutes, 2 to 3 times weekly.

Table 1
Evidence for NF for pediatric ADHD, LD, autism, and epilepsy, based on criteria by the USPSTF level of certainty of research evidence and recommendation grade

Disorder	Quality of Evidence for Children or Adolescents/Clinical Recommendation	Basis of Recommendation
ADHD	Fair to good/recommend (with reservation)	12 published RCTs (4 are sham-controlled with nonsignificant effects that did not use optimal protocols)
Autism	Fair/recommend (with reservation)	4 small RCTs (2 sham-controlled with significant effects, 1 wait-list control with several improvements, reportedly maintained over a period of 6 mo, and 1 compared with a biofeedback condition and a wait list)
Learning disorders	Poor to fair/insufficient evidence to make a recommendation	2 studies using operationalized definitions and assessments of LD, and 1 small RCT
Epilepsy	Poor/insufficient evidence to make a recommendation	There are no clinical trials specific to pediatric epilepsy, although children and adolescents have been included in trials of NF for epilepsy; 2 meta-analyses of NF reported 82% of subjects experienced >50% seizure reductions[64] & 79% statistically significant reduction in frequency of seizures[65]

The treatment would aim to reduce θ and increase β power, with manual modulation of training thresholds by the NF clinician monitoring the in-session qEEG.

NEUROFEEDBACK FOR AUTISM

NF was initially proposed for the treatment of autism because qEEG studies of autism demonstrate (1) reduced connectivity between cortical areas, especially with increasing distance; (2) a lack of hemispheric differences; and (3) a wide variety of significant and sometimes contradictory EEG differences, including decreased and increased frontal δ power; increased generalized δ activity; increased and reduced θ activity in frontal, central, and temporal regions; decreased α activity, and increased β and γ activity.[44] These diverse and variable physiologic differences in the brain probably reflect the "pervasive" functional variability that characterizes autism.

Four small RCTs and one review[45] of qEEG NF treatment of autism have been published.[46–48] The first 2 RCTs, appearing in the same article[46] as 2 separate studies, focused on decreasing μ brain-wave frequency (8–25 Hz) over the sensorimotor cortex, which is an EEG correlate of mirror-neuron activity associated with imitation abilities that are thought to be limited in autism.[49] The first study randomized 8 youths (ages 7–17) with an unverified diagnosis of high-functioning autism to either NF (N = 5, μ rhythm, right hemisphere C4, 30 half-hour sessions, 3 times weekly for 10 weeks) or a sham-NF control (N = 3). Participants and parents were blinded to the treatment assignment. Compared with sham controls, NF significantly increased sustained attention and sensory/cognitive awareness scores on subscales of the parent-rated Autism Treatment Evaluation Checklist (ATEC). The second study

Table 2
Authors' opinions regarding recommendations and advice

Diagnosis	Quality of Evidence for NF for Children or Adolescents/ Clinical Recommendation	Authors' Recommendation, Clinical Tips, and Cautions
ADHD	Fair to good/recommend with reservations	• Currently NF is not recommended for most families. • Due to lack of benefit in several sham-controlled trials, NF cannot be strongly recommended as a stand-alone treatment of pediatric ADHD at this time. • NF is an acceptable treatment for families with the time and money to invest in the treatment without diverting resources from other treatments or family needs.
Autism	Fair/recommend with reservations	• NF should not replace evidence-based practice in the treatment of autism, including applied behavior analysis, medication management for comorbid behavior problems, allied health intervention (eg, speech therapy, occupational therapy), and educational intervention. • As there are currently no evidence-based treatments for the *core symptoms of autism*, and given the positive findings in most of the controlled trials, NF is an acceptable complementary adjunctive intervention for pediatric autism.
Learning disorders	Poor to fair/not recommended	• Given small sample sizes in current literature, NF should not replace evidence-based educational intervention for children with learning disabilities. • NF may be acceptable as a complementary adjunctive intervention, particularly for children with comorbid ADHD symptoms and whose families have the resources (time, money, energy) to invest in the treatment.
Epilepsy	Poor/not recommended	• Given the lack of data, NF should not replace anticonvulsant medications for the treatment of pediatric epilepsy. In cases of uncontrolled seizures unresponsive to medication, it would be reasonable to try for those with the time and money to invest.

examined 19 youths (ages 7–17) with rigorously diagnosed autism diagnoses in a randomized (NF = 9, sham NF = 10) double-blind design involving NF training of a higher μ band (10–13 Hz). This study confirmed significant improvements in sustained attention but not in sensory-cognitive awareness and also reported significant parent-rated ATEC improvements in speech/language communication, sociability, health/physical behavior subscales, and overall score. In addition, this second study found decreases in amplitude but increases in phase coherence in μ rhythms and normalization of μ rhythm. Although both studies demonstrated normalization of the NF-targeted μ rhythm as well as improvements in a variety of behaviors associated with autism, neither study showed the expected behavioral improvements in imitation. The authors were unable to compute ESs, because means and standard deviations were not reported for either study.

The 2 most recent RCTs[47,48] were conducted by Kouijzer and colleagues as a follow-up to their nonrandomized pilot study[50,51] of 8- to 12-year-olds with PDD–not otherwise specified, in which NF led to improved executive functioning, social communication, and atypical behavior, which was sustained for 6 months after the termination of treatment; qEEG changes included significantly reduced θ and increased β power in central and frontal brain regions. In their first RCT, Kouijzer and colleagues examined 20 youths (ages 8–12) with high-functioning autism, whose diagnoses were verified by a study psychiatrist. They were randomized to individualized qEEG-guided NF treatment (N = 10) or a wait-list control (N = 10). NF involved forty 21-minute sessions, twice weekly for 20 weeks, and focused on decreasing excessive θ power in central and frontal brain areas. Excessive θ power reflects altered activity in the anterior cingulate cortex, which is thought to be involved in the social and executive problems associated with autism. Various individualized treatment protocols were used (different θ frequency bands and electrode placements), depending on each participant's baseline qEEG, which led to (1) successful reductions in excessive θ power; (2) significant improvements on a reciprocal social interactions (d = 1.61), communication (d = 1.19), initializing peer interactions (d = 1.13), nonverbal communication (d = 1.1), semantics (d = 0.93), and linguistic coherence (d = 0.71); and (3) significant improvements in neuropsychologic set-shifting and cognitive flexibility skills on the Trail Making Test (d = 0.99). The treatment gains were maintained at 6-month follow-up, and some additional treatment gains were demonstrated at 6 months for the NF group but not for the control group.

In their second small RCT, Kouijzer and colleagues[48] attempted to control for some nonspecific treatment effects by comparing NF, skin-conductance biofeedback, and a wait-list control. In this study, 38 adolescents (ages 12–18) with rigorously diagnosed autism were randomly assigned to individualized qEEG-guided NF (n = 13; forty 21-minute sessions, twice weekly for 20 weeks), skin-conductance biofeedback (n = 12; identical treatment to NF except feedback was based on skin-conductance from the index and ring fingers of the nondominant hand); or a wait list (n = 13). Subjects and parents were blinded to treatment assignment for the NF or skin-conductance biofeedback, but not for the wait list. This blinding was reported to be successful, with 58% of subjects in both treatment groups believing that they had received a combination of NF and skin-conductance biofeedback, and 33% of the NF group and 42% of the skin-biofeedback group believing that they had received NF alone. In addition, the treatment expectations of subjects and their parents were found comparable among all 3 groups and were not a significant covariate of treatment outcome.

In the NF group 54% of the NF group were classified as "EEG regulators" because they were able to significantly reduce their δ and/or θ power during treatment sessions; none of the skin-conductance biofeedback group were classified as EEG regulators. Unexpectedly, this in-session EEG regulation did not generalize beyond the training sessions and lead to pre-post EEG changes. In the skin-conduction biofeedback group, 75% were "skin-conductance regulators" who were able to significantly reduce in-session skin conductance; 38% of the NF group was also classified as "skin-conductance regulators." EEG regulators showed significant pre-post treatment improvements on laboratory measures of cognitive flexibility ($d = 0.53$), with pre-post treatment gains maintained at 6 months after the end of treatment ($d = 1.4$). However, EEG regulators did not show changes in EEG regulation beyond the training sessions, significant changes in parent-rated autistic symptoms, or clinician-rated global clinical functioning outside of the laboratory. No significant pre-post treatment differences were found on any outcome measure for the EEG non-regulators, skin-conductance nonregulators, or wait-list controls, suggesting that the change in cognitive flexibility was due to specific effects of NF and that NF did not lead to any nonspecific treatment effects on other outcomes. That is, NF-facilitated reduction of δ and/or θ power led to a highly specific improvement in cognitive flexibility in adolescents with autism.

In the 2 RCTs that provided means and standard deviations allowing calculation of posttreatment ESs (2/4, 50%), the mean ESs for NF in autism on all measures was $d = 1.11$, which is a large ES. However, 9 of the 10 ESs were derived from one study, which was the first Kouijzer RCT.[47]

Several of the studies of NF for autism include the use of randomization, some form of blinding, formal assessments of autism diagnoses, multidomain assessment, and documentation of EEG changes. Future directions for research include larger double-blind sham-controlled RCTs with follow-up, tests of the validity of the blind, use of standardized outcome measures, assessment and control of comorbidity and concomitant treatments, and monitoring/reporting of adverse effects.

Regarding clinical recommendations, applying the USPSTF Level of Certainty of Research Evidence and Recommendation Grade,[43] the quality of data-based evidence of NF for autism is rated as "fair," and according to the USPSTF guidelines, the clinical recommendation is to "recommend" NF for treating autism (see **Tables 1** and **2**). However, given that the main positive results on NF for autism derive from one small study,[47] this recommendation is again qualified with reservations and mainly relevant for families who have tried or considered conventional psychosocial treatments for autism, have the time and money to invest in NF, and follow the clinical recommendations outlined at the end of the article.

NEUROFEEDBACK FOR LD

The NF literature on LDs is confounded because many studies profess to examine participants with LD who instead have ADHD, general academic issues and/or developmental delays rather than the more specifically defined DSM-IV reading disorders, disorders of written expression, mathematics disorders, or LD–not otherwise specified. LDs, as defined by the DSM-IV,[52] require that the "individual's achievement on individually administered, standardized tests in reading, mathematics, or written expression is substantially below that expected for a particular age, schooling, and level of intelligence."

NF treatment of LDs has been suggested because the presence of more θ and less α power, compared with same-aged controls, can be viewed as suggestive of maturational delay.[53] Following early case studies of youths with poorly defined learning problems, an important but flawed series of studies was conducted by Fernández and colleagues.[54] In a 2003 controlled study using the DSM-IV operational criteria for reading, math, or writing disorders[54] in 10 youths (ages 7–11), selected for abnormally high EEG θ/α ratios for their age and no comorbid neurologic or psychiatric disorders, participants were nonrandomly assigned to either NF (n = 5, location based on initial qEEG) or sham-NF (n = 5, random feedback noncontingent on EEG), with both groups receiving twenty 30-minute sessions on a twice-weekly basis for 10 to

12 weeks. Although this study had a sham-NF control group, no comparisons of NF and sham-NF were conducted; instead, only pre-post treatment analyses were made for each treatment group separately, defeating the purpose of a controlled study. Under these circumstances, NF seemed to lead to significant improvements in both global and performance Wechsler Intelligence Scale for Children (WISC) scores and in Test of Variables of Attention (TOVA) ADHD scores, changes that were not shown by the sham control group. Both NF and sham-NF groups showed EEG improvements compatible with maturation, but the NF group showed a greater number of regions with significant EEG changes, including larger magnitudes. Without randomization or a statistical comparison of the NF and sham-NF control groups, inferences about treatment efficacy cannot be drawn.

A 2-year follow-up study of this sample[55] found significant improvements (relative to baseline and to treatment end) again in WISC performance scores and TOVA ADHD scores, for the NF group only, but again with no statistical comparison of active and control groups. Using DSM criteria at the 2-year follow-up, DSM-IV criteria for an LD were no longer fulfilled in 80% of the NF group compared with 0% of the sham-NF group. The NF group showed a further increase in EEG improvements, but the control group experienced an actual worsening on EEG, including an increase in frontal θ "reaching abnormally high values."

This study was extended further with the nonrandom assignment of 6 additional children to the NF group.[56] For this larger data set (NF increased to 11 subjects, sham-NF remaining at 5), the NF group now showed significant clinical improvements in verbal WISC-R scores but not performance WISC-R scores. A significant improvement in TOVA scores was also reported. EEG data indicated a decrease in θ/α ratio. In this study, a more advanced method called frequency domain variable resolution electromagnetic tomography was used to estimate EEG changes in cortical subregions. No immediate posttreatment changes were observed at the end of treatment, but various EEG changes were observed 2 months later in several areas involved in executive functioning: θ power was decreased in the left frontal and cingulate regions; α power was enhanced in the right temporal lobe and right frontal regions, and there was increased β power in the left temporal, right frontal, and cingulate cortex regions.

Taken together, this series of studies by Fernández and colleagues leaves numerous methodological questions. In their nonrandomized studies of NF or sham-NF in youth with DSM-IV LDs, the unorthodox statistical analyses suggested that functional improvements (WISC-R and TOVA) were accompanied by delayed EEG improvements (decrease in θ/α ratio) in cortical regions subserving executive functions. However, these changes were not observed at the end of the treatment, but instead emerged several months later, perhaps consistent with a beneficial effect on general maturation rather than a specific therapeutic effect on the DSM-IV LD. Because many of the subjects seemed to have concurrent ADHD, it is possible that some or all of the improvement in LDs may have been due to a therapeutic effect of NF on ADHD, again rather than a direct effect on LD. It is unclear whether the blinding methods were effective in these nonrandomized studies. The strongest finding suggestive of a specific effect was the apparent resolution of LD diagnoses in the NF group and not in the sham-NF group, which renders this series of studies suggestive of some possibility of effectiveness.

The most recent study on NF for LD involved 19 youths (ages 8–15) with developmental reading disorder (dyslexia, diagnosed by their remedial teacher using a structured assessment of reading and spelling), who had no other personal or family history of mental illness.[57,58] Participants were randomized to individualized qEEG-based NF (n = 10, 20 sessions over a period of 10 weeks) and a wait-list control group (n = 9). All participants also received reading and spelling remedial counseling. NF led to a small but significant (ES; $d = 0.26$) improvement in spelling; this was associated with a significant increase in α coherence, suggesting that attentional processes may have mediated the improved spelling. In contrast, there was no significant improvement in reading or any related frontocentral changes.

The mean ESs for all measures across the 2 studies[56,57] were modest ($d = 0.39$). In addition to very small sample sizes, the overall limitations of these few studies include the lack of randomization, blinding, testing of validity of blinding, testing of sham inertness, standardized outcome measures, parent/teacher ratings, functional ratings, reporting of adverse effects, reporting of or controlling for concomitant treatments, and long-term follow-up.

Regarding clinical recommendations, applying the USPSTF Level of Certainty of Research Evidence and Recommendation Grade,[43] the rating of the quality of data-based evidence for NF of LD is "poor" to "fair," and the clinical recommendation is "insufficient evidence to make a recommendation" (see **Tables 1** and **2**). The authors are not recommending NF for LDs because findings were weak and only one study[57] involved randomization. However, if NF is pursued by families of children with LD, a short trial is suggested using an individualized qEEG-based approach involving 20 sessions over a period of 10 weeks to assess whether continued treatment is worthwhile in that individual.

NEUROFEEDBACK FOR EPILEPSY

Because epileptic seizures are time-limited abnormalities in the electrical activity of the brain that disrupt normal brain functioning, NF would seem a natural treatment option for researchers to explore. In the initial work of Sterman[59] on the operant conditioning of slow-wave rhythms in the sensorimotor cortex in cats, it was found that these sensorimotor rhythms were functionally related to thalamocortical inhibitory discharges that could suppress drug-induced seizures.[60] Sterman and Friar[61] then took a similar approach in one of the first clinical applications of NF in 1972, in successfully treating a case of epilepsy. Since then, most investigators have focused on the operant conditioning of the sensorimotor rhythm (12–15 Hz over sensorimotor cortex), but others have examined NF of slow cortical potentials[62] or EEG-guided NF[63] for the treatment of epilepsy.

No randomized controlled study of NF for pediatric epilepsy has been published to date. Most published studies on the NF treatment of epilepsy have been single or multiple case studies involving adults, or a mixed sample of adults and youth, but without reporting age-related effects. Two meta-analyses concluded that 82% of subjects with epilepsy experienced a greater than 30% reduction in seizures,[64] and that 79% of subjects had statistically significant reduction in the frequency of medication-resistant seizures.[65]

The only RCT of NF in adult epilepsy, conducted by Lantz and Sterman,[66] involved 24 patients (ages 15–53) with chronic drug-refractory epilepsy who were randomized to 3 groups: (1) sensorimotor rhythm NF (30 minutes, 3 times weekly for 6 weeks), (2) noncontingent NF (specifically, a sham treatment condition in which NF was not contingent on participants' EEG but instead was yoked to the EEGs of participants in the first NF group), and (3) a wait-list control. Anticonvulsant medication doses and serum levels remained constant throughout the study. Only the NF group experienced a significant pre-post treatment reduction in seizures, with a median seizure reduction of 61% (individual responses ranged from 0% to 100%), accompanied by significant improvements in cognitive and motor functioning. Subjects with the most sizable seizure reductions had fewer pretreatment self-rated psychological problems, higher baseline problem-solving scores on a neuropsychologic test of problem-solving, more baseline motor performance deficits (presumably signifying more pretreatment sensorimotor rhythm problems), and a greater ability to learn to modulate their EEG. This study is one of the most rigorous in NF, involving randomization, control groups including both a sham-NF (that was shown to produce no change) and a wait list, objective treatment outcome measures, blinded assessment evaluators, and control of concomitant medication treatment. However, NF trainers were not blinded, and the validity of participant blinding was not examined (eg, by asking participants which treatment they think they received), so it is possible that participants' and trainers' expectations may have influenced the study outcome.

Another important study by Lubar and colleagues[67] examined 8 subjects (a 13-year-old and 7 adults) with drug-refractory epilepsy (most of whom had brain damage and intellectual disability) using a within-subjects ABA reversal design. Subjects were "subdivided" (random assignment not noted) into 3 treatment groups. In the 4 months of phase A of the ABA design, the 3 groups either were (1) trained to suppress 3 to 8 Hz (n = 3), (2) trained to enhance 12 to 15 Hz (n = 2), or (3) trained to suppress 3 to 8 Hz simultaneously and enhance 11 to 19 Hz (n = 3). Phase B consisted of 2 months during which the contingent EEG feedback was reversed for each individual protocol: for example, those originally trained to suppress 3 to 8 Hz were trained to enhance 3 to 8 Hz. Finally, for the 4 months of the final phase A, participants received their initial EEG feedback schedules again. Medication doses and verified blood levels remained constant throughout the study. Subjects in group 1 were able to complete the NF protocol and showed a decrease in seizures in phase A, an increase in phase B, and a decrease in the return to phase A. Group 2 subjects were less able to complete the NF and showed an increase in seizures in phase A, a decrease in phase B, which continued through the return to phase A. Group 3 showed a seizure decrease in all 3 phases, but only 1 of the 3 participants was able to complete the NF. This study demonstrates the effect NF can have on the frequency of seizures, with suppression of 3 to 8 Hz apparently being therapeutic. The results in group 2 also raise a question of possible seizure risk from enhancing 12 to 15 Hz, commonly done in the treatment of ADHD. This result illustrates the importance of accurate diagnosis before initiating NF.

Although both of these studies are frequently cited as strong evidence in favor of NF for epilepsy, major limitations include small samples, lack of evaluation of the blind, contradictory individual results within the ABA phases and groups of Lubar's study (although this may be associated with the ability of those participants to learn the protocol), and lack of statistical analysis to assess whether the observed changes were greater than chance alone.

Regarding clinical recommendations, applying the USPSTF Level of Certainty of Research Evidence and Recommendation Grade,[43] the authors' classification for the quality of data-based evidence for NF of childhood or adolescent epilepsy is "poor" and their clinical recommendation is "insufficient evidence" to make a recommendation (see **Tables 1** and **2**). However, in extreme cases, such as a youth with uncontrolled seizures that are unresponsive to medication, it would be reasonable to try NF as a desperation measure, following the clinical recommendations outlined in the next section. However, the lack of any controlled trials of NF in youth with epilepsy prevents any reasonable prediction of success.

SAFETY AND RISKS OF NEUROFEEDBACK

NF is usually considered a safe procedure by specialists in the field, but published research trials have not systematically monitored or reported adverse effects. Hammond[11] noted mild adverse effects can occur during NF sessions, such as fatigue, spacey feelings, anxiety, headaches, insomnia, and irritability. Although he noted that these adverse effects either usually disappear shortly after the session or can be addressed by changing the training protocol, he does warn about more serious negative effects, such as worsening of the symptoms the NF is intending to treat if the wrong frequency is reinforced or suppressed. Such effects may result from NF procedures that are not conducted or at least supervised by a certified expert or that have not been effectively individualized to the particular patient.

Unfortunately, there are no published studies that focus specifically on the adverse effects of NF, either in adults or in youth. There are no systematically collected data on their frequency, severity, or duration. There are no accepted guidelines or protocols used for collecting data on the adverse effects. Questions about possible differences in adverse effects in adults and youth have not been addressed, and there has been no discussion of a possible adverse impact on child development. It is not known whether NF can, in some vulnerable individuals, aggravate or induce depression, mania, or psychosis. There are no real discussions or proposals regarding possible contraindications to NF. Drug interactions are not adequately evaluated, but there are some suggestions that psychostimulant doses might need to be reduced following NF treatment of ADHD.[68]

The lack of such information is peculiar in a field of clinical medicine, especially one involving the treatment of minors. It is all the more troublesome that, despite the lack of this type of safety data, that some specialists have argued that placebo-controlled studies are not needed. The failure to provide routine systematic evaluation of possible adverse effects of NF may be associated with the general lack of standardization in this field, but it will need rectification before NF will be taken seriously as a viable treatment with demonstrable safety.

CLINICAL SUMMARY AND CLINICAL RECOMMENDATIONS

1. *Current status of evidence of the effectiveness of NF*: Applying the USPSTF levels of certainty of research evidence and recommendation grade. Based on these guidelines, it is currently concluded that the evidence for NF is "fair" to "good" for ADHD, "fair" for autism, "poor" to "fair" for LD, and "poor" for epilepsy. Using these criteria, the evidence technically allows a "recommend" (based on fair evidence of benefit and safety, but with reservations) for ADHD and autism, and "insufficient data" to make a recommendation for LD and epilepsy. However, a closely monitored trial could be defensible after conventional treatments have been tried or at least considered, and assuming that the families have the time and money to invest in multiple sessions.
2. *The SECS (safe, easy, cheap, and sensible) criterion*: A treatment that is SECS needs less evidence to justify an individual patient trial than one that is RUDE (risky, unrealistic, difficult, or expensive) based on basic research of EEG abnormalities and the effects of operant conditioning. NF seems to be a sensible treatment with a solid biologic rationale. Despite the lack of systematically collected data on the safety of NF, current clinical opinion supports the belief that NF is reasonably safe. However, NF usually requires 30 to 40 treatment sessions lasting 30 to 40 minutes (typically 2–3 weekly sessions for 3–5 months), so it is definitely not easy or inexpensive in time or money.

3. *Technical Procedures:*
   a. As a baseline evaluation, either an initial qEEG using 1 or 2 scalp electrodes or a comprehensive qEEG using 19 electrodes should identify specific brain-wave patterns to be targeted in the individual, to increase the likelihood of successful treatment and also to reduce the risks of adverse effects.[11] This initial EEG or qEEG evaluation should be conducted by a specialized professional trained in NF methodology. Certified professionals may be found at the EEG and Clinical Neuroscience Society (www.ecnsweb.com/provider-directory.html) or the Quantitative Electroencephalography Certification Board (www.qeegboard.org).
   b. Periodic qEEGs should be done to monitor progress and adjust the treatment target. If there is not a learning curve, the diagnosis and treatment should be re-evaluated.
   c. Similarly, for the NF treatment itself to be successful and safe, it needs to be conducted or supervised by a trained professional with expertise regarding brain function, beyond the mere ability to operate EEG equipment.[11] Certified NF professionals may be found at the Biofeedback Certification International Alliance (www.bcia.org) or the ISNR (www.isnr.org).
   d. As current evidence indicates NF works through the mechanisms of operant conditioning, clinical applications (as well as research) should follow the principles of learning theory.[24]
   e. Medical or neurologic mimics should be ruled out before initiation of NF, because they may require a different specific treatment. As a corollary, it would be important to distinguish petit mal or absence seizures from ADHD because the type of NF indicated may differ.
4. *Potential for abuse or dependence:* Unlike stimulant treatment of ADHD, there seems to be no risk of abuse using NF treatment. There are no current data regarding risks of dependence on NF treatment.
5. *Interactions of treatment:* Although not formally reported, NF experts have informally observed an apparent interaction with stimulant medication in patients with ADHD: as NF improvement builds up, a child becomes more irritable and moody, which is relieved by reducing or discontinuing the stimulant dose,[68] suggesting the possibility that NF might be used to lower the stimulant dose needed for optimal effect, or possibly even allowing discontinuation entirely. However, there has not yet been a well-controlled study specifically demonstrating this possibility.
6. *Duration of effects:* Several studies have reported persistence of benefit for up to 6 months after treatment end. If NF could be established as having a permanent effect beyond the treatment period, this would be an advantage over medication and might make it fiscally competitive by considering the initial high cost amortized over several years of saved medication.
7. *Physiologic mechanism of action of NF:* It should be noted that qEEG NF, the type of NF described in this article, is only one of several approaches, albeit the best established. Other types of NF are described by Simkin and colleagues in their article also in this issue. NF targets different aspects of brain functioning in the different conditions it can treat. In ADHD, physiologic underarousal is improved by suppressing frontal and central θ and enhancing β activity. The diversity of functional abnormalities in different individuals with autism leads to a more differentiated approach in which NF targets selective EEG abnormalities that are identified on an individual basis. Similarly, both LDs and epilepsy are treated mainly based on the specific EEG abnormalities identified at baseline evaluation, rather than by a diagnosis-specific approach. Indeed, NF may target specific features that are

characteristic of certain diagnoses, but more generally, it tends to target the individualized aspects of brain functioning that are manifest in qEEG findings rather than being a diagnosis-based intervention.

REFERENCES

1. Berger H. About the human electroencephalogram. Archives of Psychiatry and Neurological Sciences 1929;87:527–70.
2. Barry RJ, Clarke AR, Johnstone SJ. A review of electrophysiology in attention-deficit/hyperactivity disorder: I. Qualitative and quantitative electroencephalography. Clin Neurophysiol 2003;114:171–83.
3. Leins U, Goth G, Hinterberger T, et al. Neurofeedback for children with ADHD: a comparison of SCP and theta/beta protocols. Appl Psychophysiol Biofeedback 2007;32:73–88.
4. Strehl U, Leins U, Goth G, et al. Self-regulation of slow cortical potentials: a new treatment for children with attention-deficit/hyperactivity disorder. Pediatrics 2006;118:1530–40.
5. Drechsler R, Straub M, Doehnert M, et al. Controlled evaluation of a neurofeedback training of slow cortical potentials in children with attention deficit/hyperactivity disorder. Behav Brain Funct 2007;3:35.
6. Durup G, Fessard A. L'électrencéphalogramme de l'homme. Observations psycho-physiologiques relatives à l'action des stimuli visuels et auditifs. L'année Psychologique 1935;36(1):1–32.
7. Loomis AL, Harvey EN, Hobart G. Electrical potentials of the human brain. J Exp Psychol 1936;19:249.
8. Kamiya J. The first communications about operant conditioning of the EEG. J Neurother 2011;15(1):65–73.
9. Sterman MB, LoPresti RW, Fairchild MD. Electroencephalographic and behavioral studies of monomethyl hydrazine toxicity in the cat. J Neurother 2010;14:293–300.
10. Arns M. Historical archives: the beginning. J Neurother 2010;14(4):291–2.
11. Hammond DC. What is neurofeedback: an update. J Neurother 2011;15:305–36.
12. Robbins J. A symphony in the brain: the evolution of the new brain wave biofeedback. Revised edition. New York: Grove Press; 2008.
13. Nelson DV, Bennett RM, Barkhuizen A, et al. Neurotherapy for fibromyalgia. Pain Med 2010;11:912–9.
14. Arns M, de Ridder S, Strehl U, et al. Efficacy of neurofeedback treatment in ADHD: the effects on inattention, impulsivity and hyperactivity: a meta-analysis. Clin EEG Neurosci 2009;40:180–9.
15. Sherlin L, Arns M, Lubar J, et al. A position paper on neurofeedback for the treatment of ADHD. J Neurother 2010;14:66–78.
16. Sherlin L, Arns M, Lubar J, et al. A reply to Lofthouse, Arnold, and Hurt. J Neurother 2010;14:307–11.
17. Lofthouse N, Arnold LE, Hurt E. A comment on Sherlin, Arns, Lubar, and Sokhadze. J Neurother 2010;14:301–6.
18. Lofthouse N, Arnold LE, Hersch S, et al. A review of neurofeedback treatment for pediatric ADHD. J Atten Disord 2012;16(5):351–72.
19. Arnold LE, Lofthouse N, Hersch S, et al. EEG neurofeedback for ADHD: double-blind sham-controlled randomized pilot feasibility trial. J Atten Disord 2013; 17(5):410–9. http://dx.doi.org/10.1177/1087054712446173.

20. The Collaborative Neurofeedback Group. A proposed multi-site double-blind randomized clinical trial of neurofeedback for ADHD: need, rationale and strategy. J Atten Disord 2013;17(5):420–36.

21. Donovan HS, Kwekkeboom KL, Rosenzweig MQ, et al. Nonspecific effects in psychoeducational intervention research. West J Nurs Res 2009;31:983–98.

22. World Medical Association. The declaration of Helsinki 52nd WMA general assembly. Edinburgh (Scotland): Author; 2000. Available at: http://www.wma.net.

23. La Vaque TJ, Rossiter T. The ethical use of placebo controls in clinical research: the declaration of Helsinki. Appl Psychophysiol Biofeedback 2001;26:25–39.

24. Sherlin L, Arns M, Lubar J, et al. Neurofeedback and basic learning theory: implications for research and practice. J Neurother 2011;15(4):292–304.

25. Cohen J. Statistical power analysis for the behavioral sciences. 2nd edition. Hillsdale (NJ): Lawrence Erlbaum; 1988.

26. Linden M, Habib T, Radojevic V. A controlled study of effects of EEG biofeedback on cognitive and behavior of children with attention deficit hyperactivity disorder and learning disabilities. Biofeedback Self Regul 1996;21:35–49.

27. Sonuga-Barke EJ, Brandeis D, Cortese S, et al, European ADHD Guidelines Group. Nonpharmacological interventions for ADHD: systematic review and meta-analyses of randomized controlled trials of dietary and psychological treatments. Am J Psychiatry 2013;170(3):275–89.

28. deBeus R, Kaiser DA. Neurofeedback with children with attention-deficit hyperactivity disorder: a randomized double-blind placebo-controlled study. In: Coben R, Evans JR, editors. Neurofeedback and neuromodulation techniques and applications. London: Academic Press; 2011. p. 127–52.

29. Gevensleben H, Holl B, Albrecht B, et al. Distinct EEG effects related to neurofeedback training in children with ADHD: a randomized controlled trial. Int J Psychophysiol 2009;74:149–57.

30. Levesque J, Beauregard M, Mensour B. Effect of neurofeedback training on the neural substrates of selective attention in children with attention-deficit/hyperactivity disorder: a functional magnetic resonance imaging study. Neurosci Lett 2006;394:216–21.

31. Holtmann M, Grasmann D, Cionek-Szpak E, et al. Specific effects of neurofeedback on impulsivity in ADHD. Kindheit und Entwicklung 2009;18:95–104.

32. Gevensleben H, Holl B, Albrecht B, et al. Is neurofeedback an efficacious treatment for ADHD? A randomized controlled clinical trial. J Child Psychiatry 2009; 50(7):780–9.

33. Perreau-Linck E, Lessard N, Levesque J, et al. Effects of neurofeedback training on inhibitory capacities in ADHD children: a single-blind, randomized, placebo-controlled study. J Neurother 2010;14:229–42.

34. Lansbergen MM, van Dongen-Boomsma M, Buitelaar JK, et al. ADHD and EEG-neurofeedback: a double-blind randomized placebo-controlled feasibility study. J Neural Transm 2010;118:275–84.

35. Arns M, Drinkenburg W, Kenemans JL. The effects of QEEG-informed neurofeedback in ADHD: an open-label pilot study. Appl Psychophysiol Biofeedback 2012;37:171–80.

36. Monastra VJ, Monastra DM, George S. The effects of stimulant therapy, EEG biofeedback, and parenting style on the primary symptoms of attention-deficit/hyperactivity disorder. Appl Psychophysiol Biofeedback 2002;27: 231–49.

37. Lofthouse N, Arnold LE, Hurt E. Current status of neurofeedback for attention-deficit/hyperactivity disorder. Curr Psychiatry Rep 2012;14(5):536–42.

38. The MTA Cooperative Group. A 14-month randomized clinical trial of treatment strategies for attention-deficit/hyperactivity disorder. Arch Gen Psychiatry 1999; 56:1073–86.
39. American Academy of Pediatrics. Evidence-based child and adolescent psychosocial interventions. 2012. Available at: http://www.aap.org/en-us/advocacy-and-policy/aap-health-initiatives/Mental-Health/Documents/CRPsychosocialInterventions.pdf. Accessed February 15, 2013.
40. Bakhshayesh AR, Hänsch S, Wyschkon A, et al. Neurofeedback in ADHD: a single-blind randomized controlled trial. Eur Child Adolesc Psychiatry 2011;20:481–91.
41. Rivera E, Omizo MM. An investigation of the effects of relaxation training and biofeedback on attention to task and impulsivity among male hyperactive children. Except Child 1980;27:41–51.
42. Omizo MM, Michael WB. Biofeedback induced relaxation training and impulsivity, attention to task, and locus of control among hyperactive boys. J Learn Disabil 1982;15(7):414–6.
43. US Preventive Services Task Force. Level of certainty of research evidence and recommendation. 2007. Available at: http://www.uspreventiveservicestaskforce.org/uspstf/grades.htm. Accessed February 2013.
44. Coben RC, Chabot RJ, Hirshberg L. EEG analyses in the assessment of autistic disorders. In: Casanova MF, El-Bax A, Suri JS, editors. Imaging the Brain in Autism. New York: Springer; 2013. p. 349–70.
45. Holtmann M, Steiner S, Hohmann S, et al. Neurofeedback in autism spectrum disorders. Dev Med Child Neurol 2011;53(11):986–93.
46. Pineda JA, Brang D, Hecht E, et al. Positive behavioral and electrophysiological changes following neurofeedback training in children with autism. Res Autism Spectr Disord 2008;2:557–81.
47. Kouijzer ME, van Schie HT, de Moor JM, et al. Neurofeedback treatment in autism. Preliminary findings in behavioral, cognitive, and neurophysiological functioning. Res Autism Spectr Disord 2010;4(3):386–99.
48. Kouijzer ME, Hein T, van Schie HT, et al. Is EEG biofeedback an effective treatment in autism spectrum disorders? A randomized controlled trial. Appl Psychophysiol Biofeedback 2013;38(1):17–28.
49. Oberman LM, Hubbard EM, McCleery JP, et al. EEG evidence for mirror neuron dysfunction in autism spectrum disorders. Cognitive Brain Res 2005;24(2): 190–8.
50. Kouijzer ME, de Moor JM, Gerrits BJ, et al. Neurofeedback improves executive functioning in children with autism spectrum disorders. Res Autism Spectr Disord 2009;3:145–62.
51. Kouijzer ME, de Moor JM, Gerrits BJ, et al. Long-term effects of neurofeedback treatment in autism. Res Autism Spectr Disord 2009;3:496–501.
52. American Psychiatric Association. Diagnostic and statistical manual of mental disorders (DSM-IV, text rev.). Washington, DC: Author; 2000.
53. Fernández T, Thalía H, Mendoza O, et al. Event-related EEG oscillations to semantically unrelated words in normal and learning disabled children. Brain Cogn 2012;80(1):74–82.
54. Fernández T, Herrera W, Harmony T, et al. EEG and behavioral changes following neurofeedback treatment in learning disabled children. Clin Electroencephalogr 2003;34:145–52.
55. Becerra J, Fernández T, Harmony T, et al. Follow-up study of learning disabled children treated with neurofeedback or placebo. Clin EEG Neurosci 2006;37(3): 198–203.

56. Fernández T, Harmony T, Fernández-Bouzas A, et al. Changes in EEG current sources induced by neurofeedback in learning disabled children. An exploratory study. Appl Psychophysiol Biofeedback 2007;32(3–4):169–83.
57. Breteler MH, Arns M, Peters S, et al. Improvements in spelling after QEEG-based neurofeedback in dyslexia: a randomized controlled treatment study. Appl Psychophysiol Biofeedback 2010;35(1):5–11.
58. Breteler MH, Arns M, Peters S, et al. Erratum to: Improvements in spelling after QEEG-based neurofeedback in dyslexia: a randomized controlled treatment study. Appl Psychophysiol Biofeedback 2010;35(2):187.
59. Sterman MB. Brain mechanisms in sleep, Chapter 4, Conditioning of induced EEG and behavioral sleep patterns: doctoral dissertation. Los Angeles (CA): University of California; 1963. p. 80–99.
60. Sterman MB, LoPresti RW, Fairchild MD. Electroencephalographic and behavioral studies of monomethyl hydrazine toxicity in the cat. Aerospace Medical Research Laboratory; 1969. p. 1–8, 69-3.
61. Sterman MB, Friar L. Suppression of seizures in an epileptic following sensorimotor EEG feedback training. Electroencephalogr Clin Neurophysiol 1972;33:89–95.
62. Rockstroh B, Elbert T, Birbaumer N, et al. Cortical self regulation in patients with epilepsies. Epilepsy Res 1993;14:63–72.
63. Walker JE, Kozlowski GP. Neurofeedback treatment of epilepsy. Child Adolesc Psychiatr Clin N Am 2005;14:163–76.
64. Sternman MB. Basic concepts and clinical findings in the treatment of seizure disorders with EEG operant conditioning. Clin Electroencephalogr 2000;31(1):45–55.
65. Tan G, Thornby J, Hammond D, et al. Meta-analysis of EEG biofeedback in treating epilepsy. Clin EEG Neurosci 2009;40:173–9.
66. Lantz D, Sterman MB. Neuropsychological assessment of subjects with uncontrolled epilepsy: effects of EEG biofeedback training. Epilepsia 1988;29(2):163–71.
67. Lubar JF, Shabsin HS, Natelson SE, et al. EEG operant conditioning in intractable epileptics. Arch Neurol 1981;38(11):700–4.
68. Monastra VJ, Lynn S, Linden M, et al. Electroencephalographic biofeedback in the treatment of attention-deficit/hyperactivity disorder. Appl Psychophysiol Biofeedback 2005;30(2):95–114.

Meditation and Mindfulness in Clinical Practice

Deborah R. Simkin, MD, DFAACAP[a,b,c,*],
Nancy B. Black, MD, DFAACAP[b,d]

KEYWORDS

- Meditation • Mindfulness • Transcendental meditation • Anxiety • Depression
- Children • Adolescents

KEY POINTS

- Meditation and mindfulness techniques derive from traditional contemplative practices, but are applied in modern clinical settings without the original religious and spiritual overtones.
- Five types of meditation have been systematically examined in children and adolescents: focused attention, open monitoring, automatic self-transcending (transcendental meditation), mind-body techniques, and body-mind techniques.
- Only a few randomized controlled trials have been conducted in children and adolescents, and more rigorous research is needed.
- Meditative and movement techniques have been shown to produce benefits for anxiety, depressive, and other negative affects, behavioral and emotional symptoms, and somatic functioning.
- Meditation and mindfulness techniques produce neurobiological changes in the brain and physiologic improvements in body function that have been shown to be enduring for patients who continue to practice these techniques.
- No significant adverse effects have been identified.
- Providers who offer these techniques should be well trained to ensure the best results.
- Research outcome measures demonstrate that there is a direct correlation between the amounts of time spent practicing, or participating in formal guided practice, with increased effectiveness of the techniques.

[a] Attention, Memory and Cognition Center, 4641 Gulfstarr Drive, Suite 106, Destin, FL, USA;
[b] Committee on Integrative Medicine, American Academy of Child and Adolescent Psychiatry;
[c] Emory University School of Medicine, Atlanta, GA, USA; [d] National Capital Consortium, Child and Adolescent Psychiatry Fellowship, Walter Reed National Military Medical Center, Bethesda, MD 20889, USA
* Corresponding author. Attention, Memory and Cognition Center, 4641 Gulfstarr Drive, Suite 106, Destin, FL.
E-mail address: deb62288@aol.com

Child Adolesc Psychiatric Clin N Am 23 (2014) 487–534
http://dx.doi.org/10.1016/j.chc.2014.03.002   childpsych.theclinics.com
1056-4993/14/$ – see front matter © 2014 Elsevier Inc. All rights reserved.

Abbreviations	
AAP	Attention Academy Program
ABC	Aberrant Behavioral Checklist
ACT	Acceptance and commitment therapy
ACTeRS	ADD-H Comprehensive Teacher Rating Scale
ADHD	Attention-deficit/hyperactivity disorder
ADIS-C	Anxiety Disorder Interview Schedule for Children
AN	Anorexia nervosa
ANT	Attention Network Test
AR	Biofeedback
ASD	Autistic spectrum disorder
AST	Automatic self-transcending
BASC-2	Behavioral Assessment System for Children, second edition
BDI	Beck Depression Inventory
BMI	Body mass index
BN	Bulimia nervosa
BRIEF	Behavior Rating Inventory of Executive Function
CAM	Complementary and alternative medicine
CAS	Cognitive Assessment System
CBCL	Child Behavior Checklist
CBT	Cognitive-behavioral therapy
CD	Conduct disordered
CDRS-R	Child Depression Rating Scale—Revised
CFIT	Culture Fair Intelligence Test
CHIP-AE	Child Health and Illness Profile Adolescent Edition
CM	Contemplation meditation
CPRS	Child-Parent Relationship Scale
CPT II	Connor's Continuous Performance Test II
CTI	Constructive Thinking Inventory
D-KEFS	Delis-Kaplan Executive Function System
DBM	Deep-breathing meditation
DBT	Dialectical behavior therapy
DMN	Default mode network
DMT	Dance/movement therapy
EDE	Eating Disorder Examination
EDNOS	Eating disorder not otherwise specified
eLORETA or LORETA	Low-resolution brain electromagnetic tomography
EMG	Electromyographic
ES	Effect size
FA	Focused attention
fMRI	Functional magnetic resonance imaging
GABA	γ-Aminobutyric acid
GEFT	Group Embedded Figures Test
IT	Inspection time
KIDNET	Narrative Exposure Therapy for children
M-B	Mind-body
MANOVA	Multivariate analysis of variance
MAP	Mindfulness awareness practices
MASC	Multidimensional Anxiety Scale for Children
MBCT	Mindfulness-based cognitive therapy
MBI	Primary basis of mindfulness-based interventions
MBRP	Mindfulness-based relapse prevention
MBSR	Mindfulness-based stress reduction
MBST	Mindfulness-based stress reduction
MED-RELAX	Meditation-relaxation
MET	Motivational enhancement therapy
MFQ	Mood and Feelings Questionnaire
MM	Mindfulness meditation

MNS	Mirror neuron system
MT	Massage therapy
NCCAM	National Center for Complementary and Alternative Medicine
ODD	Oppositional defiant disorder
OM	Open monitoring
PE	Physical education
POMS-SF	Profile of Mood States—Short Form
PMR	Progressive muscle relaxation
PS	Parent Scale
PSI	Parent Stress Index
PSS	Perceived stress
PTSD	Posttraumatic Stress Disorder
PR	Progressive relaxation
R-VT	Relaxation videotape
RCMAS	Revised Child Manifest Anxiety Scale
RFT	Relation frame theory
RR	Relaxation response
RT	Relaxation therapy
SM	Sahaja meditation
SNAP-IV	Swanson, Nolan and Pelham Scale
SSM	Sahaja Samadhi meditation
STAI	State and Trait Anxiety Scale
STAIC	State-Trait Anxiety Inventory for Children
SYM	Sahaja Yoga meditation
TAS	Test Anxiety Scale
TAU	Treatment as usual
TCT-DP	Test for Creative Thinking-Drawing Production
TEA-Ch	Test of Everyday Attention for Children
TM	Transcendental meditation
TOL	Tower of London
USPSTF	United States Preventive Services Task Force
YEQ	Yoga Evaluation Questionnaire
YRS	Youth Self Report

INTRODUCTION

Meditation has been practiced in diverse forms for centuries in various non-Western cultures, and this long and complex history has given rise to a variety of definitions, forms, and techniques.[1] As a result, there is no single definition for meditation, although its general goal is to train the mind to achieve a particular goal.

Meditation and mindfulness interventions may enhance the individual skills of children and adolescents, specifically by helping them feel more relaxed, focused, and creative. Parents who practice these techniques may also benefit from these effects, and find that meditation can enhance their parenting skills.

Meditation in particular and mind-body medicine in general are described by the National Center for Complementary and Alternative Medicine (NCCAM) at the National Institutes of Health as "focusing on the interactions among the brain, mind, body, and behavior, and on the powerful ways in which emotional, mental, social, spiritual and behavioral factors can directly affect health" (www.NCCAM.NIH.gov).

Meditation may be divided into 5 categories for the purposes of explication in this article (**Table 1**).

Each of these techniques is described in terms of their therapeutic goals, how to use the techniques, their physiologic and neurobiological effects, and the available clinical

Table 1 Meditation-based therapy	
Types of Meditation	**Therapeutic Meditation Approaches**
Focused attention (FA) Primary basis of mindfulness-based interventions (MBI)	Mindfulness-based stress reduction (MBST) Mindfulness-based cognitive therapy (MBCT) Dialectical behavior therapy (DBT) Acceptance and commitment therapy (ACT) Mindfulness-based relapse prevention (MBRP)
Open monitoring (OM)	Sahaja meditation (SM) Sahaja Samadhi meditation (SSM) Sahaja yoga meditation (SYM)
Automatic self-transcending (AST)/Transcendental meditation (TM)	
Mind-body (M-B)	Meditation-relaxation (MED-RELAX) Progressive muscle relaxation (PMR) Deep breathing meditation (DBM)
Body-mind (B-M)	Exercise Movement therapy or dance therapy Tai Chi Qi Gong Yoga

research on their use in treating psychopathology in youth (and, in some cases, families). Readers seeking greater detail are referred to the references for these techniques.[2–6] The studies for the therapeutic approaches are presented in the final section of this article, and evidence-based outcomes are presented in the relevant section in **Table 3** according to the disorders treated.

Meditation and Mindfulness: Evolution from Buddhist Traditions to Modern Western Techniques

Focused attention (FA) and open monitoring (OM) have roots in Zen, Vipassana, and Tibetan Buddhist meditation traditions. FA (concentration training) uses explicit objects to attend to so that the mind will not wander. OM (mindfulness) involves being aware moment to moment of any thought or feeling that occurs in personal experience without focusing on an explicit object. Buddhist meditations were and are intended for healthy individuals.[7] Western clinical adaptations of these techniques are designed to target pathologic states of mind, such as anxiety.

In the tradition of Vipassana meditation, concentration training followed by mindfulness training together are used to gain insight.

- First, using concentration training, the person learns to attend to one object so as to not allow the mind to be distracted or to wander.
- Then, mindfulness is used to observe negative thoughts and feelings in a nonjudgmental way so that the person can detach from them. Doing this allows the person to observe these thoughts and feelings in an objective way without reacting to them. One gains insight or awareness.[8] As one becomes more aware, one makes further observations about these negative states (ie, what triggers them) as they arise, without reacting to them. When the mind achieves stillness, there is an enduring absence of reactivity.

- Then, an appreciation for the mind's natural state, which involves positive emotions, occurs. Thus, the technique allows the participant to be aware of positive mental states, such as patience, harmlessness, loving kindness, and empathy.[9]

Through these steps, Vipassana meditation builds a more positive state of mind.

In Western cultures, FA and OM have been blended into what is called, for the purpose of this review, mindfulness meditation (MM). MM is derived from either Vipassana or Zen meditation, but Vipassana techniques are often chosen over Zen in Western cultures.[10] Eastern traditions entail extensive training and involve both FA and OM. FA is the primary basis of mindfulness-based interventions (MBIs). Mindfulness-based stress reduction (MBSR) is the only FA technique overtly rooted in Buddhist philosophy,[11–14] more heavily based in Vipassana with some Zen influence.

FOCUSED ATTENTION MINDFULNESS-BASED INTERVENTIONS

Chiesa and Malinowski[11] described 4 therapeutic techniques that are based on FA or concentration training as MBIs. A recent addition to MBI is Mindfulness-based relapse prevention (MBRP). The 5 techniques based in MBI are:

1. Mindfulness-based stress reduction (MBSR)
2. Mindfulness cognitive-behavioral therapy (MBCT)
3. Dialectical behavior therapy (DBT)
4. Acceptance and commitment therapy (ACT)
5. Mindfulness-based relapse prevention (MBRP)

Kabat-Zinn[12,15] developed MBSR in 1990 as an easily learned type of meditation for the general Western public.

Segal[13] developed MBCT specifically as a treatment for clinical depression and its accompanying cognitive distortions.

Three different approaches of FA were subsequently adapted for clinical use with patients with 3 specific disorders; the 3 approaches use mindfulness skills, but not formal meditation techniques:

- Linehan[16] developed DBT for treating patients with borderline personality disorder, although it is often used to help a variety of patients manage their extreme affects and problems with behavioral control.
- Hayes[17] developed ACT which uses acceptance and mindfulness strategies, as well as, commitment and behavior change to increase psychological flexibility.
- MBRP was designed to target substance abusers.[18]

Goals of Focused Attention Mindfulness-Based Intervention

For MBI techniques the goal is clinically oriented. Their main aim is to relieve unwanted physical and psychological symptoms such as pain, anxiety, and depression.

MBSR, MBCT, and MBRP are specifically concerned with relief from negative symptoms by targeting negative thoughts or emotions, achieved by means of developing an enhanced way to cope with and/or relate differently to them.[9]

The goal of DBT and ACT is to help patients manage symptoms. DBT can reduce dangerous behaviors such as suicidal behaviors. ACT also helps foster acceptance of unwanted feelings and thoughts, and discourages avoidance of them.[17]

Mindfulness-Based Stress-Reduction Techniques and Approaches

Techniques used to learn to focus on a specific object can vary. For instance, participants can use a body scan (sweeping attention from head to foot focusing noncritically on any sensation of feeling) or attention breathing (for instance, emphasis on focusing on one's breathing while in a state of nonjudgmental awareness of cognition and distraction).[12,15] Programs may include 8 sessions for 2 hours per day.

Details of the techniques and outcomes are discussed in the section on studies.

Mindfulness-Based Cognitive Therapy Techniques and Approaches

MBCT, a variation on CBT, is based on the observation that the way we perceive and understand events is a large determinant of how we feel about them and how we behave in response to them. As in Buddhist philosophy, it emphasizes self-responsibility in the form of self-management, self-control, and self-improvement.[9,13] For example, children are encouraged to focus on remembering negative experiences and then to allow themselves to focus on feeling those emotions and becoming aware of the bodily sensations that accompany the memory of the experience. After several minutes they are asked to take a 3-minute "breathing space," when they are asked to focus on their breathing and what is going on in their body and mind. Then, in a relaxed state, they tell themselves that they can handle anything and then focus back on their body as a whole. MBCT encourages the use of this 3-minute breathing space to allow individuals to integrate formal practice into daily life whenever unpleasant feelings are noted.

MBSR and MBCT both emphasize the attitude one brings to the meditation experience. Both techniques emphasize a nonjudgmental, nonstriving, and noneffort approach; this develops as practice deepens, resulting in more effortless, enhanced meditation whereby one moves more easily from concentration to mental stability.[3]

Details of the techniques and outcomes are discussed in the section on studies.

Dialectical Behavioral Therapy Approaches and Techniques

DBT is derived from behavioral science, dialectical philosophy, and Zen practice. This approach is hypothesized to work by encouraging nonreinforced engagement with emotionally evocative stimuli while blocking dysfunctional escape, avoidance behavior, or ineffective responses to intense emotions. DBT teaches mindfulness-based skills, such as being nonjudgmental, to allow the participant to reach a level of acceptance and change. This approach is used with borderline personality disorders and suicidal behaviors.[16]

Details of the techniques and outcomes are discussed in the section on studies.

Acceptance and Commitment Therapy Techniques and Approaches

ACT is based on relation frame theory (RFT), which is derived from a philosophic view called functional contextualism. Functional contextualism uses the idea that cognitions gain importance mostly from the context in which they occur. Changing the context in which relationships occur is one example of how ACT works. Doing so can alter and limit behavior.[17] For instance, ACT uses mindful techniques, which include the ability to recognize an observing self that is capable of watching its own bodily sensations, thoughts, and emotions by seeing these aspects as separate from the person having them. For instance, a participant would recognize "I am having a thought that I am a bad person" rather than "I am a bad person."[17]

Mindfulness-Based Relapse Prevention Techniques and Approaches

MBRP is used to prevent relapse in individuals with substance abuse problems.[9] MBRP was developed to target substance abusers by using cognitive behavioral therapy, mindfulness and relapse prevention techniques.

Physiologic and Neurobiological Effects of Focused Attention Mindfulness-Based Interventions

The literature reflects a variety of findings according to the design and tools used. The neurobiology of traditional Vipassana (which is meant to target healthy individuals) is discussed first, followed by the neurobiological effects seen in MBI (which are used to target pathologic states).

Vipassana meditation

- Meditators showed stronger activations in the rostral anterior cingulate cortex and the dorsal medial prefrontal cortex bilaterally in comparison with controls. The involvement of the rostral anterior cingulate suggests greater attention control during meditation, and the involvement of the dorsal medial prefrontal cortex suggests detecting interference between competing responses, thus signaling the need for control so that the mind will not wander.[19]
- Meditators in another study (who had meditated an average of 20 years and had been meditating daily for at least 2 years), had magnetic resonance imaging (MRI) results indicating greater gray matter concentration in the right anterior insula, which is involved in interoceptive awareness or the ability of the mind to integrate different sensory signals from the body to produce the experience of the body as the person's own. These same mediators had greater gray matter concentration in the left inferior temporal gyrus and right hippocampus. The hippocampus is involved in modulating cortical arousal and responsiveness. The hippocampus also modulates amygdalar activity and its involvement in attention and emotional processes. The mean value of gray matter concentration in the left inferior temporal gyrus was correlated with the amount of meditation training. Thus, the greater the meditation training, the greater was the gray matter concentration seen in this region. The temporal lobe has been implicated in religious activity, which is characterized by the feeling of deep pleasure and the experience of insight.[20]

Results suggest that meditation practice is associated with structural differences in regions that are typically activated during meditation, and in regions that are relevant for the task of meditation.

- In another study of Vipassana meditators, the P3a amplitude from a distracter (white noise) was reduced during meditation. P3a is hypothesized to index frontal neural activity produced by stimulus-driven attention mechanisms. Consistent with the aim of Vipassana meditation, to reduce cognitive and emotional reactivity the state effect of reduced P3a amplitude to distracting stimuli reflects decreased automatic reactivity and the ability to evaluate and ignore irrelevant attention-demanding stimuli.[21]
- In this same study, increased oscillation over the parietal-occipital region was seen in the gamma frequency range (35–45 Hz), signifying exclusion of external stimuli, and increased frontal theta (4–8 Hz), signifying the processing of positive internal emotions.[22]

Taken together, the neurobiological evidence correlates with the sequence of events that occur in persons who perform Vipassana meditation.

1. First, during the meditation, the person focuses attention on an object (rostral anterior cingulate), and competing stimuli are avoided so as to not allow the brain to be distracted (dorsal medial prefrontal cortex).
2. Then the person is aware of negative bodily sensations, thoughts, or feelings moment to moment (right anterior insula) but without reactivity, as if they are

irrelevant (hippocampus and corresponding influence over the amygdala, reduced amplitude of P3a), thus allowing a more objective way of observing them.

3. Finally, the increase in gamma waves in the parietal-occipital areas and the increased theta in the frontal area occurs when all external stimuli are excluded and only positive internal emotions occur, such as empathy.

Mindfulness-based intervention: changing pathologic states

MRI results After 8 weeks of MBSR training, MRI data confirmed increases in gray matter concentration within the left hippocampus. Whole brain analyses also identified increased gray matter in the posterior cingulate cortex, the temporoparietal junction, and the cerebellum in the MBSR group when compared with the controls.

The results suggest that participation in MBSR is associated with changes in gray matter concentration in brain regions involved in learning and memory processes, emotion regulation, self-referential processing, and perspective taking.[23]

In another study all participants completed the 8-week MBSR program, consisting of weekly group meetings and daily home mindfulness practices. Individuals were eligible to enter the study if their score on the Perceived Stress Scale (PSS) was 1 standard deviation (SD) or more above the population mean. The PSS is a validated self-report questionnaire widely used for assessing an individual's self-perception of stress. However, in this study, individuals were excluded if they had a current psychiatric illness or medical illness, ineligibility for MRI scanning (claustrophobia, metallic implants, pregnancy, and so forth), or significant previous meditation or yoga experience. After 8 weeks of MBSR, perceived stress was rated again on the PSS. PSS scores decreased from preintervention (mean 20.7; SD 5.6) to postintervention (mean 15.2; SD 4.7; T = 3.7; df = 25; $P<.001$). Anatomic MR images were acquired before and after intervention. Larger decreases in perceived stress were correlated positively with decreases in right basolateral amygdala gray matter density.[24]

It should be noted that the effects of FA on the attention system may differ based on the experience of the meditator.

Functional MRI results One study[25] used functional MRI (fMRI) to investigate the neural correlates of FA meditation in experts and novices. In this study, FA meditation on an external visual point was compared with a rest condition. It was associated with activation in multiple brain regions implicated in monitoring (dorsolateral prefrontal cortex), engaging attention (visual cortex), and attentional orienting (eg, the superior frontal sulcus and intraparietal sulcus). Expert meditators showed stronger activation in these areas than the novices. In addition, expert meditators showed less activation than novices in the amygdala during FA meditation, and activation in this affective region correlated negatively with hours of practice in life. Although meditation-related activation patterns in the aforementioned areas were generally stronger for long-term-practitioners than for novices, activity in many brain areas involved in FA meditation showed an inverted U-shaped curve in expert meditators: that is, those with more total practice hours (mean hours = 44,000; range 37,000–52,000; mean age 52.3 years) compared with those with fewer total practice hours (mean hours = 19,000; range 10,000–24,000; mean age 48.8 years). Expert meditators who had more total time meditating showed less activation. This inverted U-shaped function provides support for the notion that after extensive FA meditation training, minimal effort is necessary to sustain attentional focus.[25]

Therefore, although long-term meditators show less reactivity because of a less reactive amygdala and more FA in comparison with novices, the variation in the total number of hours spent in meditation by expert meditators can still reveal differences between them. Expert meditators who had more total hours meditating had less activation in the attention system than meditators with less total time meditating. This finding probably is due to the fact that as a meditator progresses, less effort is needed to sustain attention.

These studies were conducted with adults. However, given these findings one might ask if FA may be helpful in children with attention-deficit/hyperactivity disorder (ADHD). The attention system in the brain involves 3 components: conflict monitoring, orienting, and alerting. FA is thought to involve 2 aspects of the attention system, namely conflict monitoring (eg, dorsal anterior cingulate cortex and dorsolateral prefrontal cortex) and orienting (eg, the temporoparietal junction, ventrolateral prefrontal cortex, frontal eye fields, and intraparietal sulcus). Many of these neurobiological components overlap with components in a previous study.[26] Youth with ADHD seem to have more problems with executive function (a part of conflict monitoring) and sustaining attention (alerting) but not orienting. The following study suggests that FA meditation may be helpful in adolescents with ADHD.

In a study in adolescents aged 13 to 15 years, the influence of concentration training (or FA) on attention bolstered sustaining alerting and conflict monitoring, but did not appear to improve orienting. The FA group had conflict monitoring scores of much smaller magnitude than those of controls ($P<.05$). Alerting revealed a main effect for both reaction times ($P<.05$) and accuracy ($P = .01$) in the concentration training group versus the control group. Therefore, FA may be a possible additional technique for use with youth with ADHD,[27–38] although more studies are needed.

OPEN MONITORING

Presented here is a brief overview of OM followed by its goals, clinical approaches/techniques, and physiologic effects. Studies related to OM for ADHD are presented later in this article.

OM is often the next step after the ability to focus attention is stabilized. During OM one aims to remain only in the monitoring state, attentive moment by moment to anything that occurs in experience without focusing on any explicit object. The person monitors any experiences that arise (thoughts, feelings, and so forth). This monitoring occurs in a nonjudgmental way so that the person can detach from experiences, be nonreactive, and gain insight or awareness.

The types of OM meditations include Sahaja meditation (SM), Sahaja Samadhi meditation (SSM), and Sahaja Yoga meditation (SYM).[39] Only SYM is discussed here because this is the only technique researched in children and adolescents.

Goals of Open Monitoring

The goal of OM is to increase awareness without automatic responses.[39,40] During OM one aims to remain only in the monitoring state, attentive moment by moment to anything that occurs in experience without focusing on any explicit object. To reach this state, the practitioner gradually reduces the focus on an explicit object in FA, and the monitoring state is correspondingly emphasized. Practitioners describe the experience of thoughtless awareness or "mental silence" as an enhancement of awareness and self-control, enabling them to attend to the demands of the present moment.[41]

Open Monitoring Techniques and Approaches

Harrison and colleagues[39] described a modified OM for SYM for children, which involved a 6-week program with twice-weekly clinical sessions and expected meditation at home. The therapy began with guided meditation sessions and sharing of experiences in the clinic combined with shorter meditation sessions conducted at home, guided by parents trained in guiding meditation.

Details of the technique and outcomes are discussed in the section on open monitoring studies.

Physiologic and Neurobiological Effects of Open Monitoring

Some of the neurobiological findings for SYM are similar to the findings discussed previously in regard of Vipassana meditation, probably because both use FA and OM, which allow one to reach a state of awareness.

Brain-wave activity

In one study, the generation of distinct meditative states of consciousness was marked by distinct changes in brain-wave activity, especially enhanced theta-band activity in the frontal areas during deep meditation. Meditators also exhibited increased theta coherence when compared with controls. Higher theta activity and coherence reflects increased attention, in addition to cognitive and affective processing during meditation. The emergence of the slow-frequency waves in the attention-related frontal regions provides strong support to the existing claims of frontal theta in producing meditative states along with increased attentional processing. Of interest, increased frontal theta activity was accompanied by reduced activity (deactivation) in parietal-occipital areas, signifying reduction in processing associated with self, space and, time.[42,43] In this way, the participant is unaware of present external stimuli.

Parasympathetic activity

Reports of direct physiologic effects of SYM include "indicators of increased parasympathetic activity such as a decrease in blood pressure, decrease in heart and respiratory rates and an increase in galvanic skin resistance as an indicator of decreased sympathetic activity."[39] Taken together, the OM meditative state appears signified by theta waves in attention-related frontal areas, deactivation of the parietal-occipital processing of self and surroundings, and reduced sympathetic activity.

AUTOMATIC SELF-TRANSCENDING OR TRANSCENDENTAL MEDITATION

Presented here is a brief overview of transcendental meditation (TM) followed by its goals, clinical approaches and techniques, and physiologic effects. Studies on TM are presented later in the article.[1]

Automatic self-transcending is commonly known as TM. TM has its roots in Indian (Vedic) or Chinese origins, and is known in the modern era as being developed by Maharishi Mahesh Yogi. It involves a profound sense of relaxing the body with a subsidence of mental activity during the session.[6]

The term "automatic" indicates that the individual is not trying to control mental activity. In contrast to FA, which requires concentration, and OM, which additionally requires being aware of experiences without reactivity, TM does not involve focused control or an awareness of experiences, instead attempting to let mental activity subside. TM entails the regular use of a relaxation exercise to attain a state of physical and psychological calmness. During the relaxation exercise, the participant repeats a mantra (words spoken silently), which is used to block distracting thoughts.[6] This technique does not require concentration, contemplation, or control of the mind. TM allows the body to effortlessly reach a level of deep calmness while alert. Although this concept may be difficult to understand at first from the Western viewpoint, in simple terms, it is used to reduce physiologic arousal yet induce increased alertness.[6,44,45]

Goals of Transcendental Meditation

From a physiologic perspective, the TM technique is intended to reduce physiologic arousal and increase alertness, achieved through an "adaptive efficiency of physiologic processes rather than reduction of somatic arousal during stress."[46] Preliminary studies of Iraq War veterans have shown promising results using TM for veterans with Posttraumatic stress disorder (PTSD).[44]

Transcendental Meditation Techniques and Approaches

Training for TM must be accomplished with a certified instructor. The 7 steps of training, documented in a study by So and Orme-Johnson,[47] are:

Step 1. One-hour introductory lecture covering research on the benefits of the practice, followed by a question and answer period

Step 2. One-hour preparatory lecture on the mechanics of the technique and a comparison with other techniques, followed by a question and answer period

Step 3. Brief personal interview with the teacher to enable the teacher and student to become better acquainted

Step 4. Personal instruction in the TM technique by a qualified teacher that takes approximately 2 hours. Students are given an appropriate mantra and taught how to use it properly, that is, to use it mentally without effort. TM practice is performed to enable the mind to settle into a quiet yet wakeful state called "pure consciousness," which has been associated with a wakeful hypometabolic physiologic state. After personal instruction, subjects are instructed to practice the technique twice a day, once in the morning and once in the afternoon

Step 5. The first 2-hour group check-in meeting to check the correctness of practice includes further instruction

Step 6. The second 2-hour group check-in meeting to discuss mind and body meditation, consciousness and physiology of the technique, and the role of thoughts and the mechanics of stress normalization

Step 7. The third 2-hour group check-in meeting to discuss the benefits of TM practice, the importance of regularity of practice, comparison of the of the physiology of waking, dreaming, sleep, TM, and a vision of the goal of a stress-free life.

Details of the technique and outcomes are discussed in the section on studies related to cognitive ability, ADHD, and anxiety and depression.

Physiologic and Neurobiological Effects of Transcendental Meditation

Although many clinicians have thought of TM as a relaxation technique, this is not the case. In fact during the session there seems to be a state of deep rest while alert.

- For instance, the oxygen consumption is as low as during deep sleep; however, there is no brain-wave activity to suggest that the person is asleep. In addition, usually some forms of deep relaxation are associated with brain-wave (electro-encephalographic [EEG]) signs of drowsiness or superficial sleep. However, EEG patterns during TM indicate a state of alertness despite the deep physiologic rest.[48]
- TM practice was analyzed using low-resolution brain electromagnetic tomography (eLORETA or LORETA) in adults. LORETA can identify brain-wave activity in

deeper structures in the brain than is ordinarily sensed by a raw EEG. LORETA analysis identified sources of alpha-1 activity in midline cortical regions that overlapped with the default mode network (DMN). The DMN is a brain circuit thought to be more commonly engaged and active when people think about the thoughts, beliefs, emotions, and intentions of others, and involves executive control. However, spontaneous self-referential thoughts involved in TM were associated with enhanced alpha activity in the DMN.[49,50] The role of the DMN in TM may differ somewhat in comparison with when someone is actively using executive function. It may be that during TM executive function is not as actively involved and, instead, the DMN may be "idling" and therefore require less executive function. More research is needed to understand the exact role of the DMN. It may be that as the participant becomes more skilled at TM, less executive function is required.

- EEG coherence (the ability of different areas of the brain to communicate more efficiently) becomes more pronounced with longevity in practice. This coherence has been found to be correlated with different measures of the quality of the functioning of the brain, including intelligence and creativity in addition to indicators of mental health.[50] TM, compared with just resting with eyes closed, had a significantly larger effect size for the physical-parameter findings of decreased heart rate, respiration rate, and plasma lactate. These same findings were seen in TM subjects before meditation in comparison with participants who were about to enter a relaxed state. The implication is that the effects of TM are probably sustained even when not in an identified session of TM.[49,50]

- TM can also have an effect on brain plasticity. Comparing adult TM meditators with controls, pronounced group differences indicating larger gyrification in meditators were evident within the left precentral gyrus, right fusiform gyrus, right cuneus, and left and right anterior dorsal insula. Positive correlations between gyrification and the number of meditation years were similarly pronounced in the right anterior dorsal insula. Given that meditators are masters in introspection and mental and emotional awareness, increased insular gyrification may reflect an integration of autonomic, affective, and cognitive processes.[51]

Some studies have included people who have been practicing TM from a very early age. However, it is unclear as to whether these changes would begin occurring during adolescence or only after the brain fully matures in the early 20s. Studies on younger subjects during adolescence who started TM at an early age would be important. Such studies would help to determine whether the use of TM can alter the normal developmental trajectory, or whether it can help change brain patterns in someone who has, for instance, an anxiety disorder.

MIND-BODY

Some methods and techniques in the reviewed literature for mind-body (M-B) techniques seem to bridge the FA and OM methods, and, in some cases, the TM methods as well; they may also include relaxation components.

Examples of M-B therapies are:

1. Relaxation techniques, including Meditation-Relaxation (MED-RELAX)[52]
2. Progressive muscle relaxation (PMR) or relaxation therapy (RT)[53–58]
3. Deep-breathing meditation (DBM) is an M-B method used for test anxiety[59]
4. A combination of posture, breathing, attention, and visualization[2]
5. Electromyographic (EMG) biofeedback (AR) as described by Eppley and colleagues[54]

Goals of Mind-Body Therapies

Catani and colleagues[52] used MED-RELAX with Sri Lankan children traumatized acutely after the 2004 Tsunami event.

PMR is used for relaxation.[54]

DBM is used to counteract the fight/flight/fright responses, and is useful for test anxiety.[59] Fisher's technique helps children be more receptive to learning in the classroom environment.[2]

MED-RELAX Techniques and Approaches

MED-RELAX as used by Catani and colleagues[52] comprises meditation and relaxation techniques. The methods discussed here are taken directly from their article.

- The first session of MED-RELAX started with psychoeducation, followed by a thorough assessment of the child's current problems, and ended with a breathing exercise of at least 15 minutes.
- Each following session started and ended with a 15-minute breathing exercise, guiding the child to achieve relaxation by attaining a conscious focus in the mind on the incoming and outgoing breath.
- The middle part of the subsequent sessions consisted of different meditation and relaxation techniques and exercises, including "inner peace meditation" (session 2, 25 minutes), "uchchadana mantra chanting" (session 3, 25 minutes), "progressive muscle relaxation" (session 4, 25 minutes), "ice cream body relaxation" (session 5, 25 minutes), and "inner light meditation" (session 6, 25 minutes). Each of these methods can be found in a detailed manual.

Each meditation and relaxation exercise was read out in the same way by the master counselors. For instance, the "ice cream body relaxation" was introduced in the following way in the manual:

'Ice Cream Body Relaxation' (20–25 minutes): Have a bed sheet or mat on the floor and ask the client to stand on it with bare feet. Have relaxation music in the background and guide the client as follows: 'Stand up and raise your hands upwards. Imagine that you are an ice cream now. In the air this ice cream will melt gradually. Likewise your body also relaxes gently. (In between the music, the instructions come very gradually and slowly). The tension of your body reduces step by step and you are melting more and more. The height of this ice cream will reduce as it melts. Likewise your height goes down slowly...- slowly...some more...some more...it melts more...and comes flat to the ground.' (Repeat the sentence slowly many times until the client lies flat on the floor and relaxes).

Children were instructed to practice the meditation techniques as homework for about 1 hour per day.

PMR or RT teaches subjects to relax and tense 8 different muscle groups, beginning with the feet and ending with the head.[53]

DBM entails several minutes of quiet time to focus breathing as a stress-management strategy. The technique involves working in a quiet environment, concentrated breathing to focus on attention, while sitting in a comfortable position and a receptive attitude.[59,60]

Fisher[2] describes FA/OM techniques for latency-age children and adolescents. He offers 4 methods that were designed to be used in the classroom setting: Posture, Breathing, Attention, and Visualization. Posture assists with body management. Breathing helps calm participants in preparation for "brainstorming or free writing."

Attention develops recall, and Visualization helps with imagination. Fisher further describes 3 components of the technique (Receptive, Generative, and Reflective). The reader is referred to the article for further explanation of these components. Methods for Posture for elementary school ages include imagining a thread holding you up. For the junior and senior high school students it includes an established, agreed-upon cue, to do a posture that was learned earlier. Methods for Breathing include alternating inhaling and exhaling, slowly and quickly. To train for Attention, he suggests playing concentration games with children. Finally, for Visualization he references his category of Generative, and suggests guided imagery.

EMG biofeedback methods are not mentioned here because biofeedback does not derive from Eastern meditation techniques that are the focus of this review.

Details of the technique and outcomes of MED-RELAX are discussed in the section on studies related to PTSD.

Physiologic and Neurobiological Effects of MED-RELAX

In Catani's post-Tsunami research, both narrative and MED-RELAX therapies showed significant and lasting decreases in symptoms associated with PTSD 6 months after a disaster.[52] The monitored confirmed DBM led to reported beneficial physiologic effects.[60]

BODY-MIND
Evolution from Buddhist, Chinese, and Indian/Vedic Traditions, and Modern Techniques

In the literature there are body-centered techniques with corresponding mental focusing, physiologic, and calming effects. Exercise, classified under Body-Mind (B-M), has many forms but is not considered to have evolved from the Buddhist, Chinese, and Indian/Vedic traditions. Dance or movement therapy is a more recent intervention, and also does not have roots in these traditions. Many of the body-centered techniques may overlap with the FA, OM, and TM categories because of the similar methods used for instruction and implementation; they may incorporate movement sequences as in Tai Chi and Qi Gong (which have Chinese origins), or postures, as in yoga (which has Indian/Vedic origins).

There are 5 B-M subtypes:

1. Exercise[61]
2. Movement or dance therapy[62,63]
3. Qi Gong[6]
4. Tai Chi[64,65]
5. Yoga[66–68]

Goals of Body-Mind Therapies

In movement therapy research conducted by Hartshorn and colleagues,[62] the goal was to reduce symptoms particular to autism. The study by Rosenblatt and colleagues[63] targeted autistic symptoms using dance and music therapy and yoga. Qi Gong's meditative effects on brain waves are presented in the review article by Travis and Shear.[6] In the Tai Chi pilot study by Hernandez-Reif and colleagues,[64] the goal was to reduce ADHD symptoms. For Wall's research,[65] the goal was to determine if middle school students could benefit from Tai Chi and MBSR. Both focused on reducing anxiety. In research by Carei and colleagues,[66] the goal was to determine if adolescents in an inpatient care setting for eating disorders could benefit from yoga as part of the intervention. In the study by Kaley-Isley and colleagues,[67] the aim was to present an overview of different yoga forms and to offer a guide to clinicians focused on developmental stages. The study by Noggle and colleagues[68] targeted psychosocial well-being in high school students.

Body-Mind Techniques and Approaches

Exercise

In a study by Doop and colleagues,[61] the effect of exercise was studied in adolescents with depression, including a 12-week intervention that had 3 supervised sessions in the first week. Supervision was done 2 times in the second week, and once per week during weeks 3 through 12. During the 12 weeks, students had to perform a total of 3 sessions per week. A target heart rate was determined for each participant, and each participant was encouraged to maintain that heart rate for 40 minutes to achieve an aerobic effect.

Movement or dance therapy

Hartshorn and colleagues[62] studied movement therapy for children with autism. The number of movement activities per session varied from 3 to 5 (each approximately 6–10 minutes). The sessions all began with a warm-up activity and ended with a cool-down activity. The warm-up activity was the therapist saying hello to each member of the group and clapping the syllables of each person's name as she greeted that member. The cool-down activity at the end of the session was a song with a specific pattern of movements that did not change. The intermediary activities for each session involved using hoops and jumping in and out of them, putting different body parts in and out of the hoops, following the therapist through an obstacle course of gym mats of differing shape and height, and moving to the rhythm of a tambourine and stopping when the tambourine stopped. Sessions occurred twice per week for 8 weeks.

A combination of dance, music, and yoga for young children with autism was studied by Rosenblatt and colleagues.[63] The efficacy of an 8-week multimodal yoga, dance, and music therapy program based on the relaxation response (RR)[60] was developed and examined. After an initial orientation and pretesting session, there were 8 treatment sessions of 45 minutes, then a final summary and posttesting session. The sessions were led by a licensed clinician with added certification in yoga and dance therapy. Each session followed the same format to create predictability and familiarity, and to reduce anxiety. Specifically, sessions involved (in sequence): breathing techniques from the RR (10 minutes), yoga postures (10 minutes), music and dance (20 minutes), and typical yoga relaxation postures (5 minutes).

Details of the technique and outcomes of exercise are discussed in the section on studies related to depression. Details of the technique and outcomes of movement and dance therapy are discussed in the section on studies related to autism, autism spectrum disorders, and behavior analysis.

Physiologic and Neurobiological Effects of Body-Mind Therapies

Exercise

In a review by Field and colleagues,[56] exercise has been shown to benefit bone growth,[69,70] motor competence, and body mass index (BMI),[71] to reduce inflammation in autoimmune diseases such as asthma and arthritis,[72,73] and to decrease symptoms of anxiety and depression.[74] No significant studies have been conducted with children and adolescents.

Some examples of the effects of yoga on physical exercise[75] have been that it improves exercise secondary to the increased motivational effects of the yoga. A few minor comparison studies have compared yoga with physical exercise[76] and African dance.[77] The former seemed to reduce symptoms of ADHD, which was thought to occur because yoga requires more attention than physical exercise. The latter study demonstrated that compared with African dance, yoga resulted in decreased anxiety and lower cortisol levels. However, the results of this study were thought to be related to the fact that African dance is more energetic and therefore may have been more arousing, and thus were judged to be inconclusive.

Movement or dance therapy

There is growing research suggesting the presence of neural circuitry called the mirror neuron system (MNS), which is similarly activated whether an individual performs an action or simply observes an action.[78] Lucy and colleagues[79] have proposed a neuro-psychological model, involving motor simulation and the MNS, which can elucidate the benefits of mirroring in dance/movement therapy (DMT) on empathy. These investigators further propose that practice engaged in mirroring leads to enhanced MNS functioning in the person mirroring, as well as in the mirrored individual. In turn, MNS activity during the observation or execution of emotional movement will enhance activation in the limbic system, leading to a greater empathic response. In addition, they propose that if a patient with a disorder involving empathy were to participate in mirroring practice, and perhaps learn the technique, this intervention may help improve empathy. All of these theories are speculative and need further research to validate them.

Qi Gong

Qi Gong is studied with a teacher and practiced on one's own. It involves the 3 elements posture (whether moving or stationary), breathing techniques, and mental focus.[6] There are no studies with children and adolescents using Qi Gong. One case study with a practitioner of 45 years is referenced in the article by Travis and Shear.[6]

In their review of the literature, Travis and Shear[6] cited

A case study of a single practitioner of Qigong tested once and then 45 years later, reported that global alpha 1 power increased immediately during Qigong practice on posttest, and remained higher at rest after the Qigong practice... Alpha 1 appears to index level of internalized attention, alertness and expectancy.

[In a study that] tested EEG patterns...frontal midline theta rhythm was higher during the concentrative Qi Gong state...frontal midline theta [theta (4–8 Hz)] is a neural index of monitoring inner processes.[6]

Tai Chi

In a study of Tai Chi by Hernandez-Reif and colleagues,[64] each session began with slow raising and lowering of the arms in synchrony with breathing exercises for 5 minutes. The adolescents were then taught to perform slow turning and twisting movements of the arms and legs, shifting body weight from one leg to the other, rotating from side to side and changing directions in a sequence of Tai Chi forms.

Wall[65] included some MBSR with Tai Chi. When Tai Chi was used in the public school, the method used was the traditional style of sequential instruction of segments of the whole movement routine so that the segments lengthened into the whole. There was a sequence of classes that also introduced including attending, breathing, and guided imagery. Classes were always voluntary, and students were allowed to participate for the entire session, observe, or depart.

For Tai Chi no physiologic or neurologic effects were reported.

Yoga

In the research by Carei and colleagues,[66] there is a description of yoga for possible use in the treatment of eating disorders. It includes a 1-hour semi-weekly class for 8 weeks and 1-on-1 instruction of Viniyoga with a certified instructor.

As described by Kaley-Isley and colleagues,[67] yoga was used for 1 hour per week in a group of 20 students. The type of yoga used varied, depending on the developmental age of the youth. The article offered a method for how to use yoga for each of the developmental stages in children and adolescents. For example, when using extracting awareness, breathing, and guided visualization, the time for preschoolers is 2 to 3 minutes per segment or 9 minutes in total. For school-aged children, the time is 3 to 5 minutes per segment for a total of 15 minutes, and for adolescents the time is 5 to 10 minutes per segment for a total of 30 minutes.

In a study by Noggle and colleagues,[68] a Kripalu-based yoga program of physical postures, breathing exercises, relaxation, and meditation was taught 2 to 3 times per week for 10 weeks. The 30-minute Yoga sessions were structured to include 5 minutes for centering, 5 minutes for a warm-up, 15 minutes of yoga postures/exercises, and 5 minutes for closing relaxation. (Durations of each segment were extended to varying degrees in the 40-minute sessions, typically by including more yoga postures/exercises.) Breathing techniques were progressively incorporated during the initial centering. In addition, slow abdominal breathing was a focus throughout the duration of all sessions. Each session had a theme or talking point that was discussed throughout the session by the instructor. Themes included a basic yoga approach and methodology (postures, breathing, relaxation, meditation, and awareness), nonviolence, M-B interactions and awareness, body systems, stress management, emotional intelligence, self-talk and critical voice, contentment, discipline, decision making, values and principles, commitment, and acceptance.

One study[80] demonstrated a 12-week yoga intervention to be associated with greater improvements in mood and anxiety than a metabolically matched walking exercise. The study also showed that increased thalamic γ-aminobutyric acid (GABA) levels are associated with improved mood and decreased anxiety. Moreover, yoga postures were associated with a positive correlation between acute increases in thalamic GABA levels and improvements in mean scores on mood and anxiety scales.[80]

Neuroimaging studies have shown that yoga meditation results in an activation of the prefrontal cortex, activation of the thalamus and the inhibitory thalamic reticular nucleus, and a resultant functional differentiation of the parietal lobe. This action decreases the flow of sensory information to the thalamus. Thus during yoga meditation, external stimuli are blocked and the mind can stay focused without being distracted. The neurochemical changes, as a result of meditative practices, involve all the major neurotransmitter systems. Such changes contribute to the amelioration of anxiety and depressive symptomatology, and in part explain the psychogenic property of meditation.[81]

Neurochemical changes induced by yoga meditation can produce an anxiolytic effect. The factors decreasing anxiety during meditation are increased parasympathetic activity, decreased locus coeruleus firing with subsequent decreased noradrenaline, increased GABAergic drive, increased serotonin, and decreased levels of the stress hormone cortisol. Increased levels of endorphins also contribute to the anxiolytic effects of meditation.[82]

STUDIES OF MEDITATION MINDFULNESS THERAPIES WITH YOUTH AND FAMILY

The following is a discussion of techniques reviewed by Burke[28] and Sibinga and Kemper[29] with additional studies. The studies are listed as clinical or nonclinical.

DBT is not reviewed because it is well known in the literature by clinicians. ACT has not been studied in children and adolescents.

Mindfulness-Based Clinical Studies

One mindfulness pilot study[30] targeted 3 adolescents with conduct disorders (13–14 years), who were at risk of school expulsion. The mindfulness intervention was administered individually in 12 sessions over 4 weeks. After this initial phase, the adolescents participated in a 25-week practice phase with monthly instructor-led sessions. The dependent variable was the self-reported number of aggressive and noncompliant acts, which showed minimal decrease in the training period, but a more substantial decrease (up to 52%) in the follow-up period, and all 3 students completed middle school without further threats of expulsion. The lack of randomization and a control group, the small sample, no statistical analysis, and self-reported data make this pilot study inconclusive as to whether the intervention or other variables (ie, the added attention these youth received) was the reason there were no further threats of expulsion.

Mindfulness-Based Stress Release

Biegel and colleagues[31] reported a randomized controlled trial (RCT) of an MBSR intervention with 102 adolescents (14–18 years), who were under current or recent psychiatric outpatient care. The subjects were recruited from an outpatient child and adolescent psychiatry department through a Kaiser Permanente hospital. The control group received treatment as usual (TAU) and the intervention group participated in TAU and an 8-week MBSR program. All disorders in the sample were based on DSM-IV-TR (Diagnostic and Statistical Manual of Mental Disorders 4th edition, text revision) Axis I diagnoses; the most common were mood disorders (49%) and anxiety disorders (30.4%). Other disorders were found in 24.5% of the sample. Most individuals in the sample (56.9%) were also diagnosed with V-codes (eg, parent-child relational problems and/or problems related to abuse or neglect). There was considerable comorbidity in the sample. Posttest measures were obtained from all available participants 8 weeks later (immediately following MBSR program completion) and at 3 months following the posttest.

The study adhered closely to the standard MBSR curriculum and structure, and was facilitated by trained, experienced mindfulness teachers. This manualized intervention consisted of 8 weekly classes, meeting 2 hours per week. Weekly homework was assigned. Frequency analyses of the group differences in specific diagnoses at post-treatment and follow-up showed that MBSR participants evidenced a significantly lower rate of mood disorder ($P<.01$). The groups did not differ significantly in the other diagnostic frequencies at the follow-up point. It should be noted that only results pertaining to sitting meditation frequency and duration are presented, as these measures showed the most frequent effects on mental health change. For example, more days of sitting practice predicted an increase in Global Assessment of Functioning (GAF) score and declines in self-reported Symptom Checklist-90 depressive symptoms (and anxiety) from baseline to follow-up, all $P<.05$. At follow-up, the group difference in GAF score (measured by blinded clinicians) favoring MBSR participants was significant ($P<.001$) and moderate in effect size ($d<0.56$). The inclusion of blind clinician ratings added objectivity. Clinical measures of mental health, made by clinicians blinded to treatment conditions, showed significant improvement in the treatment group ($P<.0001$) and at follow-up ($P<.0001$) for completers. The 3-month follow-up allowed examination of maintenance of changes. The study would be strengthened by a larger sample, longer follow-up assessments, and inclusion of more specific analysis of the effects of the individual mindfulness component, outside of the group and psychoeducation effects used in the TAU. Nonetheless the findings are promising and give evidence that MBIs can be effective as an adjunct to TAU in clinical populations of adolescents.

Much of the other research in MBSR is limited by small sample size, difficulty in teasing out the effects of other multimodal components of the studies, no randomization, and no control. The study by Bootzin and Stevens[32] was a pilot study of adolescents who received substance abuse treatment and presented with sleep problems. The study had many variables (light therapy, CBT, and MBSR) and the effects could not be isolated. Even though substance abuse seemed to decrease in completers in comparison with noncompleters 12 months later, these data were self-reported and may have been overreported. The other study by Saltzman and Goldin[33] was directed at training parents and children in MBSR. There were 2 types of home practice for parents and children: formal (eg, instructor guided sitting, body scan) and informal (eg, a meaningful pause during the day to practice mindfulness in daily life). Informal practice alone significantly correlated with improvement in self-reported depressive symptoms in adults ($P<.05$). However, formal practice, by children, did significantly explain a substantial amount of variance in post-MBSR cognitive control of attention, after accounting for baseline cognitive control ($P<.05$). Hence, MBSR may increase attention in children and improve family harmony.

Therefore, when designing treatment using MBSR, it is important to emphasize the mechanisms of MBSR practice to achieve better results. A study by Sibinga and colleagues,[34] using a manual designed for group MBSR in children from low-income households in a pediatric outpatient setting, demonstrated significant reductions in anxiety. The exercise was done for 12 weekly 45-minute sessions. Comparable pre- and post-MBSR program survey data exist for 19 of the 26 completers. MBSR program participation was associated with statistically significant reductions in hostility ($P = .02$) on the Symptom Checklist-90 (Revised), and general discomfort ($P = .01$), and emotional discomfort ($P = .02$) on the Child Health and Illness Profile Adolescent Edition (CHIP-AE). Although human immunodeficiency virus (HIV) was not necessarily described as the primary stressor in the lives of those study participants living with HIV, it was mentioned as an important concern on probing this issue. The MBSR methods seem to have a positive effect in terms of ameliorating HIV-specific stressors such as taking medicines, fearing illness and death, experiencing stigma and discrimination, and disclosing HIV status. Although these are subjective responses, MBSR may be helpful in decreasing anxiety and the general and physical discomfort associated with having a chronic illness experienced by chronically ill children.

Mindfulness-Based Cognitive Therapy

The results of a pilot study by Bogels and colleagues[35] using a modified MBCT did help reduce behavioral problems in children with disruptive disorders, but the most impressive outcome was the lasting effect it had in improving socials skills in children with autism. The study was a quasi-experimental within-participant wait-list control nonrandomized design in a community mental health setting, with 14 adolescents (aged 11–18 years) with externalizing disorders (ADHD, oppositional, and conduct disorders), and children with autistic-spectrum disorders that had externalizing behaviors. Their parents were in concurrent MBCT groups. Preintervention measures were done, followed by posttreatment measures immediately after 8 weeks of the intervention. The treatment sessions were once per week with an instructor, and there was instruction for exercises to be done at home. Another follow-up measure was done 8 weeks after the intervention ended. There were accommodations made to some of the interventions to address particular symptoms involved in the study. For instance, for the impulsivity in children with ADHD: children were given one half of a chocolate cookie and told if they did not eat it while the instructors were out of the room, they would be given the other half of the cookie when the instructors returned. The children were told to focus their attention on breathing as a means to distract them from wanting to eat the cookie. For children with ADHD, shorter concentration techniques were also used: commitments to homework assignments, attendance, or participation were rewarded with points. The posttreatment effect size in the parent-rated Children's Social Behavior Questionnaire (which measures behavior problems typically found in autistic children) was 0.8, and at follow-up was 0.6. Surprisingly, children with autism found the homework assignments easy to follow and they performed better than any other children in the study. This study provides information for future research on how to revise the interventions based on the diagnosis and age of the children involved. The highest drop-out rate was among the oppositional defiant disorder (ODD)/conduct disordered (CD) children, who tended to disturb the groups. The investigators suggested that these children might do better with individual training. Studies using MBCT also are limited by nonrandomization, no blinding, small sample size, and no control.

Finally, Semple and colleagues[36] used a cross-legged nonrandomized design. Each 12-week program consisted of one 90-minute, small-group, mindfulness training session per week, supplemented with brief daily home practice exercises. In this study, the investigators assumed that anxiety disrupts attention and interferes with affective self-regulation. MBCT-C is a manualized group psychotherapy for children ages 9 to 13 years from low-income, inner-city households, which was developed specifically to increase social-emotional resiliency (affective self-regulation) through the enhancement of mindful attention. Measures included the Child Behavior Checklist (CBCL), State-Trait Anxiety Inventory for Children (STAIC), and Multidimensional Anxiety Scale for Children (MASC). A one-group, paired-samples t-test of the pooled pretest and follow-up data found significant reductions in behavior problems over the course of the study, with a medium effect size [$t(24) = 4.35$, $P<.001$ (2-tailed), Cohen $d = 0.44$]. MBCT-C is a promising intervention as an adjunct for attention and behavior problems, and may reduce childhood anxiety symptoms.

Combination MBSR/MBCT

Limitations of the combined MBSR/MBCT studies were nonrandomization, no blinding, small sample size, and no control.

Van der Oord and colleagues[37] evaluated the effectiveness of 8-week mindfulness training for children aged 8 to 12 with ADHD and parallel mindful parenting training for their parents. Children entering the study had a DSM-IV diagnosis of ADHD established with the parent and child version of the Anxiety Disorder Interview Schedule for Children (ADIS-C). Participants had to be able to attend the first session and a minimum of 6 out of 8 sessions of treatment. Treatment was conducted in groups of 4 to 6 children and parents, and consisted of 8 weekly 90-minute group sessions. From pretest to posttest the reduction of teacher-rated inattentive behavior reached significance ($P = .10$; effect size [ES] $= 0.39$). Parental stress on the Parent Stress Index (PSI) decreased (ES $= 0.57$; medium ES) and overreactivity on the Parent Scale (PS) showed a significant reduction (ES $= 0.85$; large ES) on posttest. The PS was used to assess ineffective discipline styles on 3 subscales (laxness, verbosity, and overreactivity). Although the study demonstrated a small ES for attention in children, it improved family harmony.

In a study of combined MBSR/MBCT by Zylowska and colleagues,[38] the intervention was directed at ADHD symptoms in children and adults. The combined technique used was referred to as the Mindfulness Awareness Practices (MAP). The study was an 8-week intervention with a mixed group (N = 32) of adolescents (n = 8; mean age 15.6 years) and adults (n = 24; mean age 48.5 years) with ADHD. The study evaluation consisted of semistructured clinical interviews by trained research clinicians: Schedule for Affective Disorders and Schizophrenia—Lifetime Version for adults and Schedule for Affective Disorders and Schizophrenia for School-Age Children—Present and Lifetime Version for adolescents (sequential interviews, first with a parent and then with the adolescent). Self-report and observer (spouse or friend for adults; parent for adolescents) behavioral ratings were collected using the ADHD-IV scale (adults) or Swanson- Nolan-Pelham Scale (SNAP-IV; adolescents). The within-participant pre- to posttest intervention with no control group included weekly 2.5-hour sessions. MAP homework of 5 to 15 minutes' sitting meditation was assigned, and specific psycho-education about attention-deficit disorders was discussed. Pooled results for adults and adolescents indicated significant improvements in self-reported ADHD symptoms overall ($P = .01$), and some significant changes in neurocognitive measures. On neurocognitive task performance, significant improvements were found for measures of attentional conflict (Attention Network Test and Stroop color-word) and set-shifting (Trails A and B) (all $P<.01$) but not for measures of working memory. The Attention Network Test (ANT) is a computerized test measuring 3 aspects of attention: alerting (maintaining a vigilant state of preparedness), orienting (selecting a stimulus among multiple inputs), and conflict (prioritizing among competing tasks). The Trail-Making Test assesses attentional set-shifting and inhibition. Of note, the mean posttraining ANT score in the ADHD sample was comparable with mean scores found elsewhere in non-ADHD adults or adolescent samples. The neurocognitive finding suggests that mindfulness may specifically improve conflict attention, set-shifting, and inhibition in ADHD. These tests of attention seem to play a role in the development of inhibition and self-regulation. The study, as noted by Zylowska and colleagues, is limited by the small sample size, no control group or randomization, and the use of self-reported outcome measures. However, the strength of the neurocognitive testing results implies that this may be a helpful adjunctive treatment in children and adults with ADHD.

Napoli and colleagues[40] reported an RCT with 228 nonclinical first to third grade students in a city in the southwestern United States. Ninety-seven children were randomized to the treatment group and 97 were randomized to a control group (participated in reading). Twelve 45-minute sessions were held biweekly over 24 weeks. The Attention Academy Program (AAP) core practices of MBSR/MBCT included breathing exercises, a body-scan visualization application, a body movement–based task, and a postsession debriefing or sharing of instructor feedback with the class. Before and at the end of the 24-week AAP, each child either completed or was measured with 4 established measures: The ADD-H Comprehensive Teacher Rating Scale (ACTeRS), the Test of Everyday Attention for Children (TEA-Ch), which utilizes 5 subtests measuring sustained and selective (visual) attention, and the self-reported Test Anxiety Scale (TAS). Paired t-tests were conducted for each group on the pretest/posttest measures and showed statistically significant results for TEA-Ch selective (visual) attention subscale ($t_{diff} = 7.94$, $P<.001$), the ACTeRS Attention Subscale ($t_{diff} = -8.21$, $P = .001$), the ACTeRS Social Skills Subscale ($t_{diff} = -7.19$, $P = .001$), and the TAS ($t_{diff} = -1.34$, $P = .007$). The TEA-Ch Sustained Attention subscale showed a nonsignificant difference between groups pretest and posttest and nonsignificant pre-to-post differences. Reported ES ranged from small to medium ($d = 0.39–0.60$).

Limitations were that teachers were not blinded. The study suggests the AAP intervention is feasible in a school setting, with results lending support for a possible treatment effect on selective (visual) attention and test anxiety, but not for sustained attention, in this intervention. Although AAP included core practices of MBSR/MBCT, it differed by the absence of home practice.

Taken together, these studies demonstrate that combined MBSR and MBCT may be helpful as an adjunctive treatment for ADHD, anxiety, and improving cognitive skills. Furthermore, these techniques may improve family harmony.

SYM FOR ATTENTION-DEFICIT/HYPERACTIVITY DISORDER

Using the method as described by Harrison and colleagues,[39] SYM was used as a potential nonmedication adjunctive intervention for children with ADHD. The program was publicized by a newspaper article and an introductory lecture, which was open to parents of school-aged children with ADHD. Interested parents were invited to participate with their child in a 6-week program of twice-weekly teaching sessions. Inclusion criteria were that the children had a formal diagnosis of ADHD using the DSM-IV criteria made by a pediatrician or child psychiatrist. The program made no recommendations about medication, except that parents should monitor and adjust their children's medication as they normally would, in conjunction with their doctor or psychologist. At the midpoint and end point of the program, parents were asked about any changes they may have made to their child's level of medication. Only those children who scored above threshold for ADHD were included in the study (ie, a score of 15 and higher on the Conner Parent-Teacher Questionnaire). Most children (n = 31) were receiving medication (eg, ritalin, dexamphetamine), 14 were not medicated, and medication information was not provided for the other 3 children. Because of the requirement for personalized training in the SYM program, it was necessary to separate the children into 2 groups and run 2 sequential treatment programs.

The treatment program consisted of twice-weekly 90-minute clinics, held in large meeting rooms at the hospital. For the first 3 weeks, the clinic consisted of guided meditation sessions, with parents attending one group and the children another. The meditation process involved practicing techniques whereby participants were helped to achieve a state of thought-free awareness. Instructors directed participants to become aware of this state within themselves by becoming silent and focusing their attention inside. Parents were also asked to conduct shorter meditation sessions at home twice a day. In the clinic, there were usually 2 periods of meditation of 5 to 15 minutes each, supplemented by information about how to meditate and sharing of experiences. The parent sessions had 1 to 2 instructors, but the child sessions had a higher instructor-to-child ratio (normally 1 instructor for every 3 children). From week 4 to week 6, one of the weekly sessions was conducted as a joint parent-child meditation, which enabled instructors to train parents in guiding their child's meditation. Children and parents were asked to meditate regularly at home and to record their progress in a diary, which was checked each week to encourage compliance.

Assessments were conducted at 3 points:

Week 1: Recruitment or commencement of the meditation program
Week 3: Midway point of the program
Week 6: At the end of the program

The full schedule of assessments was completed for group 1. The second treatment program, group 2, used fewer measures and assessments were only completed at the commencement (week 1) and end of the program (week 6). The Conner

Parent-Teacher Questionnaire ADHD symptoms were assessed via parent report, using the Conner Parent-Teacher Questionnaire and the Conner parent-rated checklists, which are shorter versions of the 93-item original. Parents completed the 30-item Child-Parent Relationship Scale (CPRS), which assesses the quality of the parent-child relationship. Items on the CPRS tap 4 dimensions of child-parent attachment, namely warmth, conflict, dependence, and open communication, on a 5-point rated scale.

On the Conner Parent-Teacher Questionnaire, mean scores decreased from $M_{pre} = 22.54$, SD $= 4.61$, to $M_{post} = 14.62$, SD $= 5.15$. The average mean decrease in reported ADHD symptoms was 7.91 points (SD $= 4.91$, range 0–19), which represented an improvement rate of 35%. Statistical analysis using paired-sample t-test showed that the difference in pretreatment and posttreatment scores was highly significant ($t = 8.23$, $P<.001$). Because of the possibility that the improvement in behavior may have been due to the medication children were receiving rather than the SYM program, further comparisons were made to assess whether medication status may have contributed to this change. Results demonstrated a similar reduction in ADHD symptoms for the 20 children who were receiving medication compared with the 6 who were not, with a mean reduction in scores of 7.83 (SD $= 5.15$) and 7.95 (SD $= 4.97$), respectively ($t = -0.50$, not significant). This result suggests that the reduction in ADHD symptoms was not related to children's pharmacologic treatment. It was also noteworthy that in several cases, parents stated that they had been able to reduce their child's medication during the course of the SYM program. Of the 20 children who were receiving medication when they started the program, 11 had reduced the dose during SYM treatment—2 by less than half, 6 by half, and 3 by more than half—and 9 did not change the dose. Comparison of means indicated that the improvement in the level of ADHD symptoms was significantly greater for the 11 children who had reduced their medication ($M_{reduction} = 10.18$, SD $= 4.79$) than for the 9 who had maintained the same level of medication ($M_{reduction} = 5.22$, SD $= 3.83$; $t = 2.51$, $P = .022$).

These findings suggest that SYM treatment not only contributed to the reduction in children's ADHD behavior scores but also had the added benefit of helping children manage their own behavior with a reduced level of medication. When asked if they felt their child had benefited from the SYM program, 92% of parents agreed that they had. Particular benefits for the child that were rated highly (>3 on a 5-point scale) by parents were "more confident in him/herself" ($M = 3.35$, SD $= 0.93$), "improved sleep patterns" ($M = 3.27$, SD $= 1.42$), and "more cooperative" ($M = 3.18$, SD $= 1.01$). Similar high ratings for benefits related to school included "less difficulty with the teacher," "more able to manage schoolwork," "more able to manage homework" ($M = 3.47$, SD $= 1.33$), and "positive about going to school."

All of the parent-rated measures on the CPRS showed significant improvements. For each measure, mean pretreatment and posttreatment scores were compared using paired-sample t-test analysis. ADHD symptom scores at the midpoint and final point were significantly lower than the baseline score ($M_{pre} = 22.62$, $M_{post} = 15.94$ and 16.25, $t = 5.81$ and 5.65, respectively; $P<.001$). A similar improvement was seen in parents' reports of their children's confidence and social behavior. Child-parent relationships also significantly improved during the course of the SYM treatment. Examination of the subscale components of the CPRS showed that this change was accounted for by lower scores for relationship conflict ($M_{pre} = 3.37$, $M_{post} = 2.94$, $t = 3.08$, $P<.01$). A decrease in ADHD symptoms was strongly correlated with an increase in (CPRS) scores, that is, less conflicted (more secure) parent-child interaction ($r(14) = -0.67$, $P<.01$). Interestingly the relationship between ADHD symptoms and relationship quality at the commencement of the program was not significant (r(14) = −0.41), but at the end of the treatment the outcome scores on these measures were strongly correlated (r(14) = −0.66, P = .01), suggesting a change in family functioning processes during the treatment program. Scores for children's self-description and self-evaluation ratings of self-esteem did not change significantly from the commencement to the end of the meditation program. It should be noted, however, that the average scores were fairly high at change. Limitations to the study were no comparison to the wait-list control, no randomization, and small study size. It should also be mentioned that the results may be biased because all parents who volunteered their children to the study were seeking to find a nonpharmacologic alternative, and no corresponding teacher report forms were done. Taken together, the study shows promise in improving ADHD symptoms, in possibly helping to reduce ADHD medication, and in improving child-parent relationships. Follow-up studies to assess the lasting effects of the results found in this study should also be done.

STUDIES WITH YOUTH AND FAMILY: TRANSCENDENTAL MEDITATION

As per the data base of Black and colleagues,[83] studies reviewed were primarily youth with preexisting high normal blood pressure. However, other effects, beyond lowering blood pressure, included decreased anxiety, improved self-esteem, decreased externalizing problems, and improved school attendance. Only studies that did not use the criteria of having increased blood pressure as the initial entry are discussed, as the main focus of this article is on child and adolescent psychiatric disorders.

Attention-Deficit/Hyperactivity Disorder

A small study by Grosswald and colleagues[84] included students with ADHD and comorbidities, including general anxiety disorder, dysthymia, obsessive compulsive disorder, pervasive developmental disorder, sleep disorders, and tics, diagnosed by a psychologist or a psychiatrist. Known ADHD inventories and performance measures of executive function were administered at baseline and 3 months later. Data collection was divided into 2 categories: (1) measures of stress, anxiety, ADHD symptoms as reported by parent, teacher, and student inventories; (2) measures of executive function as measured by parent and teacher inventories, and by performance tests.

Assessments were done pretest and posttest (after practicing the technique for 3 months). The assessments used are as follows.

1. Teachers and parents completed the Achenbach Child Behavior Checklist (CBCL) inventory and the Behavior Rating Inventory of Executive Function (BRIEF). The BRIEF assesses behavioral regulation and executive functioning. The BRIEF includes 3 composite measures: Behavioral Regulation Index, Meta-Cognition Index, and General Executive Composite. The Global Executive Composite is composed of the Behavioral Regulation Index and the Meta-Cognition Index.
2. Children completed the Youth Self Report (YSR). Variables selected for analysis from the YSR were Anxious/Depressed, Withdrawn/Depressed, Affective Problems, Anxiety Problems, Attention Problems, ADHD Problems, and Total Problems. Added to these variables was the single result of the child-completed Revised Child Manifest Anxiety Scale (RCMAS).
3. Clinicians completed 4 performance tests used to measure different aspects of executive function listed below.
   a. The Cognitive Assessment System (CAS) subtest for Expressive Attention. The CAS Expressive Attention subtest is a color-word interference test. It measures higher-level complex attention and the ability to inhibit impulses.

b. Delis-Kaplan Executive Function System (D-KEFS) Verbal Fluency subtest. The D-KEFS measures verbal fluency.

c. Tower of London (TOL). The TOL measures higher-order problem-solving and is used to evaluate executive function difficulties.

d. Connor Continuous Performance Test II (CPT II). The CPT II measures sustained attention.

The anxious/depressed category of the CBCL (rated by teachers) reached statistical significance with good ES pre- and posttest (pretest mean = 10.2, SD = 6.4; posttest mean = 3.6, SD = 3.6; ES = 0.7). The YSR, rated by the students, reached statistical significance in 2 categories with good ES, anxious/depressed (pretest mean = 5.7, SD = 3.6; posttest mean = 2.7, SD = 3.7; ES = 0.8) and anxiety (pretest mean = 3.2, SD = 2.0; posttest mean = 1.6, SD = 1.9; ES = 0.8).

Teachers and parents completed the BRIEF. Repeated-measures multivariate analysis of variance (MANOVA) of the General Executive Composite indicated significant improvement in executive function from pretest to posttest, $F(1,9) = 5.5$, $P = .022$. Repeated measures by MANOVA were conducted on the scales comprising the 2 indices. These MANOVAs were also statistically significant: Behavioral Regulation Index (Inhibit, Shift, and Emotional Control), $P<.00001$; and Meta-Cognition Index (Initiate, Working Memory, Planning, Organize Material and Monitoring), $P = .0025$.

The CAS expressive attention and the CAS accuracy yielded statistically significant results with good ES. The CAS expressive attention yielded pretest mean = 36.11, SD = 10.63; post-test mean = 44.70, SD = 13.59; ES = 0.8; and the CAS accuracy yielded pretest mean = 37.70, SD = 2.21; posttest mean = 39.40, SD = 1.27; ES = 0.8. In addition, the investigators pointed out that a review of measures of executive function used for assessing ADHD suggests that tests of letter fluency are not reliable for distinguishing ADHD from controls because of the confounding presence of learning disorders. Similarly, the TOL has been found to be less consistent than other measures in distinguishing specific effects associated with ADHD from those related to learning disorders. Therefore, no statistical analysis was performed on these tests. CPT pretests and posttests were not reported because students had left school before the posttest could be completed.

Taken together, the study did show a corresponding decrease in problematic symptoms associated with working memory, planning, organization, ability to inhibit and shift, and expressive attention (often seen in ADHD) when anxiety and depression symptoms decreased. Even though a direct correlation cannot be definitively concluded at this time, because TM is easy to learn it may serve as an adjunct in the treatment of cognitive dysfunctions often found with ADHD. Although the study lacked randomization and blinding, it is important because it demonstrated improvement in ADHD symptoms and executive function across several comorbid conditions. Caution should be used in interpreting self-reports by adolescents, but the neurocognitive testing gives stronger evidence about the effect of TM on cognitive functions.

High School Setting

1. The objective of the study by Rosaen and Benn[85] was to systematically explore the first-person experience of young adolescents who practice TM for longer than a year. This study used a more subjective approach to access common themes students felt about themselves after a year of TM practice. Participants included 10 seventh-grade students from a Detroit Charter School who had practiced TM for 1 year. Researchers concluded that the state of restful alertness induced by

meditation may facilitate the growth of social-emotional capacities necessary for regulating the emotional ups and downs, and the interpersonal stresses of adolescence. Future empiric validation is needed to systematically analyze the impact of TM practice on students' social-emotional and cognitive development, and to determine whether its practice can serve a protective function, helping students to successfully meet the challenges of adolescence.

2. So and Orme-Joohnson[47] described 3 studies on 362 high school students at 3 different schools in Taiwan. This study is one of the best RCTs (which was blinded and had substantial sample numbers), and is therefore discussed in detail here. Researchers tested the hypothesis that regular practice of TM for 15 to 20 minutes twice a day for 6 to 12 months would improve cognitive ability.

The same 7 measurements were used in all studies:

1. Test for Creative Thinking-Drawing Production (TCT-DP).
2. Constructive Thinking Inventory (CTI). The CTI was designed to assess "practical intelligence," nonintellectual abilities and attitudes that predict success in work, love, social relationships, and in achieving and maintaining emotional and physical well-being.
3. Group Embedded Figures Test (GEFT). The GEFT is a measure of field independence, a cognitive style that is part of a cluster of psychological traits that cuts across many dimensions of cognitive functioning, personality, and social behavior. Field independence predicts academic achievement, controlling for fluid intelligence.
4. State Anxiety (STAI). The STAI is widely used to measure anxiety, both state anxiety (state anxiety is the temporary change in a person's emotional state due external stimuli) and trait anxiety (the anxiety that is part of a person's personality that may be due to inherited anxiety disorders).
5. Trait anxiety measured by the STAI.
6. Inspection Time (IT). IT is considered to be a framework for assessing the speed of information processing at the stage at which the stimulus is encoded or transferred into short-term memory.
7. Culture Fair Intelligence Test (CFIT). The CFIT is said to be a measure of "fluid intelligence," the ability to successfully reason in novel situations. Fluid intelligence correlates with the executive control functions of the frontal lobes, which involve keeping attention on task requirements that are understood and remembered.

The 3 studies are as follows:

• The first study consisted of all first-year senior high school students from 4 different classes at Chun-Chow Private School in Taiwan (N = 154; 78 boys, 76 girls). Subjects were given a lecture on the TM technique, and of those interested in learning, half were randomly assigned to learn the TM technique (the TM group) and the other half was randomly assigned to a wait-list control group who took naps on the same schedule as meditation (the Napping group). The latter group was included to determine if the effects that occurred for TM were the same as the effects that occurred for napping. Those not interested in learning the technique were designated as the No-interest group. The mean age was 16.5 years. The numbers (males/females) for the TM group, Napping group, and No-interest group, respectively, were 56 (25/31), 58 (28/30), and 40 (25/15). Instruction followed a standard 7-step protocol that has been used to uniformly teach more than 4 million people throughout the United States (described in "methods" under TM). Participants practiced 15 to 20 minutes twice a day for 6 months. Pretests and posttests were done by teachers who were blinded as to who was in which group.

- The second So study was of 118 junior high school students from 3 different classes at Yang-Ming National School in Taipei, in the northern part of Taiwan. The study compared TM with a contemplation meditation (CM) group and a control. The students' mean age was 14.6 years. The experimental group consisted of 37 girls, the No-treatment control group had 40 girls, and a third comparison group, of CM, had 41 girls. Like the TM technique, this CM was practiced mentally, sitting with eyes closed. However, there is a fundamental difference between the 2 types of meditation in that contemplation requires thinking about the meaning of something, which keeps the mind on the surface level of thinking. TM practice does not involve meaning and allows the mind to settle into a pure consciousness state. The procedure was essentially identical to that of Experiment 1, but the design was somewhat different. In Experiment 2, 2 groups designated for the study were randomized by class (rather than by student) to the TM technique or to the No-treatment control group. The third group took a 5-day course to learn a CM technique from the Chinese tradition taught by a class master. Exercise practice and pretest and posttest measures were the same as in the other experiments.
- So's third study consisted of 99 male vocational students from 2 classes at Nan-Ying Commerce and Industry Training School in Tainan, in the southern part of Taiwan. Subjects' mean age was 17.7 years: 17.8 years for the TM group and 17.6 years for the control group. There were 51 males in the experimental group and 48 males in the No-treatment control group. These students all majored in technical drawing. Experiment 3 was essentially the same as Experiment 2, randomized by class to the TM group or to a No-treatment control group, except that posttest was after 12 months instead of 6 months as in Experiments 1 and 2. There were only 2 groups in this study, and there was no attrition on any measure.

Results of the 3 studies included:

1. In studies 2 and 3, the TM group demonstrated significant improvement over the controls in all 7 measures (study 2 range $P<.0001$ to .052 and study 3 range $P<.001$ to .032).
2. In study 1, the TM group showed significant improvement over controls in 6 of the measures (range $P<.001$ to .005), with CFIT (executive control of attention) being nonsignificant.
3. In study 2, the contemplation group only demonstrated significant improvement over the control group on 2 measures, the GEFT (psychological traits that improve academic success, $P<.057$) and IT (time it takes to process a stimulus into short-term memory, $P<.005$). In addition, anxiety seemed to increase in the contemplation group. However, in comparison with the CM group, the TM group experienced significant improvement on the creativity measure (TCT-DP), the state and trait measure (STAI), the IT measure (time it takes to process stimuli into short-term memory), and the CTI measure (psychological factors that increase academic success).

As noted by the investigators, these 3 studies strongly support the hypothesis that the TM program improves performance on several cognitive and affective measures. The randomization, large numbers of participants, and use of blinding in these studies lends validity to the research. The use of an active comparison group for TM (the contemplation group) proves that not all meditation techniques are alike.

The average statistical ES for the 3 studies for each measurement was calculated. The creativity variable (TCT-DP) had the largest ES (0.77), followed by practical intelligence (CTI, executive control of attention) (0.62), field independence (GEFT, social behaviors, personality traits, and cognitive traits that predict academic success) (0.58), and state and trait anxiety (STAI) (0.53 and 0.52), with inspection time (IT) (0.39) and fluid intelligence (CFIT) (0.34) having the smallest ES. These results indicate that improvements in creativity, executive control of attention, psychological factors that may predict academic success are more likely involved in improving cognitive ability using TM.

As also noted by the investigators, the study demonstrated that there was a low correlation between changes in anxiety and changes in cognitive variables in all 3 studies. Therefore, anxiety alone may not be responsible for cognitive improvement. Perhaps participants who were anxious had an increase in cognitive variables once their anxiety was reduced using the technique. However, individuals who were not anxious may have still have an increase in cognition using the technique. In addition, the effects of TM may be more consistent with other physiologic changes associated with TM, such as increased EEG coherence, suggestive of a wakeful hypometabolic state.

Taken together, TM does seem to increase cognitive ability, although more research is needed.

MEDITATION-RELAXATION STUDIES WITH YOUTH AND FAMILY
PTSD Meditation-Relaxation Versus Narrative Exposure Therapy

Catani and colleagues[52] tested the efficacy of 2 pragmatic short-term interventions when applied by trained local counselors in the acute aftermath of a tsunami (conducted within the first 5 months following the tragedy). The researchers trained local counselors in the use of 6 sessions of MED-RELAX. The northeastern part of Sri Lanka had already been affected by civil war when the 2004 tsunami hit the region, leading to high rates of PTSD in the children. A randomized treatment comparison was implemented in a refugee camp in a severely affected community. The population of the initial assessment consisted of children in the age range of 8 to 14 years living in the newly erected camps. All 71 eligible children who were present in the camps on the day of the interview were interviewed. All requirements for the diagnosis for PTSD were fulfilled using the DSM-IV except for the criteria of time because the diagnosis was made within 3 weeks of the tsunami. In this study, 31 children who presented with a preliminary diagnosis of PTSD were randomly assigned to either 6 sessions of Narrative Exposure Therapy for children (KIDNET) or 6 sessions of MED-RELAX.

As noted by the investigators

> ...during the 6 KIDNET sessions, the child, assisted by the therapist, constructs a detailed chronological account of his or her personal biography. Particular attention is given to any traumatic experiences, including those related to the Tsunami, as well as those linked to violence and war situations. The autobiography is recorded by the therapist in written form and corrected and filled with details with each subsequent reading. The aim of this procedure is to transform the generally fragmented reports of the traumatic experiences into a coherent narrative.... The child is encouraged to relive these emotions while narrating.... In the last session, the participant receives a written version of the autobiography.

The complete technique used for MED-RELAX is mentioned earlier in the section on techniques and approaches.

Outcome measures included severity of PTSD symptoms, level of functioning, and physical health. In both treatment conditions, PTSD symptoms (avoidance, intrusions, and hyperarousal) and impairment in functioning were significantly reduced at 1 month after testing and remained stable over time at the 6-month follow-up. No statistical P value was given for the PTSD symptoms, but the P value for impairment in functioning was less than 0.001. The ES for the KIDNET group was 1.76 (confidence interval [CI] 0.9–2.5) at posttest and 1.96 (CI 1.1–2.8) at the 6-month follow-up. The ES for MED-RELAX were 1.83 (CI 0.9–2.6) and 2.20 (CI 1.2–3.0). At the 6-month follow-up, recovery rates were 81% for the children in the KIDNET group and 71% for those in the MED-RELAX group.

Therefore, the KIDNET and the MED-RELAX therapies were useful for the treatment of PTSD in children in the direct aftermath of mass disasters. A limitation of the study was the lack of a control group. However, with the devastating effects of this disaster and the poor living conditions, for reasons of ethical concerns the researchers decided to not use a control group.

Relaxation Therapy or Progressive Muscle Relaxation Studies

Meta-analysis

In the meta-analysis by Eppley and colleagues,[54] the relaxation techniques were less effective than TM. The study noted differences between the methods as the possible reason for the effectiveness. Participants stated that required effort or focus of some kind is needed during the relaxation methods, compared with TM, which was self-described as effortless.

Relaxation therapy for depression and anxiety

One study by Reynolds and Coats[53] involving RT, specifically PMR, was found to be as useful as CBT for depression in comparison with wait-list controls. Three rating scales were used to measure effects, and all demonstrated significant effects of PMR and CBT (Beck Depression Inventory [BDI] Rating Scale, $P<.001$; Reynolds Adolescent Depression Scale, $P<.05$; and the Beck Depression Index, $P<.001$ before and 5 weeks after treatment). However, a slightly different picture emerged in relation to anxiety. Specific pairwise comparisons revealed that the relaxation training group had a significantly lower mean score than the wait-list group ($P<.05$ on the State-Trait Anxiety Inventory [STAIC] Scale compared with the wait list). These findings suggest that depression and anxiety, although related in symptomatology, may respond to different treatments. Limitations of the study included subjects not being formally diagnosed using DSM-IV, and that the only non–self-rated measure was the BDI. Therefore, students may have rated themselves in a biased way to look better than they really were. Clinicians were not blinded.

In this study, therefore, both CBT and PMR seemed equally effective in decreasing the symptoms of depression. However, PMR seemed more effective in decreasing symptoms of anxiety than CBT.

In contrast to the Reynolds study, a study by Wood and colleagues[55] comparing RT with CBT reported that both techniques had equal effects on anxiety. Anxiety on the RCMAS decreased significantly from pre- to posttreatment for both groups ($P<.01$), both for postassessment and at the 6-month follow-up. At the 6-month follow-up, differences between the groups for the Mood and Feelings Questionnaire (MFQ) were reduced, but the initial effect of the CBT intervention was no longer significant. It was thought that this occurred in part because of a high relapse rate in the depressive disorder group, and partly because subjects in the RT group continued to recover and receive other treatments. It is not known whether this recovery was solely due to the other treatments or to the lasting effects of the relaxation technique. Limitations to the study were the small number of participants and the absence of blinding. Both studies used randomization.

Therefore, owing to the multiple variables after treatment, it is difficult to delineate whether the relaxation group continued to recover in comparison with the CBT group. However, unlike the Reynolds study, CBT and RT seem to be more effective for anxiety. The different effects on anxiety in both studies may have been due to other variables, such as the quality of the training of the clinicians.

These results should be considered with caution owing to the limitations of the studies; no solid conclusions can be drawn. In addition, the study by Reynolds measured effects 5 weeks after treatment, whereas the Wood study measured effects 6 months after treatment. To determine efficacy, future studies need to monitor which, if any, techniques continue to be used by the participants and which other variables may have occurred after the study was finalized. More studies are needed.

Relaxation therapy versus massage therapy

Two studies measured cortisol levels to draw conclusions about the outcomes of RT in comparison with massage therapy (MT).

In one of the studies, Field and colleagues[56] compared RT with MT. Thirty-two depressed adolescent mothers were randomly assigned, and received ten 30-minute sessions of either RT or MT over a 5-week period. To qualify for the study, the mothers needed to have an elevated BDI score and to be free of current medication or other treatments for depression or related disorders. The depression classification was based on a diagnosis of dysthymia on the Diagnostic Inventory Schedule and a score greater than 16 on the BDI.

Although both groups reported lower anxiety on the STAIC following their first and last therapy sessions, only the MT group showed behavioral changes and stress hormone changes, including a decrease in anxious behavior, pulse, and salivary cortisol levels. A decrease in urine cortisol levels suggested lower stress following the 5-week period for the MT group. Limitations of the study were no control group, no blinding, and a small sample size. Future studies using meditation techniques should consider salivary cortisol levels as a better indicator of decreased stress and, therefore, decreased anxiety. It may also be useful to monitor cortisol levels to compare the decrease in depression with a corresponding decrease in anxiety.

Relaxation therapy in a child and adolescent clinic

In an RT study that measured cortisol by Platania-Solazzo and colleagues,[57] the immediate effects of RT were assessed in children and adolescents recruited from a psychiatric unit. The subjects were randomly assigned to an RT group or to a control group watching a relaxation videotape (R-VT). Diagnoses were made using DSM-III-R (*Diagnostic and Statistical Manual of Mental Disorders*, 3rd edition revision) criteria for depression or an adjustment disorder. The relaxation intervention occurred twice per week in the afternoon. Pretest and posttest measures of the STAIC in the RT group were highly significant when compared with the control group ($P<.01$). Pretest and posttest behavioral scales were significant for affect ($P<.05$), anxiety ($P<.005$), and the fidgety scale ($P<.001$). Heart rate and activity level were significantly decreased compared with the R-VT control group ($P<.001$ and $P<.01$, respectively). Patients with adjustment disorder and one-third of the depressed patients showed decreases in cortisol levels following RT, whereas no changes were noted in the R-VT group. Thus, both diagnostic groups appeared to benefit from the RT class.

Following RT, a closer look at the data from the depressed group revealed that 62% had cortisol levels that were higher than their starting baseline, and 38% had lower cortisol levels than their starting baseline. These results suggest there were 2 types of depressed patients being sampled. The STAIC scores tended to decrease more following RT for the 38% with decreasing cortisol levels, compared with the 62% with the increasing cortisol levels. Hence, a decrease in anxiety in depressed patients may be necessary for cortisol levels to decrease.

Taken together, the studies by Field and Platania-Solazzo demonstrate that MT reduced anxiety when there was a corresponding decrease in cortisol, and RT caused a greater decline in depressive symptoms when there was a corresponding decrease in anxiety and cortisol. Although the use of cortisol levels may prove to be useful in differentiating the outcomes of future studies, again caution should be used when drawing conclusions from these studies because of their limitations.

Relaxation therapy versus EMG biofeedback
In an RT comparison study, Denkowski and Denkowski[58] examined whether group progressive relaxation (PR) training was as effective as individual EMG biofeedback training in facilitating the academic achievement and self-control of 45 hyperactive elementary school children. Students were randomly assigned to EMG biofeedback, RT, or a control group. All had learning disorders but none were diagnosed with ADHD using standardized instruments. Teachers were blinded as to which treatment the students received. MANOVA indicated no significant differences among the 3 contrast groups when all dependent variables were considered together. However, univariate F values and discriminant analysis disclosed locus of control to be significantly more internal for the PR condition ($P<.01$). Although teachers were blinded as to who received the different interventions, the study had small numbers and potentially discriminating information, such as diagnosis, and the study did not identify which subjects were on medication. Therefore, this study cannot conclusively demonstrate that EMG biofeedback was better than RT or vice versa.

Deep-Breathing Meditation

Test anxiety
In a study conducted by Paul and colleagues,[59] DBM is used for test anxiety in a post-college program preparing underprivileged students for premedical school exams. It is mentioned here because it involves young adults. Sessions were done over a 1-year period for 5 minutes before a scheduled lecture. Results showed increased concentration with attention and visualization, and decreased nervousness and self-doubt when testing. There was a total of 64 participants in the study.

The results were self-reported, and the study was limited by there being no randomization and no control group; however, DBM may be helpful in reducing test anxiety.

Posture, Breathing, Attention, and Visualization

Although there are no reported studies using this technique,[2] it has been suggested for use in children and adolescents to help produce productivity in a classroom situation.

STUDIES WITH YOUTH AND FAMILY: BODY-MIND
Exercise

Exercise[61] was studied to determine the effects on adolescents with depression. Although a self- report scale was used in this study (which reported positive effects), the results using a clinician rating scale are discussed here because it is thought to have more validity. The Child Depression Rating Scale—Revised (CDRS-R) was used to evaluate students who reported symptoms of depression and low levels of physical exercise. A raw score of 36 or greater was necessary gain entry to the study. Adolescents with a prior history of bipolar disorder were excluded. Thirteen adolescents fulfilled all the requirements of the program discussed under the Methods section. Ten of the 13 were overweight or obese as determined by their BMI. Of the 13 participants, 69% were in psychotherapy and/or were on psychotropic medication, and 54% were not on medication. Remission was determined if the CDRS-R scale reached a value of 28 or less. The CDRS-R was administered 3 months after intervention. Of the 13 participants, 62% achieved remission.

Limits to the study are small size, no control group, and lack of randomization. However, exercise has many health benefits and may be a useful adjunct in depressed adolescents.

Movement or Dance Therapy

Movement therapy and autism

In the study by Hartshorn and colleagues,[62] 38 autistic children (mean age 5 years) from a school setting were given movement therapy in small groups. A control group was used as a comparison whereby a movement therapy session was done once in the beginning and once at the end of the 8-week period. Behaviors were observed on the first and last days of movement classes for both groups. The movement therapy for this study is described under the Methods section. Sessions occurred 2 times per week for 8 weeks. The children were observed randomly for 1 minute 6 times during the first 18 minutes of movement therapy. During each minute, period behaviors were recorded in 10-second time-sample units. The sample units were then converted to percentage of time each behavior occurred. Interrater reliability was 80%. After 2 weeks of 30-minute biweekly sessions, in comparison with the control group the movement therapy group spent less time wandering ($P<.05$), less time showing negative responses to being touched ($P<.005$), more time showing on task passive behavior ($P<.05$) and less time resisting the teacher ($P<.01$). The increase in more time showing on task passive behavior suggested that when children were not actively engaged in a movement activity, they were engaged at least passively by watching the teacher or other children participating, rather than wandering about the room or resisting the teacher. The intervention did not help with eye contact, social relatedness, or stereotypic behaviors. Study limitations were no randomization and a small sample size.

Movement and music therapy and yoga

In the study by Rosenblatt and colleagues,[63] 24 children with a diagnosis of an autistic spectrum disorder (ASD) comprised the study group. Subjects were enrolled after referral from 2 sources: (1) children with a diagnosis of an ASD, ages 3 to 18 years, referred for treatment to the outpatient practice of the senior author, and 2 responses to a list serve notifying parents of children with a diagnosis of an ASD of the program's availability. Subjects ranged in age from 3.6 to 16.5 years (mean = 8.9). Fourteen completed the study from the outpatient practice and 10 completed the study from the list serve. To optimize the number of participants, enrollment included much diagnostic comorbidity.

The program was designed to best engage the unique sensory features of patients with ASD, and to incorporate aspects of the use of yoga and music that have shown promise for this population. Verbal instructions were complemented by pictures and examples. Tools such as pinwheels and bubbles were used to help children experience their breath. Competition was deemphasized and children were given encouragement for whatever they were able to do. By the end of the 8 weeks, most children were able to execute the 18 different postures. Imitation of both the facilitator and each other was encouraged with the goal of enhancing social interaction.

Parents were given a CD of the music from the class as well as guidelines for practicing at home.

Outcome measurements used in this study included:

1. Behavioral Assessment System for Children, Second Edition (BASC-2). This tool measures a range of psychiatric functions in children between ages 3 and 21 years. The investigators examined its 3 clinical composite indices (Externalizing Scale, Internalizing Scale, and Behavioral Symptom Index or BSI), with 9 subscales, which were also examined: (1) Aggression, (2) Anxiety, (3) Attention problems, (4) Atypicality, (5) Conduct problems, (6) Depression, (7) Hyperactivity, (8) Somatization, and (9) Withdrawal. The parent rating scale was used in this study.
2. Aberrant Behavioral Checklist (ABC), a symptom checklist for assessing problem behaviors of children and adults with mental retardation. ABC assesses irritability, lethargy, hyperactivity, stereotypy, and inappropriate speech. Internal structural and validity properties of the test have been well demonstrated in children with developmental delays, including ASD. Scores on the Irritability scale of the ABC were a priori identified as the scale of interest, as changes on this scale have become the gold standard for establishing the efficacy of medications for behavioral symptoms of children with ASD.

When all subjects were considered, of the 3 BASC-2 composite clinical scales (Externalizing, Internalizing, and BSI), only the BSI showed improvement. While the BSI scale changed for all subjects, the change was greater for the latency-aged group ($P<.01$) compared with all ages ($P<.05$). Unexpectedly, the posttreatment scores on the Atypicality scale of the BASC-2, which measures some of the core features of autism, changed significantly ($P = .003$).

Although the overall posttreatment T-score changes for the BASC-2 BSI and the Atypicality scales were significant, a subject-by-subject change score analysis revealed much intersubject variability. For example, among the latency-aged children who completed the study (outpatient and list serve), although 13 subjects showed posttreatment improvements, 3 subjects had worse posttreatment scores. To determine whether age, medication status, medical or psychiatric comorbidity, or number of sessions attended accounted for the variability in posttreatment change scores, these factors were examined for those subjects for whom such data were available. Although the data were somewhat limited (they were not available for the list-serve referred patients), there was no apparent relationship between these variables and the subjects' degree of improvement. For the entire cohort, no scales on the ABC changed. For the latency-aged children, there was a trend toward improvement on the Irritability scale of the ABC ($P = .06$).

Taken together, a movement-based, modified RR program, involving yoga and dance, showed efficacy in treating behavioral problems and some core features of autism, particularly for latency-age children. Limitations to the study were no randomization, no control group, and small sample size.

STUDIES WITH YOUTH AND FAMILY: QI GONG

No studies of Qi Gong have been done in children and adolescents.

STUDIES WITH YOUTH AND FAMILY: TAI CHI
Tai Chi and Attention-Deficit/Hyperactivity Disorder

In the pilot study by Hernandez-Reif and colleagues,[64] 13 adolescents (mean age 14.5 years) with a DSM-IV diagnosis of ADHD were recruited from a remedial school for adolescents with developmental problems. An A, B, A2 design was used. Tai Chi was done 2 times per week for 5 weeks. A Connors Teacher Rating Scale, Revised was done at baseline, on the last day of Tai Chi training and 2 weeks later without Tai Chi. Changes were significant for less anxiety ($P = .00$), less daydreaming ($P = .00$), fewer inappropriate emotions ($P = .00$), and less hyperactivity ($P = .000$). Limitations to the study were no control groups, no randomization, and small sample size.

Tai Chi may therefore have potential as an appropriate adjunctive treatment for ADHD.

Tai Chi and Mindfulness in Middle School Setting

Wall[65] reported a clinical project that combined Tai Chi and MBSR in an educational program. The 5-week program demonstrated that sustained interest in this material in middle school–aged boys and girls is possible. The total number of participants was 11, aged between 11 and 13 years. The sessions were 1 hour per week for 5 weeks. Statements the boys and girls made during the process suggested that they experienced well-being, calmness, relaxation, improved sleep, less reactivity, increased self-care, self-awareness, and a sense of interconnection or interdependence with nature. The curriculum is described in detail for nurses, teachers, and counselors who wish to replicate this type of instruction for adolescents. The project infers that Tai Chi and MBSR may be transformational tools that can be used in educational programs appropriate for middle school–aged children. There was no statistical analysis reported in this article. Recommendations are made for further study in schools and other pediatric settings.

This study helps to show that MBSR and Tai Chi may be equally effective when used to produce a more relaxed atmosphere in classrooms. Obviously, continued use may have to be implemented to sustain the effects. More research is needed.

STUDIES WITH YOUTH AND FAMILY: YOGA

There are many forms of yoga. The reader is referred to the article by Kaley-Isley and colleagues[67] for a helpful list of the various types of yoga.

Yoga and Eating Disorders

In the study by Carei and colleagues,[66] a total of 50 females and 4 males aged 11 to 21 years were recruited and randomized to an 8-week trial of standard care alone versus standard care plus yoga. The mean age of the participants was 16.52 years. Ethical guidelines required standard care for all subjects (physician and/or dietician appointments every other week assessing weight, height, vital signs, BMI, nutritional habits, and menstrual status when pertinent).

Inclusion criteria included the following: (1) between 10 and 21 years of age and (2) meeting DSM-IV criteria for anorexia nervosa (AN), bulimia nervosa (BN), and/or eating disorder not otherwise specified (EDNOS). Exclusion criteria included: (1) a resting pulse less than 44 beats per minute, (2) physical inability to participate in yoga as determined by the referring health care provider, and (3) a comorbid DSM-IV diagnosis of psychotic disorder, conversion disorder, substance-related disorder, and/or an axis II disorder.

Randomization was done after baseline measures were completed; the baseline measures included: a videotaped meal with a family member (30 minutes), an optional break (30 minutes), State-Trait Anxiety Inventory (STAIC), a Food Preoccupation questionnaire (FP), a BDI questionnaire (30 minutes), and the Eating Disorder Examination (EDE) (1.5 hours). The randomization sequence was generated independently by biostatisticians at Seattle Children's Hospital and was stratified according to diagnosis of eating disorder. The participants were randomized to the treatment groups.

The Yoga group received 1 hour of yoga semiweekly for 8 consecutive weeks (1:1 instruction). The No Yoga control group was offered yoga after completion of the study as an incentive to maintain participation.

Assessments were completed for both the Yoga and No Yoga group at 3 time points: baseline, postintervention (week 9), and at 1-month follow-up (week 12). In addition, to examine possible mechanisms for the impact of yoga, food preoccupation was measured for both groups. Participants completed the EDE, a standardized, semistructured, diagnostic, clinical interview based on DSM-IV-TR criteria. Outcomes evaluated at baseline, end of trial, and 1-month follow-up included BMI, and the EDE, BDI, STAI, and FP questionnaires.

The Yoga group demonstrated greater decreases in symptoms of eating disorders. Specifically, the EDE scores decreased over time in the Yoga group, whereas the No Yoga group showed some initial decline but then returned to baseline EDE levels at week 12. Food preoccupation was measured before and after each yoga session, and decreased significantly after all sessions. Paired t-tests revealed highly significant differences ($P<.01$) from pretest to posttest in all 16 sessions, such that participants indicated less food preoccupation after doing yoga. Seven sessions had pre-to-post differences in the medium ES range according to Cohen criteria ($0.4<d<0.8$), and the other 9 sessions had large ES ($d>0.8$). Both groups maintained current BMI levels and decreased anxiety and depression over time. No significant differences between groups in depression, anxiety, or weight were reported. However, for BMI there was a significant main effect of group, such that the Yoga group had somewhat higher overall BMI at all time points than the No Yoga group, $F(1, 31) = 4.83$, $P = .04$, $\eta^2 = 0.14$. There was also a significant main effect of diagnosis, such that those participants with BN and EDNOS had significantly higher BMI than the Anorexia group at all time points, $F(1,31) = 9.90$, $P<.001$, $\eta^2 = 0.39$. There were no other significant main effects or interactions, indicating that the yoga treatment did not adversely affect BMI over time.

These results suggest that individualized yoga therapy holds promise as an adjunctive therapy to standard care, especially for those with BN and EDNOS.[68] Limitations to the study include small sample size and no blinding.

Yoga for High School Students

In the study by Noggle and colleagues,[68] Grade 11 or 12 students (N = 51) who registered for physical education (PE) were cluster-randomized 2:1 by class, yoga versus PE-as-usual. The yoga method was as described earlier in the Body-Mind section. Participants in the PE-as-usual class period met for 30 to 40 minutes, 2 to 3 times per week over the course of the 10-week yoga program. The PE curriculum consisted of 2-week units with the first week focused on learning the history, rules, and skills for an activity, with the second week consisting of a tournaments or games. Students unable to participate directly in an activity were assigned to support roles (referee, setup, and coach/mentor), thereby still participating. Units included traditional sports such as tennis, volleyball, hockey, football, ultimate Frisbee, and baseball. Nontraditional sports and other activities were also included, such as a ropes course, backcountry living skills, stress management, first aid/cardiac pulmonary resuscitation, and planned parenthood health and wellness. Self-report questionnaires were administered to students 1 week before and after the program.

The instruments used in this study were:

1. Yoga Evaluation Questionnaire (YEQ), given to the students in the Yoga group at the end of the study. The YEQ was an internally created qualitative survey to assess feasibility of conducting a yoga program with adolescents. It was an 8-item

measure of the students' perception of the benefits, utility, and value of the yoga program using a 10-cm visual analog scale on which students marked their degree of agreement with statements from "not at all" to "very much so."

2. Primary outcome measures of psychosocial well-being were the Profile of Mood States—Short Form (POMS-SF) and Positive and Negative Affect Schedule for Children. Other measures were used for the study, but none were significant so they are not mentioned here.

Total mood disturbance in yoga students improved, but worsened in controls (P = .015). The POMS-SF Tension Anxiety Scale also worsened in controls (P = .002). In addition, negative affect significantly decreased in controls while improving in the yoga students (P = .006).

Limitations to the study were small size, self-reporting, and no blinding. These results suggest that Kripalu Yoga may be a helpful alternative to a traditional PE class.

SUMMARY OF STUDIES AND GRADING IN TABLE FORM

Tables 2–5 are based on the United States Preventive Services Task Force (USPSTF) Quality of Evidence grade, a qualitative ranking of the strength of the published evidence in the medical literature regarding a treatment: Good = consistent benefit in well-conducted studies in different populations; Fair = data shows positive effects, but weak, limited, or indirect evidence; Poor = cannot show benefit due to data weakness, no data-no information on youth. The USPSTF Strength of Recommendations is: I = insufficient data, D = recommend against (5 fair evidence of ineffectiveness or harm), C = neutral (5 fair evidence for, but appears risky), B = recommend (5 fair evidence of benefit and of safety), A = recommend strongly (5 good evidence of benefit and safety) (see **Table 2**).

Tables 2 and **3** summarizes the quality and strength of research. **Tables 4** and **5** shows the authors' personal clinical opinions based on information from the adult trials, information in this article, or personal experience.

SUMMARY

Taken together, the techniques discussed here offer a full range of possibilities from improving symptom profiles, preventing recurrences, and reducing pain to enhancing skills, and promoting health and well-being. For some patients, they may be truly transformative. Although the techniques for clinical use may be known from, or used in, religious or spiritual settings, it is important to bear in mind that the clinical use of these techniques does not mean that one has to follow any tradition from which the techniques derive, nor does the clinical use place one within any tradition.

Complementary and alternative medicine (CAM) meditation techniques may benefit patients, parents, teachers, and providers. Even the briefest intervention, such as a few minutes of focused breathing, has a beneficial effect. It can now be recognized that there are multiple physiologic and affective effects that cross-integrate areas of the brain and nervous system, reregulating patterns for long-lasting improved functioning and health. Group sessions, individual sessions, and sessions with parents that reinforce what is expected to be repeated in the home setting are significant to success. Just as the quality of CBT may be influenced by the training and skill of the treatment provider, hence, too, the training and skill of the clinician using MM techniques described here must be a necessary part of the treatment regimen. More randomized, double-blind, placebo-controlled studies are needed. However,

Table 2
Mindfulness-based therapies and Open Monitoring-Quality of Evidence/Strength of Recommendations for each treatment and indication in youth

Treatment	ADHD	Mood	Substance Abuse	Attention and Behavior	Anxiety	Family Harmony	Eating Disorder	Basis
Mindfulness-based Stress Reduction		Good/A to Fair/B		Fair/B	Good/A to Fair/B	Fair/B		1 RCT 2 non RCT
MBST/MBCT	Fair/B			Fair/B Teacher Rated	Fair/B Self rated			2 non RCT
Mindfulness-based Cognitive Therapy				Fair/B	Fair/B-dec. Test anxiety & Anxiety due to chronic illness			2 non RCT 1 cross leg Wait list
OM-Sahaja Yoga meditation	Fair/B Enabled some to reduce meds				Fair/B	Fair/B		1 non RCT

Abbreviations: ADHD, attention-deficit/hyperactivity disorder; AST, Automatic self transcending; M-B, Mind Body; CBT, Cognitive Behavior Therapy; DBM, deep breathing method; dec, decreased; inc, increased; M-B, Mind Body; MBCT-C, mindfulness-based cognitive therapy for children; MBI, Mindfulness-based Interventions; MBSR, mindfulness-based stress reduction; MED-RELAX, meditation relaxation; n, number; NET, Narrative Exposure Therapy; OM, Open Monitoring; PMR, Progressive Muscle Relaxation; RCT, randomized controlled treatment; relax, relaxation; SYM, Sahaja Yoga Meditation; tech, technique; TM, Transcendental Meditation; wks, weeks; WLC, wait list control; yo, years old.

Tables are based on the United States Preventive Services Task Force (USPSTF). USPSTF Quality of Evidence grade is a qualitative ranking of the strength of the published evidence in the medical literature regarding a treatment: Good = Consistent benefit in well-conducted studies in different populations. Fair = Data shows positive effects, but weak, limited, or indirect evidence. Poor = Can't show benefit due to data weakness, no data-no information on youth. USPSTF Strength of Recommendations: I = Insufficient Data, D = Recommend Against (= Fair evidence of ineffectiveness or harm), C = Neutral (= Fair evidence for, but appears risky), B = Recommend (= Fair evidence of benefit and of safety), A = Recommend Strongly (= Good Evidence of Benefit and Safety).

Table 3
Quality of Research/strength of recommendation of studies in youth

Treatment	Autism	ADHD	Mood	Substance Abuse	Attention and Behavior	Anxiety	Family Harmony	Eating Disorder	Basis
AST or TM		Pilot study = Fair/B	Good/A & Fair/B (mood) & creativity		Good/A & fair/B Attention & Cognitive Ability improved	Good/A & Fair/B			Pilot & 3 RCT 1 raters blinded N = 371 healthy students in 3 RCT
Mind-Body MEDITATION - RELAX						Fair/B			Randomized to MED-RELAX vs KIDNET
Mind-Body Progressive Muscle Relaxation or Relaxation Therapy			Fair/B PMR = CBT (mood)			Fair/B PMR>CBT			Non Randomized comparative study with wait list control
Mind-Body Relaxation Therapy/CBT			Fair/B CBT>Relax (mood)			Fair/B Relax = CBT			Randomized control
Mind-Body Relaxation Therapy/Massage						Fair/B Massage >relax			Randomized comparative, no control
Mind-Body Deep Breathing Meditation						FAIR/B			Pilot study
Body Mind Exercise			Fair/B						Pilot study

Category				Studies
Body-Mind YOGA	Fair/B	Fair/B	Fair/B	1 Randomized comparative control; 1 non randomized & no control study
Body-Mind Movement Therapy			Fair/B	1 non randomized Controlled study
Body-Mind Movement & Music therapy & yoga			Fair/B	1 non Randomized no control study
Body-Mind Qi Gong				No studies
Body-Mind Tai Chi	Fair/B	Fair/B		2 pilot studies

Tables are based on the United States Preventive Services Task Force (USPSTF). USPSTF Quality of Evidence grade is a qualitative ranking of the strength of the published evidence in the medical literature regarding a treatment: Good = Consistent benefit in well-conducted studies in different populations. Fair = Data shows positive effects, but weak, limited, or indirect evidence. Poor = Can't show benefit due to data weakness, no data–no information on youth. USPSTF Strength of Recommendations: I = Insufficient Data, D = Recommend Against (= Fair evidence of ineffectiveness or harm), C = Neutral (= Fair evidence for, but appears risky). B = Recommend (= Fair evidence of benefit and of safety), A = Recommend Strongly (= Good Evidence of Benefit and Safety).

Abbreviations: ADHD, attention-deficit/hyperactivity disorder; AST, Automatic self transcending; B-M, Body Mind; CBT, Cognitive Behavior Therapy; DBM, deep breathing method; dec, decreased; inc, increased; M-B, Mind Body; MBCT-C, mindfulness-based cognitive therapy for children; MBI, Mindfulness-based Interventions; MBSR, mindfulness-based stress reduction; MED-RELAX, meditation relaxation; n, number; NET, Narrative Exposure Therapy; OM, Open Monitoring; PMR, Progressive Muscle Relaxation; RCT, randomized controlled treatment; relax, relaxation; SYM, Sahaja Yoga Meditation; tech, technique; TM, Transcendental Meditation; wks, weeks; WLC, wait list control; yo, years old.

Table 4
Mindfulness-based therapies and Open Monitoring–Quality of Evidence/Strength of Recommendations for each treatment and indication in youth–personal opinion

Treatment	ADHD	Mood	Substance Abuse	Attention and Behavior	Anxiety	Family Harmony	Eating Disorder	Personal Opinion
Mind Body Stress Reduction		Good/A to Fair/B			Good/A to Fair/B	Fair/B		Adjunctive Treatment mood and anxiety and family harmony
MBSR/MBCT				Fair/B Teacher rated	Fair/B Self rated			Adjunct behavior & attention ADHD & Anxiety
Mind Body Cognitive Therapy				Fair/B	Fair/B Test anxiety & anxiety with chronic illness			Good adjunct performance anxiety & stress of chronic illness attention and behavior
OM-Sahaja Yoga Meditation	Fair/B Enabled some to reduce meds				Fair/B	Fair/B		Anxiety and Family therapy

Tables are based on the United States Preventive Services Task Force (USPSTF). USPSTF Quality of Evidence grade is a qualitative ranking of the strength of the published evidence in the medical literature regarding a treatment: Good = Consistent benefit in well-conducted studies in different populations. Fair = Data shows positive effects, but weak, limited, or indirect evidence. Poor = Can't show benefit due to data weakness, no data–no information on youth. USPSTF Strength of Recommendations: I = Insufficient Data, D = Recommend Against (= Fair evidence of ineffectiveness or harm), C = Neutral (= Fair evidence for, but appears risky). B = Recommend (= Fair evidence of benefit and of safety), A = Recommend Strongly (= Good Evidence of Benefit and Safety).

Abbreviations: ADHD, attention-deficit/hyperactivity disorder; AST, Automatic self transcending; B-M, Body Mind; CBT, Cognitive Behavior Therapy; DBM, deep breathing method; dec, decreased; inc, increased; M-B, Mind Body; MBCT-C, mindfulness-based cognitive therapy for children; MBI, Mindfulness-based Interventions; MBSR, mindfulness-based stress reduction; MED-RELAX, meditation relaxation; n, number; NET, Narrative Exposure Therapy; OM, Open Monitoring; PMR, Progressive Muscle Relaxation; RCT, randomized controlled treatment; relax, relaxation; SYM, Sahaja Yoga Meditation; tech, technique; TM, Transcendental Meditation; wks, weeks; WLC, wait list control; yo, years old.

there are no clinically reported adverse effects from these techniques, and clinicians who are well trained in the techniques may benefit from using them as adjunctive therapies. It is hoped that providers now consider themselves more informed and more able to consider these methods with confidence.

These techniques offer the potential for treating a range of symptoms and disorders in youth with psychiatric disorders, enhancing general mental and physical health in the community and conceivably increasing the general well-being of youth and society. The evidence base for these techniques ranges from less robust to more robust. An example of a stronger study is the MBSR in targeting anxiety and mood.[69] Components of studies that point to the need to continue research are found in the Sahaja Yoga Meditation study whereby medications were decreased in children with ADHD,[78] and the combined MBSR/MBCT or the AAP, whereby neurocognitive testing identified improvements in visual attention in children.[77]

TM, MB, and body-mind techniques offer the potential as an adjunct in treating a range of symptoms and disorders in youth with psychiatric diagnoses. More research is needed to determine if they can be used as stand-alone interventions. However, there is much physiologic and neurobiological evidence to suggest that these techniques may have effects that address known neurobiological and physiologic effects of psychiatric disorders. Stronger studies include the M-B MED-RELAX study as acute intervention of traumatic experiences[52] and the effect of TM on cognitive improvement.[45] There are promising studies of techniques such as yoga (demonstrating that it may be helpful in the treatment of eating disorders[66]) and Tai Chi (demonstrating that its use may reduce the symptoms of ADHD[64]). This latter study may need to be repeated in the future to include measurement of cortisol levels, to determine whether the improvements in ADHD are due to reduced anxiety as has been reported in adult studies.[86] Tai Chi may be as helpful as MBSR, but more research is needed to confirm this finding.[65] Movement[62] or a combination of music and movement therapy and yoga[63] may be especially helpful in autism. If the theory that movement therapy affects neurobiological pathways associated with empathy gains more evidence, these interventions may prove to be a useful adjunctive therapy for youth with autism. Finally, DBM may help reduce test anxiety.

Studies using PR[53,55] do show promise as an adjunct for the treatment of depression and anxiety. However, future studies should measure cortisol levels,[57] which would help delineate whether participants with depression and anxiety only seem to get better if there is a corresponding decrease in cortisol levels, and if those with depression and anxiety who do not get better do not have a corresponding decrease in cortisol. This measurement may be also helpful when designing studies using MT. Perhaps the effect of MT on anxiety can be measured if cortisol levels also decrease after the intervention.

Although many of these techniques have origins in religious or spiritual traditions, they can be applied with a secular orientation. Mindfulness can be, and has been used with other adjunctive therapies. For instance, mindfulness has been used in combination with motivational enhancement therapy (MET) with adolescents. MET has been used in many adult and adolescent studies as an intervention for substance abuse, and has been considered effective. However, adaptations of adult mindfulness methods for youth need further exploration. More rigorous clinical trials need to be available before more firm clinical claims can be made. The persistence of observed changes needs to be explored. The design matter of relevant control groups for these studies needs more thoughtful examination. The options for group sessions, individual sessions, and sessions with parents need to be explored. Any adverse effects and contraindications for these techniques still need to be delineated, underscoring the

Table 5
Quality of Research/strength of recommendation of studies in youth-personal opinion

Treatment	Autism	ADHD	Mood	Substance Abuse	Attention and Behavior	Anxiety	Family Harmony	Eating Disorder	Personal Opinion
AST or TM		Pilot study = Fair/B	Good/A & Fair/B Mood and creativity		Good/A & Fair/B Attention and cognitive ability improved	Good/A & Fair/B			Adjunctive tx anxiety & increasing cognitive ability & attention
Mind-Body MEDITATION - RELAX						Fair/B			Adjunctive Acute trauma & PTSD alone or as adjunt
Mind-Body Progressive Muscle Relaxation			Fair/B PMR = CBT (mood)			Fair/B PMR>CBT			PMR adjunctive for depression & anxiety
Mind-Body Relaxation/CBT			Fair/B CBT>Relax (mood)			Fair/B Relax = CBT			Adjunctive tx anxiety
Mind-Body Relaxation/Massage						Fair/B Massage> relax			Massage> relax, massage adjunctive for anxiety Without abuse history
Mind-Body Deep Breathing Meditation						Fair/B			Adjunct decreasing Test anxiety

Body-Mind Exercise		Fair/B		Adjunct Decreasing depression
Body-Mind YOGA	Fair/B		Fair/B	Adjunctive for eating disorders and dec mood & anxiety in school setting
Body-Mind Movement Therapy	Fair/B			Adjunctive to dec sensation to touch & inc. social interactions
Body-Mind Movement & Dance therapy & yoga	Fair/B			Adjunctive tx autism -increase social skills
Body-Mind Qi Gong				No studies
Body-Mind Tai Chi	Fair/B	Fair/B		Adjunctive dec ADHD & mood

Tables are based on the United States Preventive Services Task Force (USPSTF). USPSTF Quality of Evidence grade is a qualitative ranking of the strength of the published evidence in the medical literature regarding a treatment: Good = Consistent benefit in well-conducted studies in different populations. Fair = Data shows positive effects, but weak, limited, or indirect evidence. Poor = Can't show benefit due to data weakness, no data-no information on youth. USPSTF Strength of Recommendations: I = Insufficient Data, D = Recommend Against (= Fair evidence of ineffectiveness or harm), C = Neutral (= Fair evidence for, but appears risky), B = Recommend (= Fair evidence of benefit and of safety), A = Recommend Strongly (= Good Evidence of Benefit and Safety).

Abbreviations: ADHD, attention-deficit/hyperactivity disorder; AST, Automatic self transcending; B-M, Body Mind; CBT, Cognitive Behavior Therapy; DBM, deep breathing method; dec, decreased; inc, increased; M-B, Mind Body; MBCT-C, mindfulness-based cognitive therapy for children; MBI, Mindfulness-based Interventions; MBSR, mindfulness-based stress reduction; MED-RELAX, meditation relaxation; n, number; NET, Narrative Exposure Therapy; OM, Open Monitoring; PMR, Progressive Muscle Relaxation; RCT, randomized controlled treatment; relax, relaxation; SYM, Sahaja Yoga Meditation; tech, technique; TM, Transcendental Meditation; wks, weeks; WLC, wait list control; yo, years old.

importance of the training and skill levels of the clinicians involved in both research and clinical delivery of care.

At this point, in view of the apparently low clinical risk with few adverse effects, and despite the need for more research, some clinicians may consider some of these methods for limited clinical use as adjunctive therapies in selected cases. Nevertheless, clinicians need to be mindful that risks and potential contraindications are not yet well defined, and are advised to consider consents for these interventions.

This review has been written in the spirit of benefiting patients, families, and providers.

REFERENCES

1. Ott MJ. Mindfulness meditation in pediatric clinical practice. Pediatr Nurs 2002; 28(5):487–90.
2. Fisher R. Still thinking: the case for meditation with children. Think Skills Creativ 2006;1(2):146–51.
3. Lutz A, Slagter HA, Dunne JD, et al. Attention regulation and monitoring in meditation. Trends Cogn Sci 2008;12(4):163–9.
4. Cash M, Whittingham K. What facets of mindfulness contribute to psychological well-being and depressive, anxious, and stress-related symptomatology? Mindfulness 2010;1(3):177–82.
5. Shapiro SL. The integration of mindfulness and psychology. J Clin Psychol 2009; 65(6):555–60.
6. Travis F, Shear J. Focused attention, open monitoring and automatic self-transcending: categories to organize meditations from Vedic, Buddhist and Chinese traditions. Conscious Cogn 2010;19(4):1110–8.
7. Ivanovski B, Malhi GS. The psychological and neurophysiological concomitants of mindfulness forms of meditation. Acta Neuropsychiatr 2007;19:76–91.
8. Rapgay L, Bystrisky A. Classical mindfulness: an introduction to its theory and practice for clinical application. Ann N Y Acad Sci 2009;1172:148–62.
9. Gilpin R. The use of Theravada Buddhist practices and perspectives in mindfulness-based cognitive therapy. Contemporary Buddhism 2009;9:227–51.
10. Burke A. Comparing individual preferences for four meditation techniques: Zen, Vipassana (Mindfulness), Qigong, and Mantra. Explore (NY) 2012;8(4):237–42. http://dx.doi.org/10.1016/j.explore.2012.04.003.
11. Chiesa A, Malinowski P. Mindfulness-based approaches: are they all the same? J Clin Psychol 2011;67(4):404–24.
12. Kabat-Zinn J. Mindfulness based interventions in context: past, present and future. Clin Psychol Sci Pract 2003;10:144–56.
13. Segal ZL, Williams MG, Teasdale JD. Mindfulness-based cognitive therapy for depression: a new approach to preventing relapse. New York: Guilford Press; 2002.
14. Kabat-Zinn J. Full catastrophe living: using the wisdom of your body and mind to face stress, pain and illness. New York: Dell Publishing; 1990.
15. Kabat-Zin J. Mindfulness for beginners. Boulder (CO): Sounds True, Inc; 2012.
16. Linehan M. Cognitive behavioral treatment of borderline personality disorder. New York: Guilford Press; 1993.
17. Hayes SC. Acceptance and commitment therapy and the new behavioral therapies: mindfulness acceptance and relationship. In: Hayes SC, Follette VM, Linehan M, editors. Mindfulness and acceptance: expanding the cognitive behavioral tradition. New York: Guilford; 2004. p. 1–29.

18. Witkiewitz K, Bowen S. Depression, craving and substance use following a randomized trial of mindfulness-based relapse prevention. J Consult Clin Psychol 2010;78(3):362–74.
19. Hölzel BK, Ott U, Hempel H, et al. Differential engagement of anterior cingulate and adjacent medial frontal cortex in adept meditators and non-meditators. Neurosci Lett 2007;421(1):16–21.
20. Hölzel BK, Ott U, Gard T, et al. Investigation of mindfulness meditation practitioners with voxel-based morphometry. Soc Cogn Affect Neurosci 2008;3(1):55–61.
21. Cahn BR, Polic J. Meditation (Vipassana) and the P3a event-related brain potential. Int J Psychophysiol 2009;72(1):51–60.
22. Cahn BR, Delorme A, Polich J. Occipital gamma activation during Vipassana meditation. Cogn Process 2010;11(1):39–56.
23. Hölzel BK, Carmody J, Vangel M, et al. Mindfulness practice leads to increases in regional brain gray matter density. Psychiatry Res 2011;191(1):36–43.
24. Hölzel BK, Carmody J, Evans KC, et al. Stress reduction correlates with structural changes in the amygdala. Soc Cogn Affect Neurosci 2010;5(1):11–7.
25. Brefczynski-Lewis JA, Lutz A, Schaefer HS, et al. Neural correlates of attentional expertise in long-term meditation practitioners. Proc Natl Acad Sci U S A 2007; 104(27):11483–8.
26. Baijal S, Gupta R. Meditation-based training. A possible intervention for attention deficit hyperactivity disorder. Psychiatry (Edgmont) 2008;5(4):48–55.
27. Baijal S, Jha AP, Kiyonaga A, et al. The influence of concentrative meditation training on the development of attention networks during early adolescence. Front Psychol 2011;2:153.
28. Burke CA. Mindfulness-based approaches with children and adolescents: a preliminary review of current research in an emergent field. J Child Fam Stud 2009. http://dx.doi.org/10.1007/s10826-009-9282-x.
29. Sibinga EM, Kemper KJ. Complementary, holistic, and integrative medicine: meditation practices for pediatric health. Pediatr Rev 2010;31:e91. Available at: http://pedsinreview.aappublications.org/content/31/12/e91.
30. Singh NN, Lancioni GE, Singh Joy SD, et al. Adolescents with conduct disorder can be mindful of their aggressive behavior. J Emot Behav Disord 2007;15: 56–63.
31. Biegel GM, Brown KW, Shapiro SL, et al. Mindfulness-based stress reduction for the treatment of adolescent psychiatric outpatients: a randomized clinical trial. J Consult Clin Psychol 2009;77(5):855–66. http://dx.doi.org/10.1037/a0016241.
32. Bootzin RR, Stevens SJ. Adolescents, substance abuse, and the treatment of insomnia and daytime sleepiness. Clin Psychol Rev 2005;25:629–44.
33. Saltzman A, Goldin P. Mindfulness-based stress reduction for school-age children. In: Greco LA, Hayes SC, editors. Acceptance & mindfulness treatments for children and adolescents: a practitioner's guide. Oakland (CA): New Harbinger Publications, Inc; 2008. p. 139–61.
34. Sibinga MS, Kerrigan D, Stewart M, et al. Mindfulness-based stress reduction for urban youth. J Altern Complement Med 2011;17(3):213–8.
35. Bogels S, Hoogstad B, van Du L, et al. Mindfulness training for adolescents with externalizing disorders and their parents. Behav Cognit Psychother 2008;36: 193–209.
36. Semple RJ, Lee J, Rosa D, et al. A randomized trial of mindfulness-based cognitive therapy for children: promoting mindful attention to enhance social-emotional resiliency in children. J Child Fam Stud 2010;19:218–29.

37. Van der Oord S, Bogels SM, Peijnenburg D. The effectiveness of mindfulness training for children with ADHD and mindful parenting for their parents. J Child Fam Stud 2012;21(1):139–47.

38. Zylowska L, Ackerman DL, Yang MH, et al. Mindfulness meditation training in adults and adolescents with ADHD: a feasibility study. J Atten Disord 2008; 11(6):737–46.

39. Harrison LJ, Manocha R, Rubia K. Sahaja yoga meditation as a family treatment programme for children with attention deficit-hyperactivity disorder. Clin Child Psychol Psychiatry 2004;9(4):479–97.

40. Napoli M, Krech PR, Holley LC. Mindfulness training for elementary school students: the attention academy. J Appl Sch Psychol 2005;21:99–125.

41. Manocha R. Intervention insights: meditation, mindfulness and mind-emptiness. Acta Neuropsychiatr 2011;23(1):46–7.

42. Baijal S, Srinivasan N. Theta activity and meditative states: spectral changes during concentrative meditation. Cogn Process 2010;11(1):31–8.

43. De Dios MA, Herman DS, Britton WB, et al. Motivational and mindfulness intervention for young adult female marijuana users. J Subst Abuse Treat 2012;42(1): 56–64.

44. Rosenthal JZ, Grosswald S, Ross R, et al. Effects of transcendental meditation in veterans of Operation Enduring Freedom and Operation Iraqi Freedom with posttraumatic stress disorder: a pilot study. Mil Med 2011;176(6):626–30.

45. Grosswald S. Transcendental meditation. Bethesda (MD): Grand Rounds, Department of Psychiatry, Walter Reed National Military Medical Center; 2012.

46. Dillbeck MC, Orme-Johnson DW. Physiological differences between transcendental meditation and rest. Am Psychol 1987;42(9):879–81.

47. So KT, Orme-Johnson DW. Three randomized experiments on the longitudinal effects of the transcendental meditation technique on cognition. Intelligence 2001;29(5):419–40.

48. Travis FT. Eyes open and TM EEG patterns after one and eight years of TM practice. Psychophysiology 1991;28(3a):S58.

49. Gusnard DA, Raichle ME, Raichle ME. Searching for a baseline: functional imaging and the resting human brain. Nat Rev Neurosci 2001;2(10):685–94.

50. Raichle ME, Snyder AZ. A default mode of brain function: a brief history of an evolving idea. Neuroimage 2007;37(4):1083–90 [discussion: 1097–9].

51. Luders E, Jurth F, Mayer EA, et al. The unique brain anatomy of meditation practitioners: alterations in cortical gyrification. Front Hum Neurosci 2012;6:34. http://dx.doi.org/10.3389/fnhum.2012.00034.

52. Catani C, Kohiladevy M, Ruf M, et al. Treating children traumatized by war and tsunami: a comparison between exposure therapy and meditation-relaxation in North-East Sri Lanka. BMC Psychiatry 2009;9:22. http://dx.doi.org/10.1186/1471-244X-9-22.

53. Reynolds WM, Coats KI. A comparison of cognitive behavioral therapy and relaxation training for the treatment of depression in adolescents. J Consult Clin Psychol 1986;54:653–60.

54. Eppley KR, Abrams AI, Shear J. Differential effects of relaxation techniques on trait anxiety: a meta-analysis. J Clin Psychol 1989;45(6):957–74.

55. Wood A, Harrington R, Moore A. Controlled trial of a brief cognitive-behavioural intervention in adolescent patients with depressive disorders. J Child Psychol Psychiatry 1996;37(6):737–46.

56. Field T, Grizzle N, Scafidi F, et al. Massage and relaxation therapies' effects on depressed adolescent mothers. Adolescence 1996;31(124):903–11.

57. Platania-Solazzo A, Field TM, Blank J, et al. Relaxation therapy reduces anxiety in child and adolescent psychiatric patients. Acta Paedopsychiatr 1992;55(2):115–20.
58. Denkowski KM, Denkowski GC. Is group progressive relaxation training as effective with hyperactive children as individual EMG biofeedback treatment? Biofeedback Self Regul 1984;9(3):353–64.
59. Paul G, Elam B, Verhulst SJ. A longitudinal study of students' perceptions of using deep breathing meditation to reduce testing stresses. Teach Learn Med 2007;19(3):287–92. http://dx.doi.org/10.1080/10401330701366754.
60. Benson H. The relaxation response. New York: Avon Books; 1975.
61. Doop RR, Mooney AJ, Armitage R, et al. Exercise for adolescents with depressive disorder: a feasibility study. Depress Res Treat 2012;2012:257472. http://dx.doi.org/10.1155/2012/257472.
62. Hartshorn K, Olds L, Field T, et al. Creative movement therapy benefits children with autism. Early Child Dev Care 2001;166:1–5.
63. Rosenblatt LE, Gorantia S, Torres JA, et al. Relaxation response-based yoga improves functioning in young children with autism: a pilot study. J Altern Complement Med 2011;17(11):1029–35.
64. Hernandez-Reif M, Field TM, Thimas E. Attention deficit hyperactivity disorder: benefits from Tai Ch. J Bodyw Mov Ther 2001;5(2):120–3.
65. Wall RB. Tai Chi and mindfulness-based stress reduction in a Boston Public Middle School. J Pediatr Health Care 2005;19(4):230–7.
66. Carei T, Fyfe-Johnson AL, Breuner CC, et al. Randomized controlled clinical trial of yoga in the treatment of eating disorders. J Adolesc Health 2010;46(4):346–51.
67. Kaley-Isley LC, Peterson J, Fischer C, et al. Yoga as a complementary therapy for children and adolescents: a guide for clinicians. Psychiatry 2010;7(8):20–32.
68. Noggle JJ, Steiner NJ, Minami T, et al. Benefits of Yoga for psychosocial well-being in a US high school curriculum: a preliminary randomized controlled trial. J Dev Behav Pediatr 2012;33(3):193–201.
69. Turgut G, Kaptanoğlu B, Turgut S, et al. Influence of acute exercise on urinary protein, creatine, insulin-like growth factor-I (IGF-I) and IGF binding protein-3 concentrations in children Tohoku. J Exp Med 2003;201:165–70.
70. Hind K, Burrows M. Weight-bearing exercise and bone mineral accrual in children and adolescents: a review of controlled trials. Bone 2007;40:14–27.
71. Hands B, Larkin D, Parker H, et al. The relationship among physical activity, motor competence and health related fitness in 14-year old adolescents. Scand J Med Sci Sports 2009;19:655–63.
72. Giannini C, de Giorgis T, Mohn A, et al. Role of physical exercise in children and adolescents with diabetes mellitus. J Pediatr Endocrinol Metab 2007;20:173–84.
73. Tansey MJ, Tsalikian E, Beck RW, et al. The effects of aerobic exercise on glucose and counter regulatory hormone concentrations in children with type 1 diabetes. Diabetes Care 2006;29:20–5.
74. Larun L, Nordheim LV, Ekeland E, et al. Exercise in prevention and treatment of anxiety and depression among children and young people. Cochrane Database Syst Rev 2006;(3):CD004691.
75. Donohue B, Miller A, Beisecker M, et al. Effects of brief yoga exercises and motivational preparatory interventions in distance runners: results of a controlled trial. Br J Sports Med 2006;40:60–3.
76. Haffner J, Roos J, Goldstein N, et al. The effectiveness of body-oriented methods of therapy in the treatment of attention deficit hyperactivity disorder

(ADHD): results of a controlled pilot study. Z Kinder Jugendpsychiatr Psychother 2006;34:37–47.

77. West J, Otte C, Geher K, et al. Effects of Hatha yoga and African dance on perceived stress, affect, and salivary cortisol. Ann Behav Med 2004;28:114–8.

78. Rizzolatti G, Craighero L. The mirror-neuron system. Annu Rev Neurosci 2004; 27:169–92.

79. Lucy M, McGarry B, Russo FA. Mirroring in dance/movement therapy: potential mechanisms behind empathy enhancement. Arts Psychother 2011;38:178–84.

80. Streeter CC, Whitfield T, Owen L, et al. Effects of yoga versus walking on mood, anxiety, and brain GABA levels: a randomized controlled MRS study. J Altern Complement Med 2010;16(11):1145–52.

81. Mohandas E. The neurobiology of spirituality. Mens Sana Monogr 2008;6:63–80.

82. Newberg AB, Iversen J. The neural basis of the complex mental task of meditation: neurotransmitter and neurochemical considerations. Med Hypotheses 2003;61(Suppl 2):282–91.

83. Black DS, Milam J, Sussman S. Sitting-meditation interventions among youth: a review of treatment efficacy. Pediatrics 2009;124(3):e532–41.

84. Grosswald SJ, Stixrud WR, Travis F, et al. Use of the transcendental meditation technique to reduce symptoms of attention deficit hyperactivity disorder (ADHD) by reducing stress and anxiety: an exploratory study. Curr Issues Educ 2008;101(2).

85. Rosaen C, Benn R. The experience of transcendental meditation in middle school students: a qualitative report. Explore (NY) 2006;2(5):422–5.

86. Jin P. Efficacy of Tai Chi, brisk walking, meditation and reading in reducing mental and emotional stress. J Psychosom Res 1992;36:361–70.

Music Therapy and Music Medicine for Children and Adolescents

Olivia Swedberg Yinger, PhD, MT-BC*, Lori Gooding, PhD, MT-BC

KEYWORDS

- Music therapy • Music medicine • Child and adolescent psychiatry • Mental health
- Research

KEY POINTS

- Neuroimaging research indicates that listening to preferred music activates reward circuitry in the brain and active musical participation engages more areas of the brain than passive listening.
- Music therapy is an established health care profession in which music is used within a therapeutic relationship with a music therapist to accomplish nonmusic goals.
- Emerging research indicates probable effectiveness of specific approaches to music therapy with children and adolescent mental health consumers; however, further research is necessary.

INTRODUCTION
Defining Music Therapy and Music Medicine

The American Music Therapy Association (AMTA) defines music therapy as: "…the clinical and evidence-based use of music interventions to accomplish individualized goals within a therapeutic relationship by a credentialed professional who has completed an approved music therapy program."[1] Music therapists use music within a therapeutic relationship to attend to individuals' physical, emotional, cognitive, and social needs. Although music therapists work with various populations, including individuals of all ages with medical/surgical needs or intellectual disabilities, more music therapists work with persons who have behavioral/emotional disorders than any other single population.[2]

Funding Sources: Johnson & Johnson/Society for the Arts in HealthCare (O.S. Yinger); National Institute of Aging (L. Gooding).
Conflict of Interest: None.
University of Kentucky School of Music, College of Fine Arts, 105 Fine Arts, Lexington, KY 40506-0022, USA
* Corresponding author.
E-mail address: olivia.yinger@uky.edu

Child Adolesc Psychiatric Clin N Am 23 (2014) 535–553
http://dx.doi.org/10.1016/j.chc.2013.03.003
1056-4993/14/$ – see front matter Published by Elsevier Inc.
childpsych.theclinics.com

Music therapists must complete either a 4-year undergraduate program or a 2-year graduate equivalency program in music therapy at an AMTA-approved college or university. Music therapy degree programs include course work in musical foundations, clinical foundations, and music therapy foundations and principles, as specified in the AMTA Professional Competencies. In addition to course work, music therapy degree programs include 1200 hours of clinical training, culminating in a supervised internship, which typically lasts for 6 months. After completing an AMTA-approved degree program, prospective music therapists are eligible to take the national board certification examination to earn the credential Music Therapist-Board Certified (MT-BC). The MT-BC credential is granted by the Certification Board for Music Therapists (CBMT), a separate, accredited organization.[3] After becoming board certified, training in advanced music therapy competencies is offered through mandatory continuing education courses, with the option for training at the master's and doctorate level. Music medicine, which constitutes the bulk of the literature on the use of music to accomplish nonmusic objectives, is defined as passive listening to prerecorded music provided by medical personnel.[4,5] In music medicine treatment, listening interventions are often administered via headphones, and patients may or may not be involved in selecting the music.[5] Although music-based interventions are used in both music medicine and music therapy, it is important to understand the difference between the 2, because of variations in the level of training in musical foundations and their therapeutic applications, with music therapists receiving specialized training in these domains.[5] Although training and certification are required to practice music therapy, no such specialized training and certification exists for the practice of music medicine.

Mechanism of Therapeutic Action: Music and the Brain

To understand the reasons behind the effectiveness of music in augmenting treatment of children and adolescents receiving psychiatric treatment, it is important to first understand the effects of music on the brain. Recent research on the effects of music on cognition, emotional processing, anxiety, and stress has shed light on how music therapy can enhance mental health treatment. There is no single center for musical processing in the brain. Music listening engages multiple areas of the brain, both subcortical (including the medial geniculate body in the thalamus and the amygdala) and cortical (such as the left and right primary auditory cortex). Musical participation also engages the cerebellum, basal ganglia, and cortical motor area.[6,7]

The fact that active musical participation engages more areas of the brain than passive music listening may explain in part why numerous studies have shown music therapy to be more effective than music medicine at augmenting treatment of neuropsychiatric disorders.[7] It seems that active musical participation or engagement with the therapist are integral in the success of music therapy, in addition to the music itself. The effectiveness of music therapy is in part caused by the effects of music on the brain, and in part by the interaction between the client and the music therapist.

Stefan Koelsch[8] provided an overview of ways in which music modulates attention, emotion, cognition, behavior, and communication. Readers wishing to learn in greater detail about the effects of music, and specifically music therapy, on the brain are referred to the works of Koelsch, Lin, and Taylor, among others.[6–8]

Neuroimaging techniques are helping researchers understand ways in which music listening and participation affect neural plasticity.[6–8] Recent neuroimaging studies have shed light on the activation of the reward circuit in the brain and the role that dopamine plays in musical response. In a study by Blood and Zatorre,[9] in which participants listened to self-selected music that gave them chills while undergoing positron emission tomography (PET) scans, increases in cerebral blood flow were observed in the left ventral striatum, left dorsomedial midbrain, right thalamus, and anterior cingulate cortex. In addition, decreases in cerebral blood flow were found in the right amygdala, left hippocampus/amygdala, and ventromedial prefrontal cortex. These areas have been associated with brain reward circuitry. Chills were also associated with increases in heart rate, electromyography, and respiration. The control condition in this study consisted of participants listening to music that had been selected by others but that did not elicit chills in the participant. This study shows the importance of musical preference in eliciting desired results within music medicine or music therapy.[9]

Results from a study by Menon and Levitin[10] of 13 participants between the ages of 19 and 24 years, who listened to researcher-selected classical music while undergoing functional magnetic resonance imaging (fMRI), showed that listening to music strongly modulates activity in mesolimbic structures responsible for reward processing, such as the nucleus accumbens (NAc) and the ventral tegmental area (VTA), along with the hypothalamus and insula. Correlations between responses in the NAc and the VTA found in this study indicate that dopamine response may be associated with musical response. The activation of the hypothalamus corroborates what has been previously documented, that music listening has an impact on physiologic responses controlled by the autonomic nervous system. Although the music used in this study was not selected by participants and it is unclear whether it gave them chills, the musical excerpts were rated as highly pleasant by a sample of similar individuals.

Results from a more recent study by Salimpoor and colleagues[11] support the findings of Menon and Levitin. In Salimpoor and colleagues'[11] study, 8 participants between the ages of 19 and 24 years listened to self-selected music that gave them chills while undergoing PET scans. Endogenous dopamine release was found in the striatum during music listening at the time of peak emotional arousal. Follow-up fMRI revealed that the caudate was more involved during anticipation, whereas the NAc was more involved during peak emotional arousal. Physiologic responses measured during music listening showed a relationship between increases in heart rate, skin conductance, and respiration, along with decreases in temperature and blood volume pulse amplitude as the reported intensity of chills increased. Research showing the role of music listening in activating the reward circuitry in the brain has important implications for treatment of addictions, although more research remains to be done in this area. Because music activates reward circuitry in the brain that is also activated by food, drugs, and sex, future research should explore whether music can be used as a substitute for potentially harmful addictive behavior, or as a cue for adaptive coping behavior as an alternative to addictive behavior.

In addition to addiction, music neuroscience research has implications for psychiatric treatment with other various disorders, including disorders typically diagnosed in childhood (such as autism), affective disorders, and eating disorders. Research on the neurophysiologic effects of music for each of these populations are discussed. Diagnostic terminology used in this article reflects that used by the investigators of the individual studies reported, which may be based on the *Diagnostic and Statistical manual of Mental Disorders, Third Edition* (DSM-III), DSM-IV, or DSM-IV Text Revision, depending on when and where the article was published. Readers wishing to know more about diagnostic criteria for participants in the studies reviewed are referred to the original articles. Although awareness of a client's diagnosis is an important component of music therapy research and guides treatment planning, music therapy treatment is designed based on the individual needs of the client, regardless of their diagnosis. For this reason, several studies reviewed here include descriptions of music therapy treatment of groups of clients with various diagnoses that have similar needs.

Autism

A recent study by Emanuele and colleagues[12] compared dopamine receptor expression in peripheral blood lymphocytes in adult healthy musicians with age-matched and gender-matched nonmusicians (controls) and adults with autism spectrum disorders (ASD). Significant differences in DRD4 mRNA expression were found between the control group and both experimental groups (musicians and adults with ASD; $P<.05$). No significant differences in DRD4 mRNA levels were found between musicians and adults with ASD, nor were any significant differences found between groups in DRD3 mRNA levels ($P>.05$).[12] The finding that adults with ASD were similar to musicians in their levels of DRD4 mRNA may help explain the pronounced interest in music that many individuals with ASD display and provides a rationale for further research into the use of music therapy with this population. Wan and colleagues[13] proposed that music may serve as an effective treatment of social communication in individuals with ASD by activating the mirror neuron system, although more research in this area remains to be done.

Affective disorders

In a study by Field and colleagues,[14] 28 depressed adolescent females showed increased activation of the right frontal lobe (a characteristic of chronic depression) during pretest electroencephalography (EEG). Fourteen participants were randomly assigned to listen to upbeat rock music while undergoing EEG. The other 14 participants served as a control group and were asked to relax their minds and their muscles for the same period of time that the treatment group listened to music. The treatment group showed significantly decreased right frontal lobe activation and increased left frontal lobe activation during and after listening to the music ($P<.05$), both of which are more typical of those without depression. The treatment group also showed significantly decreased salivary cortisol after listening to rock music ($P = .02$), although their observed and reported mood did not change significantly ($P>.05$). The control group did not show significant changes on any of the measures. The 3 participants in the treatment group whose EEGs showed frontal lobe shifts further to the right while listening to rock music reported preferring classical music over rock. When these 3 participants were tested again while listening to classical music, they showed frontal lobe shifts to the left. This study shows the importance of considering preference when designing music interventions.[14]

Koelsch and colleagues[15] speculated that changes in anterior hippocampal activity induced by music listening are relevant for individuals with depression or posttraumatic stress disorder, who show reduced hippocampal volume. In their 2010 study, Koelsch and colleagues[15] showed that participants who participated in socially directed music-making showed improvements in mood compared with control participants, who maintained a steady beat but lacked both the rich musical experience and the social experience within the study condition. The results of the study by Koelsch and colleagues may indicate the role of dopamine in socially directed music-making. In animal research, zebra finches showed significant increases in dopamine after socially directed singing compared with no singing or singing that was not directed at another finch ($P<.05$).[16] Although further research is necessary examining the role of dopamine in socially directed music-making in humans, current findings generally support the use of group music therapy over individual music therapy when treating individuals with affective disorders. Information regarding group music therapy is highlighted in relation to specific disorders later in the text.

Eating disorders

In a study by Uher and colleagues,[17] women with eating disorders and healthy controls were asked to rate line drawings of underweight, normal weight, and overweight.

Women with eating disorders showed weaker responses in the lateral fusiform gyrus and the parietal cortex (measured by fMRI) when compared with healthy controls while viewing line drawings of underweight, normal weight, and overweight female bodies. Activity in the right medial apical prefrontal cortex was positively correlated with ratings of fear and disgust reported by the participants with eating disorders.[17] Because decreases in ventromedial prefrontal cortex activity have been noted when participants listen to preferred music that gives them chills, further research regarding the effectiveness of music therapy in treating eating disorders is warranted, as is research into the therapeutic mechanism of music specific to treating this population.[9]

Although more neuroimaging research studying children and adolescents with specific psychopathologies is warranted, the current research suggests that the ability of certain preferred music to activated neural reward circuits supports the use of music therapy in mental health care. **Box 1** summarizes important considerations when using music in music therapy or music medicine, based on current neuroimaging research.

Music Therapy and Mental Health Overview

Approximately 20% of music therapists report working in mental health settings; this number represents the single largest specific client population category in music therapy.[18] Individual music therapists may approach treatment from different psychological orientations, including cognitive-behavioral, behavioral, humanistic, or psychodynamic. For a more thorough description of different approaches to music therapy treatment, readers are referred to the text by Darrow.[19] According to a survey conducted by Silverman,[18] many psychiatric music therapists use behavioral techniques with mental health consumers, most psychiatric music therapists use cognitive-behavioral or psychodynamic approaches, and most psychiatric music therapists believe that the cognitive-behavioral approach will be most used in the future.[20] Common goal areas included socialization, communication, self-esteem, coping skills, and stress management/reduction. Commonly used music-based interventions include music-assisted relaxation, improvisation, songwriting, lyric analysis, and movement to music. These music interventions are often paired with common psychotherapeutic techniques, including humor, redirection, reinforcement, empathy, and affirmation.[18] **Table 1** categorizes the effectiveness of music therapy approaches with children and adolescent mental health consumers, based on current research.

The research literature suggests that group work is the predominant delivery model for music therapy in mental health settings, that music therapy can be effectively incorporated in both inpatient and community-based settings, and that group work is effective in promoting group cohesion, interaction, and emotional expression.[18,56–59] In terms of treatment duration, slight improvements can be seen with a few sessions (3–10), but larger gains are found with more frequent sessions or longer courses of music therapy.[58]

Box 1
Summary of recommendations based on music neuroscience research

- Musical preference is an important consideration when designing music therapy or music medicine interventions
- Active musical participation engages more areas of the brain than passive music listening and enhances mood to a greater degree
- The social aspect of making music in a group enhances mood to a greater degree than individual music-making

Table 1
Evidence-based treatment evaluations

Treatment/Approach	Abuse/Trauma	ADHD	Aggressive Behavior	At-Risk	Autism	Bereavement	Eating Disorders	Emotional/Behavioral Disorders	Intellectual/Developmental Disabilities	Juvenile Delinquents	Substance Abuse	Various Psychopathologies[a]	Basis in Youth (Best Available Data)
Active music therapy (no psychotherapeutic approach given)	Fair/insufficient[21]	[b]	Fair/insufficient[22]	Fair/rec.[23]	Fair/rec.[24]		Fair/rec.[25]	Fair/rec.[26–28]			Fair/rec.[29]	Fair/rec.[30]	Randomized controlled study Controlled clinical trial Case study Qualitative case study
Cognitive-behavioral music therapy						Fair/rec.[31]		Fair/rec.[32–34]		Fair/rec.[35]	Fair/rec.[36]	Fair/rec.[37]	Controlled clinical trial Case study
Eclectic music therapy		Fair/rec.[38]			Fair/rec.[38–40]		Fair/no data[41]		Fair/rec.[42]		Fair/rec.[43]	Fair/rec.[30,38,44,45]	Meta-analysis Systematic review Content analysis Controlled clinical trial Case study
Humanistic music therapy (creative/Nordoff-Robbins; Orff; improvisational)		Fair/rec.[46]	Fair/rec.[47]			Fair/rec.[48]	Fair/no data[49]	Fair/insufficient[50,51]				Fair/rec.[38,52]	Meta-analysis Controlled clinical trial–case study Outcomes research Pilot study
Passive music therapy (music listening)		Fair/rec.[53]										Fair/rec.[54]	Controlled clinical trial
Psychodynamic music therapy (analytical)	Fair/insufficient[55]												Case study

Abbreviation: Rec, recommend.

[a] Studies placed under the heading of Various psychopathologies consisted of subjects with differing diagnoses. Only clinical studies were included.

[b] Blank cells indicate no data.

Music therapists work with individuals of all age groups and with a wide range of diagnoses, including children and adolescents with attention deficit/hyperactivity disorder (ADHD), posttraumatic stress disorder (PTSD), developmental delays/learning difficulties, and anxiety disorders, patients with chronic mental illness, adults with substance abuse disorders and chemical dependence, victims of intimate partner violence, and couples in counseling.[37,46,47,57,60–65] Music therapists work in a variety of settings, including inpatient (acute and chronic), outpatient, and community venues.[37,61,62,65,66] Music therapists are often asked to work in situations in which psychopharmacologic treatments have shown limited success. These situations include working with individuals who present with negative symptoms, poor social interactions, low motivation, and flattened or blunted affect.[58,67] Referrals are often made for patients with low motivation, and music therapy has been consistently shown to be effective with individuals considered to be poor candidates for verbal group therapies. Research suggests that this situation is in part caused by the activation of basic perceptual and arousal mechanisms, which are associated with an emotional response from individuals. The therapist can then use this "affective-motivational nature of music"[57(p69)] to guide therapeutic change or behavioral change.[57,67–69]

Music therapy can facilitate symptom management and allow individuals to express feelings related to their experiences.[68] Research increasingly shows its effectiveness in several areas of mental health treatment, including increased participation, improved compliance, increased motivation during treatment, and improved attendance (A Davis, unpublished master's thesis, State University of New York at New Paltz, 2008).[58,61,68] It has even been found to reduce symptoms, increase competencies, and improve quality of life.[44] Patients themselves often have a positive response to music therapy. When surveyed, inpatients valued the use of music therapy and found it helpful in improving aspects of psychiatric deficit areas.[59,62,70] Music therapy has been rated as more pleasurable than other forms of treatment, and has been viewed by participants as an effective tool for recovery (A Davis, unpublished master's thesis, State University of New York at New Paltz, 2008).[71]

Studies can be found involving music therapy treatment with a wide range of disorders usually first diagnosed in childhood (including behavior disorders, ADHD, intellectual disabilities, learning disabilities, and autism), as well as chemical dependence/substance abuse, mood/anxiety disorders, and eating disorders. The next section provides an overview of research on music therapy for children and adolescents with mental health needs.

Effectiveness Research

Disorders typically diagnosed in childhood
According to a meta-analysis conducted by Gold and colleagues,[38] music therapy has a medium to large positive effect ($d = .61$, $P<.001$) on clinically relevant outcomes, and children and adolescents with behavioral disorders, developmental disorders, and multiple psychopathologies may benefit from music therapy. Specific goal areas for individuals with childhood disorders are also addressed in the research literature, including the effect of music therapy on attention and hyperactivity symptoms, the impact of music therapy on self-esteem, and the impact of music therapy on self-expression.[22,30,33,38,50,53,72] Additional areas studied include the impact of music therapy on social skills development, the effect of music therapy on aggressive behaviors, and the effectiveness of music therapy in improving symptoms and quality of life.[22,26,32,37,52]

Results from the literature have shown music therapy to be effective with a wide variety of childhood diagnoses in[22,23,26,28,30,32,37,50,52,53]:

1. Reducing aggression and hostility
2. Reducing motor activities and increasing on-task behavior
3. Improving social functioning
4. Increasing attention and motivation
5. Improving self-concept
6. Improving symptoms and quality of life

The results of several key studies in this area are summarized here.

Aggressive behaviors

Choi and colleagues[22] studied the effects of group music intervention on aggression and self-esteem in children with highly aggressive behavior using a pretest/posttest control group design. Significant differences were found between posttreatment groups in scores of aggression ($P<.001$) and self-esteem ($P<.05$). A study by Montello and Coons[30] found that preadolescents with emotional, learning, and behavioral disorders who received passive music therapy for 12 weeks followed by active music therapy for 12 weeks showed significant improvements in attention, motivation, and hostility (all $P<.024$). Participants who received active music therapy followed by passive music therapy showed an initial increase in hostility ($P<.05$) during the active music therapy phase, followed by a significant decrease in hostility during the passive music therapy phase ($P<.05$). Because the groups in this study were made up of preadolescents with diverse needs, the results indicate that the type of music therapy treatment should be tailored to the individual needs of the clients.

ADHD

Cripe[53] used a repeated measures factorial design to study the effects of rock music on 8 males between the ages of 6 and 8 years with attention deficit disorder (the diagnostic terminology used at the time; most likely from DSM-III). Although no significant changes in attention span were observed, participants showed significant reductions in the number of motor activities performed during the music periods of the study ($P<.05$). Gooding[37] studied the effects of a music therapy-based social skills intervention program on social competence of children and adolescents with a variety of diagnoses including ADHD (using the DSM-IV definition) through 3 experiments with participants in school, residential, and after-school care settings. Results indicated significant improvements in on-task behavior in all 3 settings after 5 sessions, as measured by behavioral observations ($P<.05$). Participants from all 3 settings also showed improvements in social functioning as measured by either self-report or the report of the researcher or a case manager ($P<.05$).

General emotional and behavioral disorders

Chong and Kim[26] investigated the effects of an after-school education-oriented music therapy (EoMT) program on students' emotional and behavioral problems and academic competency. A paired-samples t-test revealed that students showed significant improvements between pretest and posttest in 3 areas of social skills (assertiveness, self-control, and cooperation; all $P<.0001$) and problem behavior ($P = .004$), but not in academic competency ($P>.05$). Johnson[35] studied the effects of incorporating objective and concrete evidence of goal achievement within music-related activities for residents of a juvenile detention center. Participants were randomly assigned to either a treatment group that received the above treatment, or a control group that participated in subjective music-related activities with no reinforcement. Participants in the treatment group showed significant improvements in self-concept ($P<.025$) relative to the control group, and perceived significantly fewer rebellious and distrustful traits in themselves ($P<.05$).

A pilot study by Gold and colleagues[52] described the music therapy treatment given to 5 children between the ages of 4 and 11 years with mental and behavioral problems. Children who received music therapy treatment (4–31 sessions over the course of 2–5 months) showed improvements in symptoms, competencies, and quality of life, although the small sample size precluded the use of statistical analyses. Taken as a whole, the results of the aforementioned studies suggest that music therapy can be a valuable medium in treating children and adolescents with mental health needs.

Autism
Research on music therapy for children with autism has received much attention from music therapy researchers in recent years.[24,40,73–77] In 2011, Reschke-Hernández[77] published a historical review of music therapy treatments from 1940 to 2009 for children with autism, which indicated that although research in this area has improved, there is a need for more high-quality studies. Although it included few studies, a meta-analysis conducted by Whipple[40] suggests that music therapy is an effective treatment of children and adolescents with autism, with an overall effect size of $d = .77$. Outcomes of music therapy treatment of children with autism included improvements in social behaviors, communication, and cognitive skills. Five of the 10 studies included in Whipple's meta-analysis were conducted by music therapists, whereas the other 5 were conducted by occupational therapists, educators, or psychologists using music medicine techniques. Two studies used a group treatment approach, whereas the remaining 8 provided individual treatment. Four studies used a developmental social pragmatic approach; 4 studies used a discrete trial-traditional behavioral approach, and 2 studies used a contemporary applied behavioral analysis approach. In this meta-analysis, all 3 approaches (developmental social pragmatic, discrete trial-traditional behavioral, and contemporary applied behavioral analysis) were found to be equally effective when incorporating music therapy treatment.[40] Regardless of the positive outcomes noted in Whipple's meta-analysis, further research on the use of music therapy in treatment of children and adolescents with autism is warranted, given the small number of studies.

Intellectual or learning disabilities
Jellison[78] surveyed the music therapy literature published between 1975 and 1999 and conducted a content analysis of music research with children and adolescents who have disabilities. Her analysis revealed that most of the research in this area focused on children with intellectual disabilities or learning disabilities. Jellison's content analysis included studies in which music educational objectives were targeted, as well as studies in which a music therapist addressed nonmusical objectives. When addressing nonmusical outcomes, Jellison describes 3 functions of music: (1) as a stimulus cue or prompt to facilitate learning, (2) as a structure or activity to provide a desired learning outcome, or (3) as a contingency. Outcomes of music therapy treatment included improvements in social, academic, motor, and verbal skills.[78] In an updated systematic review of literature on children and adolescents with disabilities between 1999 and 2009, Brown and Jellison[39] found that 34% of experimental studies on the effects of music therapy on social, motor, academic, and communicative objectives reported effective results and 47% of studies reported partially effective (mixed) results. Because of the variety of populations and dependent variables included in the studies in these systematic reviews, statistical procedures to determine the degree of effectiveness

were not appropriate. Most of the studies that reported effective or partially effective results used music therapy to address social skills (81%) or academic skills (19%).

Substance abuse
According to current research, music therapy is effective in engaging patients in substance abuse treatment regardless of age (25 years and younger vs 25 years and older) and substance use (alcohol only vs other drugs).[79] When asked if they would continue participation, 83% of individuals in a study conducted by Dingle and colleagues[79] said "Yes," with no differences because of age in motivation to participate ($X^2_{(4)}$ = 7.44, not significant). Jones[80] also found that music therapy can be effective in evoking emotional change in substance abuse patients ($P<.05$). In addition, the data suggest that music therapy can promote a healthy attitude toward self and recovery.[29] James[29] found that music therapy activities positively influenced adolescents' perceived locus of control and facilitated positive attitudes toward themselves and recovery. He studied the effects of values clarification within music therapy on adolescents with substance abuse or dependency diagnoses, using a pretest-posttest control group design. Significant differences between the experimental and control groups were found in posttest scores ($P<.05$).[29] Music therapy has even been shown to be effective in promoting on-task behaviors (off-task during music = 1%; 1.3%) in women and adolescents with chemical addictions.[36] Music therapy has been linked to longer treatment stays. In a study by Ross and colleagues[43] of dually diagnosed patients, those who attended more than 6 music therapy sessions had significantly longer treatment stays ($P<.05$) than those who attended 6 or fewer, with attendance being predictive of successful follow-up.

Mood/anxiety disorders
In 2008, Baker and Bor[81] examined the relationship between music preference and mental status in adolescents. The investigators concluded that there is limited support for a connection between music preference and mental health status, stating that music preference may indicate emotional vulnerability. There has also been some research that suggests that music-based interventions can positively affect mood and attitudes. Wooten[54] examined the effects on adolescents of listening to preferred music and found significant increases in positive affect after listening to preferred music only ($P = .038$). Likewise, James[29] found that music therapy activities positively influenced adolescents' perceived locus of control and facilitated positive attitudes toward themselves and recovery.

Music therapy as an intervention for individuals with specific mood or anxiety disorders has also been addressed in the literature. Hilliard[31,48] examined the impact of music therapy groups on mood and behavior in grieving children. Results of his studies suggest that music therapy was effective in reducing grief symptoms. In his 2007 study on the effects of Orff-based music therapy and social work groups on childhood grief symptoms and behaviors, Hilliard reported that a Wilcoxon signed rank test revealed that children randomly assigned to a music therapy group showed significant improvements in behaviors and grief symptoms ($P<.05$), whereas children who participated in a social work group showed reductions in behavioral problems ($P<.05$) but not grief symptoms ($P>.05$), and children in a wait-list control group did not improve significantly in either area ($P>.05$). Likewise, Gardstrom[51] investigated the use of clinical music improvisation with adolescents ages 12 to 17 years with PTSD, bipolar disorder, major depressive disorder, and other diagnoses in a partial hospitalization program, in a qualitative study. She concluded that music was effective in evoking emotions and allowing expression of feelings. Henderson[27] studied the effects of a music therapy program on mood awareness, group cohesion, and self-esteem in adolescents diagnosed with adjustment reaction to adolescence. He found significant improvements in use of group pronouns (as opposed to personal pronouns; $P<.05$) and agreement on mood or emotion expressed in music ($P = .01$) for participants in the music therapy treatment group.

Eating disorders

Research on music therapy and individuals with eating disorders is limited but shows promise in using music therapy as an intervention for individuals with eating disorders. In her 1994 article, Justice[82] highlighted ways in which music therapy can be used to treat individuals with anorexia and bulimia in inpatient treatment, including providing support, facilitating self-regulation and coping, and promoting awareness. Robarts[41] discussed the use of improvisation within music therapy to help adolescents with anorexia develop assertiveness and a sense of self. McFerran[49] highlighted how music therapy can be used during group work to promote expression among individuals with anorexia nervosa. In a retrospective study using a modified content analysis approach, McFerran and colleagues[25] identified themes discussed in songs written by adolescents with anorexia that support the idea that songwriting can be used to develop a sense of identity and positive self-talk. The themes most commonly used by participants in this study during songwriting were identity formation (28.2% of lyrics), relationship dynamics (17.4% of lyrics), and emotional awareness (17.2% of lyrics). These investigators noted that songs were often effective in eliciting information from participants that had not been disclosed to other team members. Participants were more willing to self-disclose information during music therapy sessions than at other times during treatment.[25] Results from a study investigating the effect of cognitive-behavioral music therapy on females ages 14 to 45 years with eating disorders suggest that music therapy was well received by patients, families, and professionals, that music therapy was motivating, and that music therapy enhanced patients' positive affect about the treatment process.[83] The research that could be found on the use of music therapy to treat eating disorders consisted of outcomes research with a qualitative measure. Future research in this area should include the use of control groups or conditions and quantitative measures.

SUMMARY

In music therapy for mental health treatment of children and adolescents, the strongest outcome findings are currently for children with intellectual disabilities, emotional and behavioral disorders, and learning disabilities, but mainly because there is less research in other areas of child and adolescent mental health, such as autism, mood/anxiety disorders, substance abuse, and eating disorders.[38,39,77,78] Research indicates that the most effective clinical treatments using music tend to be those implemented by music therapists, compared with approaches using music medicine treatments.[7] Although music may be used successfully by other health care professionals to augment mental health treatment, this treatment should be carried out with the utmost care or, as Taylor says, "If administered independently of its relationship to the therapist, it [music] may serve to intensify the pathology with which the patient is afflicted".[6(p83)] Given that musical choices may indicate mental health status and emotional vulnerability, it is advisable for the health care professional or therapist to screen patients' self-selected music before therapeutic intervention.[81]

Some music therapists provide consultations for other health care professionals on ways in which to use music in mental health treatment. The CBMT Web site, http://www.cbmt.org, has a feature that allows anyone to search for board-certified music

Table 2
Authors' recommendations

Treatment/ Approach	Abuse/ Trauma	ADHD	Aggressive Behavior	At-Risk	Autism	Bereave-ment	Eating Disorders	Emotional/ Behavioral Disorders	Intellectual/ Develop-mental Disabilities	Juvenile Delinquents	Substance Abuse	Various Psychopa-thologies	Investigators' Opinion
Active music therapy (no psycho-therapeutic approach given)		Fair/rec.		Fair/ insufficient	Fair/rec.			Fair/rec.				Fair/rec.	Can be used to address self-concept self-regulation, cognitive functioning, and social/emotional functioning Active music therapy in adults has been shown to improve attendance, participation, percep-tions of helpfulness, and learning
Cognitive-behavioral music therapy						Fair/rec.		Fair/rec.		Fair/rec.		Fair/rec.	Can be used to address self-esteem, social skills deficits, developmental objectives, self-confidence, communication, behaviors, self-esteem, cognitive functioning; and motor skills Cognitive-behavioral MT research in adults suggests that it is highly effective across a broad range of objectives

							Comments
Eclectic music therapy	Fair/rec.		Fair/rec.		Fair/rec.	Fair/rec.	Can be used to address communication, behaviors, cognitive functioning, musical or motor skills, and psychosocial functioning. The most mental health-based music therapists report use of an eclectic approach.
Humanistic music therapy (creative Nordoff-Robbins; Orff; improvisational)	Fair/insufficient	Fair/rec.	Fair/rec.	Fair/insufficient	Fair/no data	Fair/insufficient	Can be used to address joint attention, social/emotional functioning, and motivation. Can be used to decrease aggression and improve self-esteem
Passive music therapy (music listening)	Fair/rec.					Fair/rec.	Can be used to address self-regulation, behavior. Research suggests that music therapy is more effective when patients actively participate
Psychodynamic music therapy (analytical)	Fair/insufficient						All studies that used psychodynamic approaches in children also used other approaches or provided case study data only; as a result, recommendations for use of a psychodynamic-only approach cannot be made

Abbreviation: Rec, recommend.

therapists in their state. The authors offer the following evidence-based recommendations for health care professionals seeking to use music in mental health treatment of children or adolescents:

- Use high-quality, client-preferred music. Ask them what kind of music they like and bring music as close to their preference as possible.
- Allow clients to bring in their own music (listen to it before playing it for the group to screen for appropriateness of content) or give them a choice of several artists or genres.
- If you are uncomfortable performing music, use professional recordings. Become familiar with copyright restrictions to ensure compliance for you and your practice/facility.

The strengths of music therapy as a treatment of children and adolescents with mental health concerns include the fact that music therapy is known to benefit clients with a wide variety of diagnoses and can be effectively administered in group format, making it a safe, cost-efficient treatment. An increasing number of insurance providers offer reimbursement for music therapy as a biopsychosocial treatment.[84,85] One weakness of music therapy treatment of children and adolescents is that the mechanism by which it is effective is not completely understood and requires more research with randomized controlled studies. The bulk of the neuroimaging research that seeks to understand how music listening and participation affect the brain has focused on adults, so caution must be taken when interpreting results of this research with regards to children and adolescents. Although future research will better illuminate how music therapy functions, the existing research on music therapy treatment overwhelmingly indicates that music therapy does function in mental health treatment of children and adolescents. In addition, it requires a trained professional (music therapist) to effectively administer treatment; without effective administration, the use of music in mental health treatment may serve to worsen patients' conditions.[6] Music therapy may be contraindicated for individuals with profound hearing loss, who have musicogenic seizures (a rare occurrence), or who can no longer actively participate in music because of health constraints. Many individuals with mild, moderate, or even severe hearing loss do enjoy listening to music and can benefit from music therapy.[86] In addition to the aforementioned contraindications, certain types of music may be contraindicated for certain populations. For instance, an individual receiving treatment of substance abuse would be advised not to listen to music that they once listened to while getting high, because this type of music may serve to intensify cravings caused by evaluative conditioning.[6]

Although there is a growing body of research on music therapy in adult mental health treatment, further research is needed on the use of music therapy in treating child and adolescent psychiatric disorders, particularly autism, mood and anxiety disorders, substance abuse, and eating disorders in children and adolescents through randomized controlled studies. Double-blind placebo studies are not possible in music therapy because interaction with the therapist is an inherent part of the treatment and there is no way to blind participants as to whether or not they receive music therapy. However, single blind studies in which the researcher does not know which participants received music therapy are desirable. Using a variety of measures simultaneously (self-report, behavioral observation, and physiologic measurements) in research on the effects of music therapy is also recommended to help eliminate the possibility of bias. This research is warranted given the effectiveness of music therapy with adults who have these disorders and the promising nature of initial pilot studies on children and adolescents. **Table 2** summarizes recommendations based on the current clinical research and the authors' clinical experience.

Music is a useful tool in treating children and adolescents with psychiatric disorders because of the engagement of multiple areas of the brain that occur during music listening. Music therapy treatment involves active musical participation and the inclusion of therapeutic techniques by a music therapist, which provide additional levels of neural engagement and lead to successful outcomes for children with various needs in the social, behavioral, emotional, cognitive/academic, motor, and verbal domains.

REFERENCES

1. American Music Therapy Association. What is music therapy? 2011. Available at: http://www.musictherapy.org/about/musictherapy/. Accessed September 8, 2012.
2. American Music Therapy Association. AMTA 2011 member survey and workforce analysis. 2011. Available at: http://www.musictherapy.org/assets/1/7/statprofile11. pdf. Accessed September 8, 2012.
3. American Music Therapy Association. Professional requirements for music therapists. 2011. Available at: http://www.musictherapy.org/about/requirements/. Accessed September 8, 2012.
4. Dileo C, Bradt J. Medical music therapy: a meta-analysis and agenda for future research. Cherry Hill (NJ): Jeffrey Books; 2005.
5. Gooding LG. Using music interventions in perioperative care. South Med J 2012;105:486.
6. Taylor D. Biomedical foundations of music as therapy. St Louis (MO): MMB Music; 2004.
7. Lin ST, Yang P, Lai CY, et al. Mental health implications of music: insight from neuroscientific and clinical studies. Harv Rev Psychiatry 2011;19:36–46.
8. Koelsch S. A neuroscientific perspective on music therapy. Ann N Y Acad Sci 2009;1169:374–84.
9. Blood AJ, Zatorre RJ. Intensely pleasurable responses to music correlate with activity in brain regions implicated in reward and emotion. Proc Natl Acad Sci U S A 2001;98:11818–23.
10. Menon V, Levitin DJ. The rewards of music listening: response and physiological connectivity of the mesolimbic system. Neuroimage 2005;28:175–84.
11. Salimpoor VN, Benovoy M, Larcher K, et al. Anatomically distinct dopamine release during anticipation and experience of peak emotion to music. Nat Neurosci 2011;14:257–64.
12. Emanuele E, Boso M, Cassola F, et al. Increased dopamine DRD4 receptor mRNA expression in lymphocytes of musicians and autistic individuals: bridging the music-autism connection. Act Nerv Super Rediviva 2009;51:142–5.
13. Wan CY, Demaine K, Zipse L, et al. From music making to speaking: engaging the mirror neuron system in autism. Brain Res Bull 2010;82:161–8.
14. Field T, Martinez A, Nawrocki T, et al. Music shifts frontal EEG in depressed adolescents. Adolescence 1998;33:109–16.
15. Koelsch S, Offermanns K, Franzke P. Music in the treatment of affective disorders: an exploratory investigation of a new method for music-therapeutic research. Music Percept 2010;27:307–16.
16. Sasaki A, Sotnikova TD, Gainetdinov RR, et al. Social context-dependent singing-regulated dopamine. J Neurosci 2006;26:9010–4.
17. Uher R, Murphy T, Friederich HC, et al. Functional neuroanatomy of body shape perception in healthy and eating-disordered women. Biol Psychiatry 2005;58: 990–7.

18. Silverman MJ. Evaluating current trends in psychiatric music therapy: a descriptive analysis. J Music Ther 2007;44:388–414.

19. Darrow AA. Introduction to approaches in music therapy. Silver Spring (MD): American Music Therapy Association; 2004.

20. Cassity MD. Psychiatric music therapy in 2016: a Delphi Poll of the future. Music Ther Perspect 2007;25:86–93.

21. Choi CM. A pilot analysis of the psychological themes found during the CARING at Columbia-music therapy program with refugee adolescents from North Korea. J Music Ther 2010;47:380–407.

22. Choi AN, Lee MS, Lee JS. Group music intervention reduces aggression and improves self-esteem in children with highly aggressive behavior: a pilot controlled study. Evid Based Complement Alternat Med 2010;7:213–7.

23. Snow S, D'Amico M. The drum circle project: a qualitative study with at-risk youth in a school setting. Can J Mus Ther 2010;16:12–39.

24. Boso M, Emanuele E, Minazzi V, et al. Effect of long-term interactive music therapy on behavior profile and musical skills in young adults with severe autism. J Altern Complement Med 2007;13:709–12.

25. McFerran K, Baker F, Patton GC, et al. A retrospective lyrical analysis of songs written by adolescents with anorexia nervosa. Eur Eat Disord Rev 2006;14:397–403.

26. Chong HJ, Kim SJ. Education-oriented music therapy as an after-school program for students with emotional and behavioral problems. Arts Psychother 2010;37:190–6.

27. Henderson SM. Effects of a music therapy program upon awareness of mood in music, group cohesion, and self-esteem among hospitalized adolescent patients. J Music Ther 1983;20:14–20.

28. Kivland MJ. The use of music to increase self-esteem in a conduct disordered adolescent. J Music Ther 1986;23:25–9.

29. James MR. Music therapy values clarification: a positive influence on perceived locus of control. J Music Ther 1988;25:206–15.

30. Montello L, Coons EE. Effects of active versus passive group music therapy on preadolescents with emotional, learning, and behavioral disorders. J Music Ther 1998;35:49–67.

31. Hilliard RE. The effects of music therapy-based bereavement groups on mood and behavior of grieving children: a pilot study. J Music Ther 2001;38:291–306.

32. Eidson C. The effect of behavioral music therapy on the generalization of interpersonal skills from sessions to the classroom by emotionally handicapped middle school students. J Music Ther 1989;26:206–21.

33. Haines JH. The effects of music therapy on the self-esteem of emotionally-disturbed adolescents. Music Ther 1989;8:78–91.

34. Hanser S. Group contingent music listening with emotionally disturbed boys. J Music Ther 1974;11:220–5.

35. Johnson ER. The role of objective and concrete feedback in self-concept treatment of juvenile delinquents in music therapy. J Music Ther 1981;18:137–47.

36. Howard AA. The effects of music and poetry therapy on the treatment of women and adolescents with chemical addictions. J Poetry Ther 1997;11:81–102.

37. Gooding LF. The effect of a music therapy social skills training program on improving social competence in children and adolescents with social skills deficits. J Music Ther 2011;48:440–62.

38. Gold C, Voracek M, Wigram T. Effects of music therapy for children and adolescents with psychopathology: a meta-analysis. J Child Psychol Psychiatry 2004; 45:1054–63.

39. Brown LS, Jellison JA. Music research with children and youth with disabilities and typically developing peers: a systematic review. J Music Ther 2012;49: 335–64.
40. Whipple J. Music in intervention for children and adolescents with autism: a meta-analysis. J Music Ther 2004;41:90–106.
41. Robarts JZ. Music therapy and adolescents with anorexia nervosa. Nord J Music Ther 2000;9:3–12.
42. McQueen C. Two controlled experiments in music therapy. Br J Mus Ther 1975; 6:2–8.
43. Ross S, Cidambi I, Dermatis H, et al. Music therapy: a novel motivational approach for dually diagnosed patients. J Addict Dis 2008;27:41–53.
44. Gold C, Wigram T, Voracek M. Effectiveness of music therapy for children and adolescents with psychopathology: a quasi-experimental study. Psychother Res 2007;17:289–96.
45. Gold C, Wigram T, Voracek M. Predictors of change in music therapy with children and adolescents: the role of therapeutic techniques. Psychol Psychother 2007;80:577–89.
46. Rickson D. Instructional and improvisational models of music therapy with adolescents who have attention deficit hyperactivity disorder (ADHD): a comparison of the effects on motor impulsivity. J Music Ther 2006;43:39–60.
47. Rickson DJ, Watkins WG. Music therapy to promote prosocial behaviors in aggressive adolescent boys–a pilot study. J Music Ther 2003;40:293–301.
48. Hilliard RE. The effects of Orff-based music therapy and social work groups on childhood grief symptoms and behaviors. J Music Ther 2007;44:123–38.
49. McFerran K. Dangerous liaisons: group work for adolescent girls who have anorexia nervosa. Voices: a world forum for music therapy. Vol. 5. 2005. Available at: https://normt.uib.no/index.php/voices/article/view/215/159. Accessed September 8, 2012.
50. McIntyre J. Creating order out of chaos: music therapy with adolescent boys diagnosed with a behavior disorder and/or emotional disorder. Music Therapy Today 2007;8:56–79.
51. Gardstrom S. An investigation of meaning in clinical music improvisation with troubled adolescents. 2003. Available at: http://www.barcelonapublishers.com/QIMTV1/QIMT20041(4)Gardstrom.pdf. Accessed September 8, 2012.
52. Gold C, Wigram T, Berger E. The development of a research design to assess the effects of individual music therapy with mentally ill children and adolescents. Nord J Music Ther 2001;10:17–31.
53. Cripe F. Rock music as therapy for children with attention-deficit disorder. J Music Ther 1986;23:30–7.
54. Wooten MA. The effects of heavy metal music on affects shifts of adolescents in an inpatient psychiatric setting. Music Ther Perspect 1992;10:93–8.
55. Strehlow G. The use of music therapy in treating sexually abused children. Nord J Music Ther 2009;18:167–83.
56. Cassity MD. The influence of a music therapy activity upon peer acceptance, group cohesiveness, and interpersonal relationships of adult psychiatric patients. J Music Ther 1976;8:66–76.
57. de l'Etoile SK. The effectiveness of music therapy in group psychotherapy for adults with mental illness. Arts Psychother 2002;29:69–78.
58. Gold C, Solli HP, Kruger V, et al. Dose-response relationship in music therapy for people with serious mental disorders: systematic review and meta-analysis. Clin Psychol Rev 2009;29:193–207.

59. Goldberg FS, McNeil DE, Binder RL. Therapeutic factors in two forms of inpatient group psychotherapy: music therapy and verbal therapy. Behav Sci 1988;12:145–56.

60. Ulrich G, Houtmans T, Gold C. The additional therapeutic effect of group music therapy for schizophrenic patients: a randomized study. Acta Psychiatr Scand 2007;116:362–70.

61. Silverman MJ. The effect of lyric analysis on treatment eagerness and working alliance in consumers who are in detoxification: a randomized clinical effectiveness study. Music Ther Perspect 2009;27:115–21.

62. Silverman MJ. Perceptions of music therapy interventions from inpatients with severe mental illness: a mixed-methods approach. Arts Psychother 2010;37: 264–8.

63. Silverman MJ. The effect of songwriting on knowledge of coping skills and working alliance in psychiatric patients: a randomized clinical effectiveness study. J Music Ther 2011;48:103–22.

64. Teague AK, Hahna ND, McKinney CH. Group music therapy with women who have experienced intimate partner violence. Music Ther Perspect 2006;24:80–6.

65. Gallant W, Holosko M, Gorey KM, et al. Music as a form of intervention with outpatient alcoholic couples: a quasi-experimental investigation. Can J Mus Ther 1997;5:67–84.

66. Schwantes M, McKinney C. Music therapy with Mexican migrant farmworkers: a pilot study. Music Ther Perspect 2010;28:22–8.

67. Mossler K, Assmus J, Heldal TO, et al. Music therapy techniques as predictors of change in mental health care. Arts Psychother 2012;39:333–41.

68. Edwards J. Music therapy in the treatment and management of mental disorders. Ir J Psychol Med 2006;23:33–5.

69. Slotoroff C. Drumming technique for assertiveness and anger management in the short-term psychiatric setting for adult and adolescent survivors of trauma. Music Ther Perspect 1994;12:111–6.

70. Silverman MJ. Immediate effects of a single music therapy intervention with persons who are severely mentally ill. Arts Psychother 2004;31:291–301.

71. Heaney J. Evaluation of music therapy and other treatment modalities by adult psychiatric patients. J Music Ther 1992;29:70–86.

72. Jackson N. A survey of music therapy methods and their role in the treatment of early elementary school children with ADHD. J Music Ther 2003;40:302–23.

73. Kaplan RS, Steele AL. An analysis of music therapy program goals and outcomes for clients with diagnoses on the autism spectrum. J Music Ther 2005; 42:2–19.

74. Kim J, Wigram T, Gold C. The effects of improvisational music therapy on joint attention behaviors in autistic children: a randomized controlled study. J Autism Dev Disord 2008;38:1758–66.

75. Kim J, Wigram T, Gold C. Emotional, motivational and interpersonal responsiveness of children with autism in improvisational music therapy. Autism 2009;13: 389–409.

76. Gold C, Wigram T, Elefant C. Music therapy for autistic spectrum disorder [review]. Cochrane Database Syst Rev 2006; Issue 2. Art. No.: CD004381. DOI: 10.1002/14651858.CD004381.pub2.

77. Reschke-Hernández AE. History of music therapy treatment interventions for children with autism. J Music Ther 2011;48:169–207.

78. Jellison JA. A content analysis of music research with disabled children and youth (1975-1999): applications in special education. In: American Music Therapy

Association, editor. Effectiveness of music therapy procedures: documentation of research and clinical practice. 3rd edition. Silver Spring (MD): American Music Therapy Association; 2000. p. 199–264.

79. Dingle GA, Gleadhill L, Baker FA. Can music therapy engage patients in group cognitive behavior therapy for substance abuse treatment? Drug Alcohol Rev 2008;27:190–6.

80. Jones J. A comparison of songwriting and lyric analysis techniques to evoke emotional change in a single session with people who are chemically dependent. J Music Ther 2005;42:94–110.

81. Baker F, Bor W. Can music preference indicate mental health status in young people? Australas Psychiatry 2008;16:284–8.

82. Justice RW. Music therapy interventions for people with eating disorders in an inpatient setting. Music Ther Perspect 1994;12:104–10.

83. Hilliard RE. The use of cognitive-behavioral music therapy in the treatment of women with eating disorders. Music Ther Perspect 2001;19:109–13.

84. Simpson J, Burns DS. Music therapy reimbursement: best practices and procedures. Silver Spring (MD): American Music Therapy Association; 2004.

85. Standley JM, Rushing J, Swedberg O, et al. Reimbursement for evidence-based NICU-MT. In: Standley JM, Walworth DD, editors. Music therapy with premature infants: research and developmental interventions. 2nd edition. Silver Spring (MD): American Music Therapy Association; 2010. p. 116–43.

86. Darrow AA. The role of music in deaf culture: implications for music educators. J Res Music Educ 1993;41:93–110.

Omega-3 Fatty Acid and Nutrient Deficits in Adverse Neurodevelopment and Childhood Behaviors

CrossMark

Rachel V. Gow, PhD[b], Joseph R. Hibbeln, MD[a],*

KEYWORDS

- Omega-3 fatty acids • Eicosapentaenoic acid • Docosahexaenoic acid
- Arachidonic acid • Child neurodevelopment • Attention-deficit/hyperactivity disorder
- Conduct disorder • Learning disorders

KEY POINTS

- Omega-3 highly unsaturated fatty acids (HUFAs) are critical for both structure and function of the brain.
- The omega-3 HUFA docosahexaenoic acid (DHA) and the omega-6 HUFA arachidonic acid (AA) are especially critical for the development of the central nervous system.
- Omega-3 and omega-6 fatty acids have distinct roles and require a balance of omega-3/-6 for optimal physical and mental health. An excessive intake of one type of fatty acid may inhibit the conversion of the other.
- EPA-rich formulas are linked to improvements in mood and symptoms of attention-deficit/ hyperactivity disorder (ADHD).
- The American Psychiatric Association Task Force on Complementary and Alternative Medicine recommends that the dietary intake of omega-3 for patients with poor impulse control, mood disorders, or psychotic disorders should include eicosapentaenoic acid + docosahexaenoic acid at a daily dose of approximately 1 gram.
- Lower concentrations of omega-3 fatty acids have been present in both plasma and red blood cells of children and young adults with ADHD in comparison with healthy controls.
- Supplementation with omega-3 HUFAs in clinical trials have found some improvement in learning capacity and behavior in youths who are academically underachieving, have ADHD-like symptoms, and/or have severe misconduct.
- The relationship between nutritional deficiencies, in particular of omega-3 fats, and symptoms of mental ill-health, warrants closer examination by clinicians and mental health practitioners.

Funding Sources: Intramural Research Program, National Institute of Alcohol Abuse and Alcoholism (NIAAA) and Barlean's Organic Oils, LLC.
[a] Section of Nutritional Neurosciences, Laboratory of Membrane Biochemistry and Biophysics, National Institute of Alcohol Abuse and Alcoholism, National Institutes of Health, 5625 Fishers Lane, Room 3N-01, Rockville, MD 20892, USA; [b] Section of Nutritional Neurosciences, Laboratory of Membrane Biochemistry and Biophysics, National Institute of Alcohol Abuse and Alcoholism, National Institutes of Health, 31 Center Drive, Building 31, Room 1B54, Rockville, MD 20892, USA
* Corresponding author.
E-mail address: jhibbeln@mail.nih.gov

Abbreviations	
AA	Arachidonic Acid
ADHD	Attention Deficit Hyperactivity Disorder
ALA	α-Linolenic Acid
ALSPAC	Avon Longitudinal Study of Parents and Children
CDRS	Childhood Depression Rating Scale
CESD	Center for Epidemiologic Studies Depression Scale
CGI	Clinical Global Impression
CPRS	Conners Parents' Rating Scale
CTRS-L	Conners' Teacher Rating Scale
DHA	Docosahexaenoic Acid
EPA	Eicosapentaenoic Acid
ERP	Event-Related Potential
FDA	Food Drug Administration
fMRI	Functional Magnetic Resonance Imaging
GLA	Gamma-Linolenic Acid
GRAS	Generally Recognized as Safe
HUFA	Highly Unsaturated Fatty Acids
LA	Linoleic Acid
LPC	Late Positive Component
NAFLD	Non-Alcoholic Fatty Liver Disease
NIAAA	National Institute on Alcohol Abuse and Alcoholism
PCBs	Polychlorinated Biphenyls
PUFA	Polyunsaturated Fatty Acid
RA	Reaction Time
RCT	Randomized Clinical Trial
SAMe	S-adenosyl-L-methionine
SMD	Standard Mean Difference

INTRODUCTION

Anyone who has observed children knows that their behavior changes dramatically when they are hungry. However, an important consideration is that children today may be consuming adequate or excessive calories, but their brains nonetheless can be starved of vital nutrients critical for optimal brain function, thus increasing the risk for behavioral disorders and adverse developmental trajectories. Among these vital nutrients are iodine, folate, B vitamins, iron, zinc, micronutrients, and omega-3 essential fatty acids. The US Department of Agriculture publication *Dietary Guidelines for Americans, 2010*[1] addresses both specific nutrients and patterns of healthy eating for optimization of physical health outcomes. Similarly, this article considers both specific nutrients and multiple interactive nutrients for optimization of mental health outcomes.

The primary focus of the article is the effects of deficits in the dietary intake of omega-3 highly unsaturated fatty acids (HUFAs); the associated potential increase in risk for attention-deficit/hyperactivity disorder (ADHD) and similar behavioral disorders; and the hypothesis that omega-3 HUFAs have some treatment efficacy. Deficits in omega-3 HUFAs in depressive and aggressive disorders are also especially relevant to children; however, the main body of observational data and treatment studies has been conducted in adults. The proposition that nutritional insufficiencies in early development may have residual behavioral and cognitive deficits merits critical consideration.

The first part of this article introduces the reader to nutritional requirements for optimal brain development and the impacts of nutritional inadequacy during pregnancy on adverse long-term developmental outcomes. Next, basic science issues related to neurologic function and essential fatty acid metabolism underlying these findings are addressed in the context of the dramatic differences between current dietary patterns and those during hominid evolution. Finally, observational and treatment studies are assessed for the plausibility of the efficacy of nutritional treatments for psychiatric disorders in children and adolescents.

ESSENTIAL NUTRIENTS AND THE RISK OF DEFICIENCIES

The peak vulnerability to harm from nutritional deficiencies occurs during pregnancy, when the central nervous system is first developing. The quality of the maternal diet is particularly dependent on the intake of micronutrients (such as vitamins A and B, choline, and folate), trace elements (such as iodine, iron, zinc, and copper), and HUFAs, especially docosahexaenoic acid (DHA) and the omega-6 HUFA arachidonic acid (AA). These nutrients are especially critical during the fetal and early postnatal stage, when most areas of the brain are undergoing their most rapid development.

It is well established that nutritional deficiencies (and excesses) may affect the infant brain and alter subsequent development and behavior permanently.[2-4] For example, the link between iodine deficiency and mental retardation is widely documented. In developing countries, approximately 38 million children are born at risk of iodine-associated mental retardation every year.[5] Deficiencies in iodine and iron (ie, anemia) during infancy have been linked to a range of suboptimal developmental outcomes, including:

1. Abnormal neuronal development[6]
2. Disruptions in regulatory processes, such as the sleep-wake cycle[7]
3. Suboptimal performance in global measurements of cognition, motor skills, and social-emotional behavior[8-12]
4. Mental retardation and cognitive deficits associated with reductions in learning capacity and productivity[6]

In animal models of nutritional deficiencies, a similar pattern of cognitive, motor, and behavioral changes is observed, along with alterations in dopaminergic function and lower dopamine levels in the cerebrospinal fluid in comparison with controls.[13] Iron deficiency also affects other neurotransmitters and other neuronal processes, including metabolism in hippocampus and striatum, myelination, dendritogenesis, and both gene and protein profiles.[14-16] HUFAs, including the omega-3 DHA, are similarly proposed to play a critical role during sensitive periods of neurodevelopment during early childhood, and also in the regulation of cognitive function throughout the life span.[17,18] The beneficial effects of eicosapentaenoic acid (EPA) and DHA for cardiovascular diseases and stroke are well established, but their potential for preventing mild cognitive dysfunction and reducing the risk for Alzheimer disease require further evaluation in large, long-term clinical trials.[19]

THE LIPID SUBSTANCE OF THE BRAIN

About 50% to 60% of the dry weight of an adult brain is composed of lipid, and at least 35% of the lipid content is made up of HUFAs. Given the high brain content of HUFAs, it is remarkable that these fatty acids are dietarily essential. HUFAs cannot be synthesized de novo, but must be either ingested directly from dietary sources or metabolized from essential polyunsaturated fatty acid (PUFA) precursors.[20-22] These fatty acids are highly specialized, with very specific metabolic functions and unique biophysical properties.

The biosynthetic pathways (see **Fig. 1**) and metabolic interactions among the omega-3 and omega-6 series of fatty acids are complex. The parent compounds for the large number of HUFAs are 2 PUFAs: α-linolenic acid (ALA) is the precursor for the omega-3 fatty acids, and linoleic acid (LA) is the precursor for the omega-6 fatty acids.[23] These 2 precursor nutrients are the only fatty acids that are definitely essential, in the sense that the human body has no way to synthesize them and they must be ingested in the diet. Until the 1950s, ALA and LA were collectively known as vitamin F.

LA, the omega-6 precursor, is the most abundant PUFA in the Western diet. In addition to its role in the brain, the omega-6 series is vital for mammalian reproduction.[24] LA is primarily sourced from practically every commercially manufactured food in the market place; in particular, it is sourced from soybean oil (the most frequently consumed oil), corn oil, and sunflower oil.[25] Typical dietary intake of omega-6 PUFAs in Western diets are excessive, and thought to be in the region of 12 to 17 g daily.[26] LA is a metabolic precursor to γ-linolenic acid (GLA) and AA,[26] having been converted by an elongase and 2 desaturase enzymes. AA is particularly abundant in the lipids of inner cell membranes, is important in the vasculature,[24] and plays a crucial role in the production of eicosanoids. Although AA can be synthesized from LA, the main dietary sources of AA are red meat and dairy products including eggs.[27]

The omega-3 precursor ALA is metabolized into EPA and DHA, which are considered the 2 major omega-3 fatty acids. ALA is readily available in vegetable sources (especially green leafy vegetables, plants, vegetable oils, and nuts and seeds such as flax and canola). The richest direct source of EPA and DHA is marine fish (such as mackerel, salmon, herring, and sardine) and seafood.[23] These 2 omega-3 fatty acids, EPA and DHA, are associated with many important functions related to neural activity, such as cell membrane fluidity, neurotransmission, ion channels, enzyme

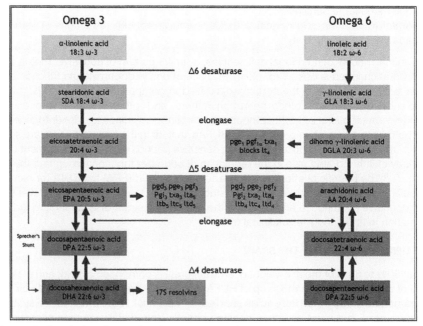

Fig. 1. Biochemical pathways for the omega-3 and omega-6 fatty acids.

regulation, gene expression, and myelination.[20,28] DHA alone makes up approximately 30% of the phosphoglycerides in the gray matter of the brain[29,30] and is essential for optimal neuronal functioning.[31] Within brain tissues, DHA preferentially accumulates in growth cones, astrocytes, synaptosomes, myelin, and microsomal and mitochondrial membranes.[32,33] Omega-3 fatty acids mediate a variety of key neurotransmitter functions, including serotonergic responsivity, signal transduction, and phospholipid turnover.[21,34,35]

The eicosanoids, which can be derived from either omega-3 or omega-6 fatty acids, are a variety of compounds involved in the regulation of blood flow (vasodilatory prostacyclin), halting of blood flow in the case of injury (anti-thrombotic thromboxanes), the resolution of inflammation (anti-inflammatory prostaglandins), and tissue homeostasis.[24,26] Diets depleted in omega-3 result in reductions of DHA in the brain and a simultaneous increase in the turnover of AA to eicosanoids.[36] These effects can be reversed by adding omega-3 to the diet.

Eicosanoids have varying crucial yet complex functions in the brain, and exercise control over numerous bodily systems. A growing body of evidence suggests that inadequate omega-3 fatty acid levels during critical stages of neurogenesis may alter parameters of cell signaling, including within neurotransmitter systems, resulting in impairments in behavior, learning, and cognition.[37–40] Eicosanoids have been shown to be involved in long-term potentiation, synaptic plasticity, spatial learning, and sleep induction; they also reduce neuroinflammation and have neuroprotective properties.[35]

EXCESS LINOLEIC ACID AND THE DIETARY BALANCE OF OMEGA-3 AND OMEGA-6 HUFAS

Both omega-3 and omega-6 fatty PUFA precursors are metabolized to their respective HUFAs by common enzyme pathways, which are influenced by many factors including diet, oxidative stress, alcohol, smoking, age, and genetic factors.[41–45] These common pathways can be overloaded, leading to a bottleneck in the metabolism of both omega-3 and omega-6 HUFAs.[46,47] The dietary balance of the ratio of omega-6 to omega-3 PUFAs therefore has important metabolic implications. For instance, excessive intake of the omega-6 LA, may inhibit the synthesis of the omega-3 ALA to EPA and DHA, and thereby reduce the availability of EPA and DHA. An excessive dietary intake of the proinflammatory omega-6 HUFAs may reduce the synthesis and functioning of anti-inflammatory omega-3 compounds, leading to a tilt toward inflammatory processes such as cardiovascular disease, metabolic disorders, immunologic conditions, and cancer.[48,49] Similarly, in the brain, an excessive intake of omega-6 or an insufficient intake of omega-3 can potentially increase the risk of depression, speculatively by altering serotonergic and catecholaminergic neurotransmission.[39,50–52]

The imbalance of omega-3 and 6 fatty acids present in modern diets is a focal point of much scientific debate. Recent calculations estimate that omega-6 to omega-3 ratios in dietary intake have risen from about 1:1 to 2:1 to approximately 20:1.[53] It has been suggested that these ratio increases are predominantly a result of the increased consumption of linoleic-rich soybean oil during the last century.[25] In a randomized clinical trial in which the intake of LA was selectively increased (N = 221) from approximately 6% to 15 % of dietary energy, increased mortality was observed from both cardiovascular disease (hazard ratio [HR] 1.70, 95% confidence interval [CI] 1.03–2.80; $P = .04$) compared with controls (n = 237) and coronary heart disease (HR 1.74, 95% CI 1.04–2.92; $P = .04$), which are findings consistent with other linoleic-selective trials (see the Sydney Diet Heart Study updated meta-analysis for more information).[54] Therefore, reducing omega-6 LA intake to ensure a good dietary balance of omega-3 and omega-6 fatty acids may be a key factor in optimal health outcomes.

IMPACT OF INADEQUATE DHA INTAKE ON BRAIN DEVELOPMENT IN ANIMALS

A large body of research has confirmed the essential role of DHA in the development and function of the brain. The negative impact of inadequate DHA during critical periods of brain development has been well studied in animals and, to a lesser extent, in humans. Maternal nutritional deficiencies during neurogenesis and angiogenesis have long been associated with behavioral impairments in both animal models[55–57] and humans.[39,58,59] It appears that HUFA insufficiency during lactation can lead to some irreversible changes,[60] presumably because of impaired connectivity.

In animal studies, prenatal and postnatal DHA insufficiency has been associated with a variety of structural changes, such as delayed neuronal migration, disrupted dendritic arborization, abnormal neuronal development in the hippocampus,[51] and abnormalities in timed apoptosis. Neurochemical studies have shown alterations of several neurotransmission systems, including the dopaminergic and serotonergic systems.[61] The resulting altered or impaired connectivity may result in permanent disturbances.[62] Subsequent functional deficits include cognitive impairments, such as memory and learning,[55] in addition to deficits in emotional regulation and behavior, such as depression, anxiety, and aggression, in animal models.[63,64] Repletion of both omega-3 and omega-6 fatty acids into the diet during lactation in animals restores the composition of brain fatty acid and some parameters of neurotransmitter function,[60] but only partially.

In humans, DHA insufficiency in utero has been hypothesized to be linked to impaired magnocellular neurite growth associated with dyslexia.[65] Some studies have also reported findings of abnormal omega-3 HUFA levels in the erythrocytes of children and young adults with ADHD.[66–73] In addition, a growing body of clinical research has reported improvements in symptoms of ADHD,[74–76] depression,[77] learning difficulties, and/or dyslexia[78] following supplementation with omega-3/-6 fatty acids relative to placebo.

There is very little research, however, investigating the potential effects of omega-3 intervention in healthy control children. One functional magnetic resonance imaging (fMRI) study reported changes in cortical attention networks in healthy boys following DHA supplementation.[79] A recent randomized placebo-controlled study reported that DHA supplementation improved both reading and behavior in healthy but underperforming schoolchildren,[80] although another clinical trial reported little or no effect of HUFA intervention compared with placebo on the cognitive ability and behavior of schoolchildren.[81] A more detailed review of the randomized placebo-controlled clinical trials in this area is provided later in this article.

Omega-3 interventions are more likely to demonstrate benefits among children with omega-3 deficiencies than among healthy children with omega-3 sufficiency. The collective findings from both animal and human studies has led researchers to postulate that deficits of omega-3 HUFAs during critical periods of brain development may increase the risk for neurodevelopmental disorders, such as ADHD, and possibly predispose toward the later appearance of depressive and aggressive behaviors.[39,82,83]

A DIETARY EVOLUTION: UNFORTUNATE CONSEQUENCES OF AGRICULTURAL DEVELOPMENTS

Crawford and others have argued that the fossil evidence indicates that the lacustrine (lake and shore) and marine food chains were being extensively exploited during the period when cerebral expansion took place, suggesting that the transition from the archaic to modern humans took place at the land/water interface. At these interfaces, in regions of hominid evolution, diets consumed from wild foods were lower in saturated fats (range 11–12 in percentage energy [en%]), higher in omega-3 HUFAs (2.26–17.0 g/d), lower in the omega-6 LA (range 2.3–3.6 en%), and a lower ALA/LA ratio (range 1.12–1.64 g/d), indicating a lower omega-3/omega-6 ratio than is present in contemporary diets.[53] The paleolithic diet is a modern dietary regimen that seeks to mimic the presumed diets of preagricultural hunter-gatherers. Arguably, compared with modern Western diets consumed today, the paleolithic diets of our ancestors provided more DHA, which is a known key omega-3 constituent of the brain (and visual photoreceptor signaling systems). The shore-based theory has provided considerable evidence for our ancestors settling along the river banks in Africa, with fish, clams, frogs, and seafood as their stable diet. Stephen Cunnane from the University of Sherbrooke and Kathy Stewart from the Canadian Museum of Nature in Ottawa have extensively studied fossil material excavated from numerous *Homo habilis* sites in eastern Africa, which have revealed a bevy of chewed fish bones, particularly catfish.[84,85] Their theory is that a rich and secure shore-based diet fueled and provided the essential nutrients to make our brains what they are today. Crawford and colleagues[86] have also proposed that the availability of DHA was crucial to permit evolution of the human brain.[87] DHA is both conserved and irreplaceable in neuronal signaling, and is involved in the expression of several hundred genes,[88] highlighting its unique and dominant place in brain evolution and biology in general.

The most dramatic and unfortunate changes from our paleolithic heritage of whole and unrefined foods are direct consequences of the Agricultural Revolution. Between the seventeenth and the end of the nineteenth century, and then continuing with a second wave after the World War II, new farming and technological changes brought the advent of mass food production, which has resulted in the problematic "modern refined diet" consumed today.[48,89–91] Contemporary Western diets also have low quantities of key micronutrients (minerals, vitamins, and trace elements), amino acids, antioxidants, fiber, and helpful phytochemicals, and are overloaded with sodium, refined sugars, and grain products that carry a high glycemic load.[89]

Even seemingly healthy parts of the modern Western diet have progressively lost their nutrient value. In the 1970s, poultry and eggs were the major land-based sources of protein and omega-3 fatty acids, especially DHA, and poultry was considered a healthy lean alternative to fatty red meat.[92] However, a laboratory analysis of modern supermarket chickens revealed that their energy from fat now actually exceeds energy from protein, and that their omega-6/omega-3 ratio is 9:1 rather than the recommended 2:1 ratio.[93] The loss of omega-3 HUFAs from chicken may result from feeding farm animals with soy-based products that are relatively deficient in omega-3 HUFAs, and the use of severely cramped bird cages that prevent exercise and reduce mitochondria-rich muscle mass.[93] This shift toward excessive omega-6 and insufficient omega-3 HUFAs in the human diet is argued to have adverse health consequences.[94]

Despite their critical biological role, essential fatty acids cannot be synthesized or stored by the body for very long periods of time and therefore must be obtained in the diet, so that these modern dietary changes have significant biological consequences. The recent increase in obesity[95] and diabetes (Word Health Organization [WHO], 2002) in both children and adults is likely a consequence of both the sedentary lifestyle and the excessive consumption of energy-dense refined foods rich in salt, sugar, and fats. Type B malnutrition is now recognized as a new type of malnutrition directly resulting from multiple micronutrient depletion and very likely deriving from the globalization of the Western food systems.[24] Several scientific and governmental bodies have made dietary recommendations, including the *Dietary Guidelines for*

Americans, 2010, to increase intake of fish and seafood during pregnancy to prevent suboptimal brain development in utero and residual problems in cognitive and visual development.[1] In view of the prediction by the WHO of a 50% increase in child mental ill-health by 2020, the promotion of optimal nutrient requirements for the developing brain warrants examination as a means to reduce the risk of potential developmental and functional consequences.

INADEQUATE HUFA INTAKE DURING PREGNANCY ON HUMAN DEVELOPMENTAL OUTCOME

Fish and seafood are the richest sources of omega-3 fats in the human diet, but also contain multiple nutrients that are beneficial to optimal brain development. Two major studies of inadequate seafood intake during pregnancy are offered here as examples to provide an overview of the potential impact of intrauterine nutrient inadequacies on behavioral and cognitive deficits later in childhood.

The Avon Longitudinal Study of Parents and Children (ALSPAC) is a longitudinal study of health care outcomes with pregnant mothers and their children conducted at Bristol University in the United Kingdom. In 1991 more than 14,000 mothers were enrolled during pregnancy, and the developmental and health trajectory of their children has been charted ever since.[96] Among the numerous nutritional factors examined, the effects of the 2004 US Food and Drug Administration (FDA) advisory to limit seafood intake during pregnancy was directly evaluated to determine whether eating seafood (ie, exposure to trace methyl mercury) or avoiding seafood (risk of nutritional deficiencies) was associated with greater harm.[97] One purpose of the advisory was to protect against impaired verbal development. However, detrimental effects on verbal development were found among children whose mothers consumed less than 12 oz (340 g) of seafood per week (odds ratio = 1.48 for greater risk of low verbal IQ). Low maternal seafood intake during pregnancy was also associated with suboptimal outcomes for fine motor skills, communication, prosocial behavior, and social development scores.[96] A net effects analysis by the WHO[98] and the FDA[99] found that the nutritional benefits of fish far exceed the toxicologic effects of methyl mercury. These findings may result in an update of the 2004 FDA advisory on EPA.[97]

Another longitudinal study conducted in Australia, known as the Raine Study,[100] followed 2868 live births to age 14 years and then assessed the adolescents for dietary patterns and ADHD diagnosis. Data were available for 1799 adolescents, including 115 with a diagnosis of ADHD. The 2 main dietary patterns were assessed and categorized as "Healthy" and "Western." The Western dietary pattern was correlated with higher intakes of total and saturated fat, salt, and refined sugars, and was inversely correlated with intake of folate, fiber, and omega-3 fatty acids.[100] By contrast, the Healthy dietary pattern was positively correlated with fiber, folate, and omega-3 fatty acid intake, and inversely correlated with the amount of refined sugars and the total fat/saturated fat ratio.[100] The results showed that an increased likelihood of an ADHD diagnosis was significantly associated with the Western dietary pattern, after adjustment for potential confounding variables from pregnancy to adolescence. The ADHD diagnosis was not associated with the Healthy dietary pattern. Clearly, firm conclusions cannot be drawn regarding the causal nature of dietary patterns on the likelihood of ADHD because of the cross-sectional nature of the study design. The observations may also be bidirectional; that is, the diagnosed ADHD may indicate poorer food choices, or the Western diet may have promoted the expression of attention deficits. However, this study does highlight the necessity for a closer inspection of the role of dietary patterns in ADHD.[100]

EFFECT OF HUFA SUPPLEMENTATION IN HEALTHY CHILDREN

Early dietary intake of HUFAs, specifically during pregnancy and breastfeeding, have been associated with subsequent improvements in an array of functions, including visual acuity at age 12 months,[101,102] problem-solving ability in infants,[103] and alterations in cortical attention networks in schoolchildren.[79]

For example, the effects of DHA supplementation on attention networks in the brain have been examined in 38 healthy boys (ages 8–10 years) using fMRI.[79] Participants were randomly allocated to receive DHA (n = 12, dose: 400 mg or n = 14, dose: 1200 mg) or placebo (n = 12), although 5 children were lost to follow-up, withdrawal, or noncompliance. Their cortical brain activity was recorded at baseline and 8 weeks later. The results found that DHA erythrocyte membrane composition increased by 47% to 70% at 8 weeks in comparison with the placebo group.[79] Both DHA dose groups had increased activation of the dorsolateral prefrontal cortex and greater reductions in activation in the occipital and cerebral cortex during a sustained attention task when compared with controls. Decreases in cerebellar activation were larger in the 1200-mg group than in the 400-mg group.[79] DHA erythrocyte levels were positively associated with dorsolateral prefrontal cortex activation and negatively associated with reaction time, which improved (ie, faster reaction) as brain function increased. This study was the first to demonstrate that dietary intake of DHA changed cortical attention networks in healthy boys.

Osendarp and colleagues[104] assessed the effects after randomization of a fortified drink containing either (1) a mix of micronutrient intervention (zinc, iron, vitamins A, B_6, B_{12}, and C, folate) alone, (2) DHA 88 mg and/or EPA 22 mg daily alone, (3) the micronutrient intervention plus DHA 88 mg and/or EPA 22 mg daily, or (4) placebo. Two groups of 6- to 10-year-old schoolchildren were enrolled and classified as well nourished (a group in Adelaide, Australia; n = 396) or marginally nourished (a group in Jakarta, Indonesia; n = 384).[104] A total of 120 children completed the study. The micronutrient treatment resulted in significant increases in verbal learning and memory in the Australian group (estimated effect size: 0.23; 95% CI: 0.01–0.46), and a similar effect was observed among Indonesian girls (estimated effect size: 0.32; 95% CI: −0.01 to 0.64). No effects were found on tests measuring general intelligence or attention. No effects of DHA + EPA on the cognitive tests were observed.[104] Overall, the investigators concluded that micronutrient intervention can have beneficial effects on cognitive performance, even in well-nourished children. The failure of EPA and DHA to produce significant effects on cognitive function, especially in marginally nourished schoolchildren, may be accounted for by the very low combined dose of EPA and DHA in this study (DHA 88 mg and EPA 22 mg daily), compared with daily doses in the region of 1000 mg used in other supplementation trials.

Together, these 2 early reports on HUFA supplementation in healthy children provide preliminary evidence that DHA might result in increased activation of the dorsolateral prefrontal cortex, thus improving the functioning of cortical attentional networks, and improving reaction times. Micronutrients, including vitamins and minerals, may improve verbal memory and learning in healthy children, but might not improve attentional functions.

HUFA ABNORMALITIES IN ADHD

In children and adults with ADHD, abnormalities in fatty acid blood profiles have been reported,[66,69–73] but it is unclear whether the observed irregularities in omega-3 and omega-6 HUFAs are due to low dietary intakes of HUFAs in ADHD or an abnormality in HUFA metabolism.

For example, Stevens and colleagues[68] reported that in 6- to 12-year-old boys with ADHD, levels of both AA and DHA were significantly lower than in matched controls (n = 43); in addition, approximately 40% (n = 53) had excessive thirst and skin problems, which are classic signs of fatty acid deficiency from the animal literature. Combining the ADHD and controls and then classifying them into low or high omega-3 and omega-6 groups, the researchers found that lower omega-6 concentrations were associated with several signs of fatty acid deficiency, such as excessive thirst, skin problems, frequent urination, rough and dry skin/hair, frequent colds, and antibiotic use. The group with low omega-3 was also found to have learning and behavioral difficulties, such as hyperactive-impulsive behavior, anxiety, temper tantrums, and conduct disorder symptoms.[105]

Another study by Antalis and colleagues[66] compared 35 young adult males with ADHD with healthy controls, and found that the ADHD group had a higher total omega-6/omega-3 ratio (ie, the sum of total omega-6 over the total of omega-3) and a 36% higher ratio of AA/EPA in erythrocytes in comparison with the controls. Erythrocyte levels of AA were also approximately 10% greater in the ADHD group than in the control group. DHA levels were 53% lower in plasma and 36% lower in erythrocytes in the ADHD group in comparison with controls. An identical pattern was also observed for total omega-3 ratio. Plasma ALA levels were greater in the ADHD group, but all ALA metabolites were lower. Correlational analysis was conducted to assess the strength of the relationships between behavior and omega-3 fatty acid levels. The percentage of DHA in the phospholipid fraction of blood correlated with the ADHD symptoms (inattention $r = -0.47$, impulsivity/hyperactivity $r = -0.45$, and *Diagnostic and Statistical Manual of Mental Disorders,* 4th edition [DSM-IV] total ADHD scores $r = -0.047$). Similar trends were observed for total omega-3 fatty acid levels in both plasma phospholipids and erythrocytes. These findings suggest that lower omega-3 levels were associated with greater severity of ADHD-like symptoms.

Colter and colleagues[73] also assessed 11 adolescents with ADHD and 12 healthy controls for fatty acid levels and severity of behavioral symptoms. The ADHD group self-reported more checklist symptoms of fatty acid deficiency. Intake of both total fat and saturated fat was positively associated with scores of oppositional, problematic, and hyperactive behaviors. Adolescents with ADHD had lower blood concentrations of DHA and total omega-3 (ALA, DHA, EPA, and docosapentaenoic acid) levels, and higher levels of the omega-6 LA. DHA levels were negatively correlated and total omega-6 levels were significantly positively correlated with inattention, behavioral problems, oppositional behavior, restlessness, and total DSM-IV symptoms on Conners Parent Rating Scale (CPRS) scores. The diet records did not reveal any differences in total omega-3 fatty acid consumption, potentially suggesting that the lower DHA levels in ADHD may be due to higher oxidative metabolism rather than dietary intake.[73] Confounding variables in this study were group differences in vitamin and mineral supplementation (50% of the ADHD group, 25% of the controls) and in gender, which is relevant because males and females can differ in their metabolism of PUFAs.[106]

Researchers in Taiwan have examined 58 children (aged 4–12 years) with a clinical diagnosis of ADHD in a comparison with 52 controls. No differences were found in dietary patterns of the children with ADHD, except for higher intake of iron and vitamin C. The ADHD children were found to have lower LA, AA, and DHA fatty acid levels in red blood cells (and higher iron levels in their blood) compared with controls.[69]

Across these studies on HUFA abnormalities in ADHD, ADHD and ADHD behaviors in youth appear to be characterized by physical symptoms characteristic of essential fatty acid deficiency, low levels of DHA and other omega-3 HUFAs, and a high levels of omega-6 HUFAs. Patients with low DHA levels were associated with more severe symptoms of inattention and hyperactivity/impulsivity, the hallmark symptoms of ADHD, and showed more learning problems and symptoms of conduct disorder. Findings on AA and omega-6 levels were more mixed, but there was a suggestion that the omega-6/omega-3 ratio may be a marker for more ADHD symptoms. However, generalized essential fatty acid deficiencies are unlikely, as these subjects were replete with omega-6 LA. These studies raise the question of whether omega-3 fatty acid supplementation, even in the face of adequate omega-6 fatty acid levels, might ameliorate symptoms of ADHD and some associated physical signs of essential fatty acid insufficiency.

Most supplementation studies have used mixtures of omega-3 HUFAs and omega-6 GLA, making it difficult to isolate the potential effects of individual fatty acids. Some of the early research in children with ADHD focused on supplementation with DHA alone, and showed little or no therapeutic effect.[107,108] Other clinical trials that have investigated supplementation with evening primrose oil or formulas rich in omega-6 in children with ADHD have also reported little or no effect on ADHD.[109–111] Very few trials used comparable experimental designs, supplements, doses, or duration of supplementation, and most studies were not adequately powered, so their nonsignificant findings and wide variations in findings are often difficult to interpret.

Differential Effects of EPA and DHA in the Brain

Little is known about the biological role of EPA in the brain, especially regarding its impact on cognition and mood. There are some preliminary research studies reporting differential effects of EPA and DHA in relation to cognitive and emotional responses.[112,113]

Resting-state electroencephalogram
Sumich and colleagues[112] reported differential associations between DHA and EPA erythrocyte levels and electroencephalogram (EEG) components in children and adolescents with ADHD: DHA levels were associated with more rapid activity (alpha activity during eyes-open and beta activity during eyes-closed resting states), and EPA levels were associated with more slow activity (theta activity during both eyes-open and eyes-closed resting states). No associations were found with omega-6 HUFA levels. Alpha activity was found to be positively associated with performance for language fluency involving semantic memory, whereas theta activity was negatively associated with verbal memory performance.[112]

Emotion-elicited event-related potentials
Gow and colleagues[113] have reported the relationship between erythrocyte HUFA levels and event-related potential (ERP) responses to the presentation of happy, sad, and fearful faces during an emotional processing task in a small sample of adolescent boys with ADHD. The investigators created an ERP cognitive bias paradigm based on 2 premises: (1) Beck's theory of depression, which postulated that individuals with depression gravitate toward negative schema and stimuli; and (2) evidence suggesting that children with ADHD have difficulty correctly identifying the emotional expression of others, especially in relation to fear and anger.[114] The investigators therefore hypothesized that EPA (because of its association with regulating and improving mood) would be positively associated with a bias in the overt P300 response toward facial expressions of happiness relative to fear or sadness. The happy-fear cognitive bias was calculated by subtracting the midline frontal P300

amplitudes to fearful faces from those of happy faces (P300$_{H-F}$). A similar calculation was made for a happy-sad bias (P300$_{H-S}$). The findings showed there was a significant positive association between EPA levels and a cognitive bias oriented toward overt expressions of happiness, relative to both sad and fearful faces, as indexed by midline frontal P3 amplitude. By contrast, DHA levels were associated with the right temporal N170 response to fear.

Memory-related event-related potentials in healthy fish-eating children

To the best of the authors' knowledge, only one study has investigated HUFA status and ERPs in healthy children. Boucher and colleagues[115] examined the prenatal omega-3 fatty acid intake of the mothers of 154 children in the fish-eating Inuit community, and compared the cord plasma concentrations to the child's subsequent memory functioning evaluated at a mean age of 11.3 years. This prospective longitudinal study used neurophysiologic data (ERPs during a continuous visual recognition task) and neurobehavioral measures of memory (Wechsler Intelligence Scales for Children, 4th edition, and the California Learning Test Children's Version). Children with higher prenatal concentrations of DHA (as measured in cord plasma) displayed, at age 11, a shorter N4 ERP latency deflection and larger late positive component, which is a positive-directed ERP component derived from EEG recordings that is thought to be associated with recognition memory processes. Elevated DHA measures were related with enhanced N4 amplitudes, and positive associations were also observed between cord DHA and neurobehavioral performance on memory tasks.

Collectively, these 3 EEG studies provide preliminary evidence to suggest that EPA and DHA may be implicated in different functional roles related to features of cognitive and affect processing in ADHD.

Milte and colleagues[116] examined 75 children (ages 7–12 years) with symptoms of ADHD with or without learning difficulties in the context of a larger study. This study reports data only from the baseline time point (after controlling for covariates). Pearson correlational analysis examined associations between literacy (word reading, spelling, and vocabulary) and behavior (using the CPRS), and found that higher DHA (omega-3) predicted better word reading ($P<.001$) whereas higher omega-6 predicted poorer levels of reading, vocabulary, spelling, and attention.[116] Higher levels of total omega-6 and AA levels at baseline also predicted lower anxiety/shyness after 4 months. In a similar fashion, both increased levels of EPA and total omega-3 were associated with decreased anxiety/shyness. However, a key limitation of this study is that the correlation analyses were used with no statistical correction for multiple testing, so it is possible that these were spurious findings. The findings are provocative enough to warrant replication, using correction for multiple testing.

INDIVIDUAL HUFA SUPPLEMENTATION TRIALS IN YOUTH WITH ADHD OR ADHD-TYPE SYMPTOMS

Several dietary supplementation trials with omega-3 and omega-6 fatty acids have reported some improvement in ADHD symptoms, typically using either the parent-rated or teacher-rated Conners scales and/or the Clinical Global Impression (CGI) scales as primary outcomes.[74,76,78,117,118]

Omega-3/-6 in Relation to Learning, Behavior, and Motor Skills

The Oxford-Durham study (2005) was arguably the landmark study linking omega-3 or omega-6 supplementation to improvements in behavior and concentration in underachieving mainstream schoolchildren.[74] Although not primarily concerned with ADHD, this examination of ADHD-like symptoms in children was a pivotal study in this field. This placebo-controlled, double-blind, randomized clinical trial (RCT) examined 117 schoolchildren, aged 5 to 12 years, with untreated DSM-IV developmental coordination disorder (also known as dyspraxia, or informally as clumsiness). Although none of the children recruited had previously received a clinical diagnosis of ADHD, cognitive and behavioral ADHD-like symptoms are frequently associated with developmental coordination disorder, and 31% of the sample at baseline scored 2 standard deviations above the mean on the DSM-IV total score on the Conners Teacher Rating Scale (CTRS-L, which assessed each of 59 items of child behavior on a 4-point scale). The participants were treated with either fish oil (n = 60) or placebo (n = 57) for 3 months. The daily dose of 6 capsules provided a combination of omega-3 fatty acids (EPA 558 mg and DHA 174 mg) and omega-6 fatty acid GLA 60 mg, and vitamin E 9.6 mg (in the natural form, α-tocopherol). Placebo treatment consisted of olive-oil capsules, which were carefully matched to the active treatment in both appearance and flavor. After 3 months, the placebo group was crossed over to the active supplement, and the active group continued with active treatment, for another 3 months.[74] Outcome variables included learning, literacy (including word reading and spelling), motor skills, and teacher ratings of behavior linked to ADHD.

Fish-oil supplementation for 3 months did not improve motor skills in these children with developmental coordination disorder, but fish oil was found to produce significant improvements in reading, spelling, and ADHD-like symptoms. The mean achievement scores at baseline for reading and spelling were 1 year below chronologic age in both fish-oil and placebo groups. Compared with controls, the fish-oil group showed significant gains in reading age (9.5 $\pm$ 13.9 months vs 3.3 $\pm$ 6.7 months for placebo, z = 2.87; P<.004), gains in spelling age (6.0 $\pm$ 11.4 months vs 1.2 $\pm$ 5.0 months for placebo, z = 3.36; P<.001), and improved behavior (CTRS-L scores decreased from 75 $\pm$ 27 to 58 $\pm$ 28; P<.05) over 3 months of treatment. When the placebo group was crossed over to the active treatment they showed similar improvements, and the active group continued to improve up to the end of the 6-month trial. Improvements for those children continuing on active treatment between 3 and 6 months were characterized by a gain in reading age of 13.5 $\pm$ 11.9 months and a gain in spelling age of 6.2 $\pm$ 6.8 months. Those children in the active treatment group demonstrated improvements above their chronologic age (reading age gain 10.9 $\pm$ 11.8 months; spelling age gain 5.3 $\pm$ 6.9 months). The placebo-to-active crossover group demonstrated behavioral improvements in teacher ratings (CTRS-L global scales) at 6 months, comparable with those of the active group after 3 months.

The findings from the Oxford-Durham trial suggest that omega-3/-6 supplementation may help children with ADHD-like behavioral symptoms and educational difficulties associated with developmental coordination disorder.

RANDOMIZED, DOUBLE-BLIND, PLACEBO-CONTROLLED CLINICAL TRIALS IN SCHOOLCHILDREN

Other trials have attempted to replicate the findings of the Oxford-Durham study in either children with symptoms of ADHD or children with actual clinical diagnoses of ADHD, with less success. For example, in the well-known Adelaide trial, Sinn and Bryan[76] conducted a randomized, placebo-controlled, double-blind study of 7- to 12-year-olds who did not have a clinical diagnosis of ADHD but were entered into the study if they scored 2 standard deviations above the mean on the Conners Abbreviated ADHD Index.[76] These psychostimulant-free children were randomly allocated into 1 of 3 groups: (1) an active group (n = 41) who were given the same fish-oil supplements used in the Oxford-Durham trial but with an additional multivitamin/mineral supplement containing daily recommended amounts; (2) a fish-oil only group (n = 36); and (3) a placebo group (n = 27). There were no significant differences between any of the treatment groups on CTRS scores at either 15 or 30 weeks, but several differences were observed on the CPRS. Parent ratings at 15 weeks showed mostly moderate effect sizes in the 2 HUFA groups compared with placebo in 9 of 14 symptom subscales, including DSM-IV inattentive subscale (effect size: 0.61), Conners ADHD Index (effect size: 0.59), CPRS cognitive problems and inattention (effect size: 0.52), DSM-IV total (effect size: 0.49), Conners Global Index restless/impulsive (effect size: 0.45), Oppositional (effect size: 0.43), Conners Global total (effect size: 0.39), DSM-IV hyperactive/impulsive subscale (effect size: 0.20), and CPRS hyperactivity (effect size: 0.17). The effects on hyperactivity/impulsivity were statistically significant despite small effect sizes, especially in comparison with the larger effect sizes on cognitive measures. When the placebo group crossed over to the active fish oil plus micronutrient treatment at week 15, parent ratings showed additional significant improvements between weeks 15 and 30 (on 9 of 14 subscales), but once again no improvement was observed by the teachers. There were no significant differences in children treated with or without the supplemental micronutrients on parent or teacher ratings, suggesting that the therapeutic effects on ADHD were due to the fish oil, and that the vitamin-mineral supplementation did not add to the fish-oil effect. However, the doses of micronutrients were somewhat low (at or below recommended daily allowances), which may have accounted for the negative findings. The investigators interpreted the parent ratings as more reliable than the teacher ratings for several reasons, including: (1) a high teacher turnover, (2) classrooms being taught by different teachers on different days, (3) long vacations and service leaves, and (4) children moving to different schools during their enrollment in the study.

During the Adelaide trial, Sinn and colleagues[75] also conducted neuropsychological assessments of cognition in the same sample of children. In the HUFA-treated groups, significant improvements were observed in the ability to switch and control attention (as measured by the Creature Counting Task) at 15 weeks when compared with placebo (effect size: 0.43), and a similar change was seen in the placebo group after switching to active treatment between 15 and 30 weeks (effect size: 0.93; $P<.001$). The observed improvements in cognitive performance were found to mediate the parent-rated improvements in hyperactivity/impulsivity and attention scores. However, no significant improvements were noted in any other cognitive test in a large assessment battery.

In short, the Oxford-Durham study found that fish oil did not improve motor skills in children with developmental coordination disorder, but did improve reading, spelling, and ADHD-like symptoms such as inattention, hyperactivity, and oppositional behavior. The Adelaide trial, which was the replication by Sinn and colleagues in children with symptoms of ADHD, confirmed that fish oil improved both inattention and hyperactivity/impulsivity symptoms, but neuropsychological testing showed only very limited areas of cognitive improvement.

Johnson and colleagues[118] conducted a randomized, placebo-controlled clinical trial of 75 youths (8–18 years old, 64 boys) with ADHD (35 with the combined type and 40 with the inattentive type) to evaluate the efficacy of omega-3/-6 fish-oil supplementation in reducing core symptoms of ADHD, and to establish subtypes of responders based on a detailed evaluation of symptoms and comorbid problems. The study used the same formula and dose of fish oil, as well as the 1-way crossover (the placebo group was crossed over at 3 months into the active group for another 3 months) used in the Oxford-Durham and the Adelaide studies. There were 37 randomized to the active group and 38 to the placebo group. The investigators carried out a medical examination including psychiatrists' assessment of diagnosis and co-morbidity using DSM-IV criteria. The 2 primary outcome measures were the investigator-rated ADHD Rating Scale IV—Parent version (which has been validated as a clinician-rated parent interview to allow evaluation of symptom severity across different settings in addition to clinician's overall experience of the patients) and the CGI severity scales.[118] Overall the findings of this study were negative, with a lack of statistically significant differences in either of the outcome measures between active and placebo groups at 3 or 6 months. In a post hoc analysis of the diagnostic subtypes, a higher number of responders were found in the inattentive subtype group ($P = .03$) compared with the ADHD combined type group. The inattentive group was more likely to have a comorbid developmental disorder (eg, reading and writing disor-der, learning disability, or autistic traits). None of the responders had comorbid conduct disorder, oppositional defiant disorder, depression, or anxiety.[118] It is unclear why the subgroup of children with inattentive-type ADHD benefited from the omega-3/-6 intervention, but a similar pattern was observed in the Adelaide trial, warranting closer examination in future clinical trials of this potential finding of improved attention.

Omega-3/-6 Relation to Dyslexia

Richardson and Puri[78] conducted an earlier 12-week randomized, double-blind, pla-cebo-controlled study of 41 previously undiagnosed children (ages 8–12 years) with high ADHD symptom ratings (according to DSM-IV criteria) and specific learning dif-ficulties, including dyslexia.[78] The active treatment group (n = 22) received omega-3 (EPA 186 mg, DHA 480 mg) and omega-6 (GLA 96 mg, cis-LA 864 mg, AA 42 mg) HUFAs, vitamin E 60 IU, and thyme oil 8 mg; and the placebo group (n = 19) received olive oil. At the end of 12 weeks, the treatment group had significantly lower scores than the placebo group on inattention (effect size: 0.61) and a global behavioral scale (effect size: 0.58), but not on other measures. However, given the large number of measures, very few positive findings, lack of adequate power, and a questionable con-trol (the olive-oil placebo contained bioactive properties), it is unclear whether any firm conclusions can be drawn from this study.

Omega-3/-6 Studies Relating to Attention and Behavior

Stevens and colleagues[119] conducted a randomized, double-blind, placebo-controlled study with omega-3 or omega-6 HUFA supplementation in 50 children (ages 6–13 years) with either a clinical or suspected diagnosis of ADHD. The parents completed a fatty acid deficiency questionnaire, and children who were rated as hav-ing 4 or more symptoms of fatty acid deficiency were recruited for the study. The fatty acid deficiency questionnaire included thirst, frequent urination, dry hair, dandruff, dry skin, brittle nails, and follicular keratosis, which parents rated on a scale of 1 to 4; Ste-vens and colleagues[68] had previously used this questionnaire and found significantly higher scores ($P = .0009$) in an ADHD group in comparison with a control group. The children with both ADHD and fatty acid deficiency symptoms were randomized to receive either an active treatment (DHA 80 mg, EPA 80 mg, AA 40 mg, GLA 96 mg, and vitamin E 24 mg daily) or placebo (olive oil 6.4 mg) for 4 months. HUFA sup-plementation resulted in a 50% increase in plasma and erythrocyte levels of EPA, DHA, and vitamin E. HUFA treatment was significantly better than placebo on only 2 of 16 measures: parent-rated conduct problems (-42.7% vs -9.9%, n = 47; $P = .05$) and teacher-rated attention (-14.8% vs $+3.4\%$, n = 47; $P = .03$). There were significant correlations between higher EPA levels and reduced parent-rated disruptive behavior scores ($r = 0.38$, n = 31; $P \leq .05$) and, similarly, correlations between higher EPA or DHA levels with reduced teacher-rated disruptive behavior ($r = 0.49$, n = 24; $P \leq .05$).

Oppositional behavior scores also showed significant improvements. Although these findings were not strong, this study suggests that HUFA supplementation may improve both attention and behavior in children with ADHD or ADHD-like symptoms.

PHARMACOLOGIC INTERVENTION AND OMEGA-3 HUFAS FOR ADHD

There are few studies comparing omega-3 with standard pharmacologic treatment or exploring the plausibility of HUFAs as an adjunctive therapy for ADHD. Perera and colleagues[120] recruited 98 children (ages 6–12 years) whose parents reported that methylphenidate produced no improvement in either behavior or learning, and randomly assigned them to receive either an omega-3/-6 combination (fish oil 296 mg, evening primrose oil 181 mg) (n = 48) or placebo (n = 46) containing sunflower oil in an identical capsule. The children continued their methylphenidate treatment (0.7–1.0 mg/kg/d) and home-/school-based behavioral interventions throughout the 6-month study period. Both treatment groups also took unspecified micronutrients to guard against any other potential deficiencies. HUFA treatment improved parent ratings of both ADHD behavior symptoms (aggressiveness, fighting, restlessness, inattention, easy anger, impulsiveness waiting for turn, cooperation) and learning (completing work, academic performance) more than placebo in 5 of 11 measurements at 3 months and in all 11 measurements at 6 months. However, HUFA treatment did not improve distractibility scores. The largest significant improvements in behavior were reported for aggressiveness (effect size: 0.98) and restlessness (effect size: 1.11).

Harding and colleagues[121] recruited 20 children (ages 7–12 years) with a clinical diagnosis of ADHD and nonrandomly allocated them (by parental choice) to methylphenidate (n = 10) or a dietary supplementation (n = 10) consisting of essential fatty acids, vitamins, minerals, amino acids, phospholipids, probiotics, and phytonutrients for a period of 4 weeks. Mean daily doses of methylphenidate were not reported, and parent ratings were collected but not reported. A nonstandard continuous performance test was used. No differences were found between methylphenidate and the dietary supplementation, and the investigators inferred that the dietary supplementation and methylphenidate were equivalent in effectiveness. However, because there was no placebo group, it is possible that the nonstandard continuous performance testing was unable to measure any clinical change, even by the methylphenidate. This small open-label study does not permit any inferences about effectiveness.

META-ANALYSES AND REVIEWS OF CLINICAL EFFICACY OF OMEGA-3 HUFAS IN ADHD

To examine the clinical efficacy of omega-3 and omega-6 interventions in child ADHD, Bloch and Qawasmi[122] conducted a recent meta-analysis of 10 well-designed trials involving 699 children. To represent effects sizes, the standard mean difference (SMD) was chosen as the summary statistic for meta-analysis, and calculated by pooling the standardized mean improvement of each study using RevMan 5 (The Cochrane Collaboration). The exact methodology was applied for the secondary analysis to test the effect of omega-3 HUFAs on symptoms of inattention and hyperactivity/impulsivity independently.

This meta-analysis found that omega-3 supplementation had a small but statistically and clinically significant effect on the treatment of ADHD (effect size SMD = 0.31, 95% CI 0.16–0.47, z = 4.04; $P \leq .001$). The meta-analysis also demonstrated similar effect sizes of omega-3 supplementation in the treatment of both the inattention (SMD = 0.29, 95% CI 0.07–0.50, z = 2.63; $P \leq .009$) and hyperactivity/impulsivity symptom clusters (SMD = 0.23, 95% CI 0.07–0.40, z = 2.78; $P \leq .005$). When the different omega-3 fatty acids were considered separately, higher doses of EPA (which collectively ranged from 80 to 750 mg daily), in comparison with ALA and DHA, were significantly but modestly correlated with omega-3 efficacy in the treatment of ADHD ($\beta = 0.36$, 95% CI 0.01–0.72, $t = 2.30$; $P = .04$, $R^2 = 0.37$).[122] Doses of other omega-3 HUFAs such as DHA and ALA were not significantly related to efficacy (DHA: $\beta = 0.24$, 95% CI 0.54–1.02, $t = 0.70$, $P = .50$; ALA: $\beta = -1.71$, 95% CI -4.62 to 1.19, $t = -1.33$, $P = .22$). The effect size of 0.2 to 0.3 for omega-3 fatty acid supplementation was modest in comparison with standard pharmacologic interventions for ADHD: The effect size for psychostimulants is approximately 0.8 (where 0.2–0.3 is small, 0.3–0.5 is medium, and 0.6–0.8 or more is large).

Bloch and Qawasmi[122] raised a critical point regarding adequate power and sample size, noting that to have sufficient power ($\beta = 80\%$, 2-tailed $\alpha = 0.05$) to detect a significant benefit (effect size of 0.31), clinical trials of omega-3 intervention compared with a placebo would need a sample size of approximately 330 children. Therefore, the actual sample sizes in the clinical trials to date are considerably underpowered and are likely to account for the inconsistent findings in the literature to date. Taking into consideration the relatively mild side-effect profile, the investigators concluded that it may be reasonable to use omega-3 fatty acid supplementation to augment traditional pharmacologic interventions or to treat youth whose families decline other psychopharmacologic options, despite the evidence of only moderate efficacy.[122]

In summary, these clinical studies have been criticized by reviewers, such as the Cochrane Collaboration, as both inconsistent and fragmentary.[123] This article has reviewed several randomized, placebo-controlled, double-blind trials, and open-label or pilot studies, of omega-3 supplementation in child literature. The authors recognize the wide variation in design and methodological issues, as well as a range of formulations, doses, and durations of supplementation: All of these factors have implications for interpretation and replication. Some improvements in behavior, concentration, and literacy have been reported following supplementation with HUFA in various populations, including underachieving mainstream schoolchildren with developmental coordination disorder and associated ADHD-like symptoms,[74] community samples of children with ADHD symptoms,[75,76] and youth with verified clinical diagnoses of ADHD.[120] The neurophysiologic and imaging research on HUFAs in children is extremely limited,[77,105–107] with only 2 studies on ADHD. Some evidence suggests abnormal erythrocyte fatty acid levels in children and young adults with ADHD.[66,69–73] To the best of the authors' knowledge, there are no published HUFA supplementation trials in adults with ADHD. Despite several reports of HUFA benefits for symptoms of ADHD in children, 5 trials have found little or no effect.[107–111] The recent meta-analysis by Bloch and Qawasmi,[122] which found some efficacy of EPA in improving ADHD symptoms in children, highlighted the valid point that available studies have small sample sizes and lack the statistical power to demonstrate a substantive effect size.

Future recommendations include carefully designed clinical trials with longer supplementation periods (ie, 6 months or more) and adequate sample sizes conducted in both children and adults with ADHD. Sensitive measures, such as event-related potentials combined with fMRI (owing to their temporal and spatial precision, respectively) may be better suited to capture changes in cortical function.

HUFAS AND YOUTH WITH AGGRESSIVE OR CONDUCT-DISORDERED RELATED BEHAVIORS

In addition to the putative role of HUFAs in ADHD, there is accumulating evidence that omega-3 HUFA and other micronutrient (vitamins and minerals) deficits may also be linked to antisocial and aggressive behaviors.[124–128] Given the comorbidity of conduct disorder in ADHD and the overrepresentation of ADHD in incarcerated adults,[129] the use of HUFAs for treating aggressive and delinquent behaviors deserves serious examination.

In a recent clinical study, Gow and colleagues[130] recruited a sample of 29 male adolescents (ages 12–16 years) with ADHD, and found a significant association between low EPA levels and high scores of callous-unemotional traits ($r = -0.597$, $P = .009$), as assessed by the Inventory of Callous-Unemotional Traits.[131,132] The ADHD group also showed correlations between high callous-unemotional scores and oppositional behaviors (CPRS subscale: $r = 0.464$, $P = .011$) and low total omega-3 levels ($r = -0.498$, $P = .027$). Though not quite statistically significant, the ADHD group also showed a trend toward a correlation between low DHA levels and high callous-unemotional scores ($r = -0.436$, $P = .054$) and a trend toward an association of low total omega-3 levels and antisocial behaviors (measured by the Antisocial Process Screening Device). This study suggests a link between low levels of EPA and high callous-unemotional behavior related to conduct disorder in male children with ADHD. Callous-unemotional personality traits are known to represent a distinct developmental vulnerability to persistent antisocial behavior.[133,134] Further research is needed to investigate whether early intervention with EPA may benefit youth with callous-unemotional traits, and help prevent the subsequent emergence of conduct disorder.

HUFAs and Young Adult Prisoners

Gesch and colleagues[124] conducted a randomized, double-blind, placebo-controlled trial on the effects of combined supplementation of HUFAs and micronutrients in a population of 231 young adult prisoners (ages ≥18 years) treated for a minimum of 2 weeks (mean duration 142 days). The nutrient supplementation consisted of LA 1260 mg, GLA 160 mg, EPA 80 mg, DHA 44 mg daily, and a broad spectrum of vitamins and minerals at recommended daily levels. The results revealed that nutrient supplementation (N = 172) at routine low daily doses produced a marked reduction (35%–37% vs 7%–10% in the placebo group) in antisocial behavior and violent offenses for the active group in comparison with baseline. This landmark study demonstrated that a nutrient supplement combining HUFAs and micronutrients can have a pronounced effect on the problem behaviors in a prison population of young adults (≥18 years). This study is instructional in showing that nutritional supplementation can affect major antisocial and aggressive behaviors, but does not isolate the role of HUFAs in producing this benefit. The findings of Gesch and colleagues[124] were later replicated and confirmed in a randomized controlled trial in the Netherlands of 221 young adult prisoners (mean age 21.0, range 18–25 years) who received comparable nutritional supplementation (N = 115) over a period of 1 to 3 months.[135] This study produced similar findings of a nearly 30% reduction in major behavioral and conduct incidents.[135]

The efficacy of nutritional supplementation, especially the combination of HUFAs with vitamins and minerals at routine doses, in producing relatively rapid reductions in major misconduct has now been shown in these 2 large randomized, double-blind, placebo-controlled studies in young adult prisoners. Future studies of HUFA and micronutrient supplementation in prison populations could assess for comorbid ADHD and mood disorders, and thus determine whether HUFAs produce a direct effect on conduct and aggression or whether the observed HUFA effects are mediated by improvements in ADHD or mood. These findings highlight the critical importance of nutrition and the potentially powerful impact that simple dietary interventions involving HUFAs (and micronutrients) can have in improving antisocial and major misbehavior in young adult prisoners. However, more clinical research is needed in youth with ADHD and/or comorbid conduct disorder to establish whether HUFAs with or without micronutrients may be a safe and effective intervention in youth at risk for the development of more serious delinquent, violent, and criminal behaviors.

OMEGA-3 HUFA SUPPLEMENTATION TRIALS IN YOUTH AND ADULTS WITH DEPRESSION

Several lines of evidence in adults support the notion that low omega-3 HUFA deficits are associated with depression and that omega-3 HUFA supplementation can treat depression.[77,136,137] Other ecologic studies by the authors' research group on negative affect in adult populations are informative, but do not establish causation because of their correlational nature.[138–140] For example, a cross-national ecologic study reported a highly significant association between low seafood consumption and low maternal milk DHA composition, with a 50-fold greater risk for postpartum depression ($r = -0.81$, $P = .0001$).[140] More broadly, in comparing countries with the lowest and highest consumption of seafood, low omega-3 HUFA intake is associated with a 65-fold higher lifetime risk for depression ($r = -0.84$, $P = .0001$),[141] a 30-fold higher risk for bipolar disorder ($r = -0.80$, $P = .0003$),[142] and a 10-fold higher risk for death from homicide ($r = -0.63$, $P = .0006$).[143]

Dietary Intake in Youth with Depressive Symptoms

Only one study provides comparable data in youth. A cross-sectional study evaluated dietary intake data from food-frequency questionnaires among 3067 boys and 3450 girls (ages 12–15 years) in relation to their depression rating scores using the Center for Epidemiologic Studies Depression Scale.[144] Boys with depressive symptoms had a lower mean value of EPA, DHA, vitamin B_6, and folate. It is uncertain why this was not observed in girls, but possibilities include a greater heterogeneity of contributing causes to girls' depressive symptoms or a more efficient endogenous conversion of ALA to EPA among females in comparison with males.[106] For girls, higher intake of B vitamins was positively associated with EPA and DHA intake. Fewer depressive symptoms also appeared to be associated with higher dietary intakes of riboflavin (in girls), folate, pyridoxine (vitamin B_6), and (in girls) riboflavin (but not with vitamin B_{12}). In girls, but not in boys, higher riboflavin intakes were associated with fewer depressive symptoms (odds ratio 0.85, 95% CI 0.67–108; P for trend = .03). In boys and girls, higher folate and pyridoxine (vitamin B_6) intakes were associated with lower risk for depressive symptoms. No clear association was seen with vitamin B_{12} intake.[144] These findings suggest that lower EPA and DHA levels are associated with depressive symptoms in boys but not girls, and that combined vitamins and mineral status may be important than HUFAs in preventing depressive symptoms in youth. In another study, an apparent association between HUFAs and depression scores in an adolescent population disappeared after adjusting for lifestyle confounders.[145]

Omega-3 in Children with Depression

The only randomized, double-blind, placebo-controlled monotherapy study thus far to investigate omega-3 HUFAs in child depression was conducted by Nemets and colleagues.[77] These researchers examined omega-3 HUFAs (EPA 400 mg and DHA 200 mg daily) in 20 children (ages 6–12 years) who completed at least a 1-month trial and were treated for a total of 16 weeks. The findings reported strong statistically significant effects of omega-3 fatty acids. By week 8, omega-3 HUFA treatment was superior to placebo (olive oil) on several depression scales: Greater than 50% reductions in Childhood Depression Rating Scale (CDRS) scores were observed in 7 of 10 children treated with omega-3 HUFAs and in none of the 10 placebo-treated children ($P = .003$,

Fisher exact test); and remission (CDRS score of <29 at the study end point) was observed in 4 of the omega-3 HUFA-treated children (P>.05). Further research in children and adolescents is needed with larger sample sizes to pursue this promising lead.

Omega-3 in Adults with Depression

Studies in adult depression have examined the use of omega-3 HUFAs as monotherapy or adjunctive therapy.[146–148] In addition, several meta-analyses and review articles have evaluated the efficacy of omega-3 HUFAs in reducing depressive symptoms.[148–154] The overall conclusion is that, much as reported in the ADHD literature, significant heterogeneity is reported in the omega-3 HUFA formulation, depression severity, experimental design, and study populations in most of these studies.[149] In these studies, only preparations containing more than 50% EPA appear to be consistently effective.[151,154,155] Another source of heterogeneity in several meta-analyses may be the inclusion of negative trials of subjects without clinically significant depression; the severity of depressive symptoms at study entry is a major determinant of the ability to detect efficacy of any antidepressant treatment.[156] Meta-analyses of omega-3 HUFA trials that distinguish clinical and nonclinical populations report antidepressant effects among those subjects who have significant depressive symptoms.[153] Given the heterogeneity in design and dose formulation, it is difficult to determine whether omega-3 fatty acids are effective as monotherapies alone or only as adjunctive therapies in treating major depression.

Ultimately, monotherapy with omega-3 HUFAs may be attractive for child and adolescent populations in view of their general health benefits, low side-effect profile, and reports of efficacy in treatment-resistant depression, but caution should be exercised, as data are insufficient to support a recommendation for treating major depression in youth.

Omega-3 and Suicide

Several studies in adults suggest that omega-3 HUFAs might have some clinical value in reducing suicidal thinking and attempts.[157,158] Sublette and colleagues[159,160] demonstrated that low levels of DHA plasma strongly predicted future suicide risk, and were associated with both hyperfunction of the limbic forebrain and hypofunction of the parietal and temporal cortex. In a case-control study of 1600 active-duty US Military personnel, low DHA status was a significant risk factor for suicide death.[158] All US Military personnel in this study had low omega-3 HUFA levels in comparison with North American, Australian, Mediterranean, Chinese, and other Asian civilian populations. These military personnel had a significantly higher odds of a suicide attempt (odds ratio 4.8, 95% CI 1.7–14.3; P<.0003) compared with the highest quartile[161] of the Chinese population. In view of these promising data in adults, a $10 million trial on the efficacy of omega-3 HUFAs (4 g daily) for the prevention of significant suicidal behaviors among US Military veterans is currently being conducted at the Medical College of South Carolina; it is being conducted in collaboration with the National Institute on Alcohol Abuse and Alcoholism (NIAAA), and funded by the Defense Medical Research Program at the US Department of Defense. To the best of the authors' knowledge, no trials of omega-3 fatty acids in relation to attempted suicide have yet been conducted in youth.

OMEGA-3 HUFA AND PREVENTION OF PSYCHOSIS IN HIGH-RISK YOUTH

Among the most interesting new developments is the potential for omega-3 HUFA treatment to prevent adolescents at high risk for psychosis from transitioning to schizophrenia. In a study of 81 adolescents at ultra-high risk for psychotic disorder,[162] participants were randomized to omega-3 PUFA (1.2 g daily) or placebo for a 12-week active intervention period, followed by a 40-week monitoring period. At the end of the 12-month study, transition to a psychotic disorder occurred in only 2 of 41 individuals (4.9%) in the omega-3 group, but in 11 of 40 (27.5%) in the placebo group ($P = .007$). For example, the reduction in transition to psychosis was reduced by 22.6% in that 12-month period (95% CI 4.8–40.4). The omega-3 HUFA intervention significantly reduced positive symptoms ($P = .01$), negative symptoms ($P = .02$), and general symptoms ($P = .01$), and improved functioning ($P = .002$) in comparison with the placebo group. Changes in intracellular phospholipase A_2 (PLA_2) activity (key enzymes in phospholipid metabolism that release fatty acids from the second carbon group of glycerol) and erythrocyte membrane fatty acids comparing the omega-3 HUFAs and placebo groups were investigated as a potential mechanism of action. The levels of membrane omega-3 and omega-6 PUFAs, and PLA_2 (from pre- to post-treatment) were significantly related to functional improvement, as indicated by increased Global Assessment of Functioning scores between baseline and the study end point at 12 weeks. Supplementation with omega-3 PUFA also resulted in a significant decrease in PLA_2 activity. This study is the first to demonstrate that a 12-week intervention trial with omega-3 fatty acids significantly reduced the transition rate from the prodromal stage to psychosis, and furthermore resulted in significant functional and symptomatic improvements during the entire follow-up period of 12 months.[162] Replication of these findings is currently being attempted in a multinational multisite trial.

CLINICAL RECOMMENDATIONS IN RELATION TO HUFAS

Clinicians can currently be guided by the 2006 treatment recommendations of a subcommittee of the Committee on Research on Psychiatric Treatments of the American Psychiatric Association that adults with major depression and other psychiatric illnesses should minimally consume 1 g daily of omega-3 HUFAs or consume seafood 2 to 3 times per week, if only because these patients are at high risk for cardiovascular and other medical illnesses.[148] In a more recent 2010 report of the Task Force on Complementary and Alternative Medicine of the American Psychiatric Association,[120] certain alternative treatments for adults with major depressive disorder showed promising results, such as omega-3 fatty acids, hypericum (St John's wort), S-adenosyl-L-methionine (SAMe), folate, acupuncture, mindfulness psychotherapies, light therapy, and exercise. In relation to omega-3 fatty acids, this review recommended that more research is necessary to clarify whether EPA is more effective than EPA plus DHA, optimum doses, and the value of fresh fish intake versus capsules. It also highlighted the need for preventive studies and the evaluation of omega-3 as a treatment intervention in recurrent major depressive disorder both as an adjunct and monotherapy. The American Psychiatric Association report also highlighted concerns about confounding variables, such as smoking (which can inhibit absorption of omega-3s into red blood cells) and methods to control for total omega-3 intake obtained from the diet in research trials.[120]

CAUTIONARY FINDINGS ON OMEGA-3 SUPPLEMENTATION

Not all research is clear-cut, of course, and negative findings can be as important and insightful as positive outcomes. Several studies that have investigated HUFAs in behavior, ADHD symptoms, school attendance, and physical aggression in youth have reported little or no effect of omega-3 supplementation.[107–111]

Hirayama and colleagues[108] conducted a randomized, double-blind, placebo-controlled study in 40 children (aged 6–12 years) with ADHD who were placed on a specific diet (fermented soybean milk, steamed bread, and bread rolls) that was fortified with either fish oil (n = 20, containing DHA 514 mg daily) or placebo (n = 20, olive oil 1300 mg daily). At baseline and 2 months later, measurements were obtained of DSM-IV ADHD symptoms (hyperactivity, impulsivity, inattention), aggression (reported by teachers and parents), visual perception, visual and auditory short-term memory, visual-motor integration, a continuous performance task measuring sustained attention, and impatience. After 2 months of treatment, the DHA treatment group did not improve on any ratings of ADHD-related symptoms in comparison with the olive-oil group. In fact, the DHA group showed significantly less improvement on commission errors on the continuous performance test (a marker of impulsivity) and on visual short-term memory. These negative results highlight several methodological issues:

- The selection of fatty acid supplement. Although the dose of DHA was moderate, previous studies using DHA-rich oils have also been found to be ineffective at improving cognitive functioning and ADHD-type symptoms. It seems that DHA alone may not be effective in ameliorating ADHD symptoms. The dose of EPA (100 mg daily) in the fish-oil group was extremely low and unlikely to have any noticeable effect.
- Choice of placebo. Olive oil is bioactive, with known anti-inflammatory and antioxidant effects, so its use as a control treatment is questionable. There was no indication of the amount of DHA or EPA that was received by the placebo-treated group in their fortified diet or olive oil.
- Bioavailability of the fatty acids. Arguably the fortification process may have lowered the bioavailability of the fatty acids, whereas a direct source of HUFAs would be more potent.
- Short duration of treatment. Without knowing the presupplementation levels of blood fatty acids, it is difficult to know whether a trial longer than 2 months was needed to correct a nutrient deficiency.
- There is such wide variation of EPA and DHA that researchers would be advised to measure it in finger-prick blood tests so as to allocate a more appropriate dose.

Itomura and colleagues[163] conducted a randomized, double-blind, placebo-controlled trial to test whether fish oil could reduce aggression in a normative population of 166 schoolchildren (ages 9–12 years). Similarly to the study by Hirayama and colleagues,[108] the participants were randomized to receive fortified foods with fish oil (bread, sausage, and spaghetti containing DHA 514 mg plus EPA 120 mg daily) or placebo (n = 83) for 3 months. A self-rated questionnaire did not identify an effect of fish oil on physical aggression (although physical aggression ratings increased in girls in the control sample). When aggressive tendencies were assessed by psychological testing, fish oil had the unexpected effect of appearing to increase aggressive responses, whereas the controls remained unchanged. When DSM-IV ADHD behavioral impulsivity symptoms were assessed by parents, fish oil appeared to reduce impulsivity in girls (relative to controls) but not in boys. The findings paint a somewhat mixed and confusing picture, and suggest a variety of methodological problems, especially in the assessment instruments, in addition to the questions raised by the Hirayama study. Furthermore, in this study the investigators mention that a control sausage contained EPA 40 mg and DHA 80 mg, but clearly control foods should not have contained any of the active omega-3 intervention at all. Otherwise, this means that the placebo was not a true placebo, a problem that was not adequately discussed by the investigators. Furthermore, both groups received the omega-6 LA

(514–1114 mg daily). The addition of LA in the fish oil group is a major confounder, because omega-3 and omega-6 compete for incorporation into the red blood cells, and a higher amount of one would suppress the absorption of the other. In this case, omega-6 would have likely been the dominant fatty acid in the diet.

Both of these studies are extremely problematic from a methodological point of view, so it is difficult to know how seriously to accept their somewhat contraintuitive and inconsistent findings; nevertheless they are mentioned here, mainly for completeness.

A final study by Hamazaki and colleagues[164] examined the effects of DHA-rich fish oil on behavior and school attendance in a randomized, double-blind, placebo-controlled trial in schoolchildren (aged 9–12 years) in Indonesia, who received either omega-3 supplementation (DHA 650 mg and EPA 100 mg, n = 116) or placebo (soybean oil capsules, n = 117). Omega-3 supplementation did not appear to improve measures of aggression or impulsivity relative to placebo treatments. However, interestingly school absenteeism appeared to be reduced in the children treated with DHA-rich fish oil relative to the control group (odds ratio 0.40, 95% CI 0.23–0.71; $P = .002$). Although the effects of nutritional supplementation on endemic diseases might conceivably have been a mediating factor, this particular finding warrants further exploration because school absenteeism is often linked with depression and anxiety in Western populations.

Collectively, these studies suggest that DHA-rich formulas show little or no effect in improving aggressive behaviors, ADHD symptoms, or cognitive performance, although these studies are particularly problematic from a methodological point of view. The fortified food studies seemed the least promising, and it is probably preferable to use more directly quantifiable sources of omega-3 fatty acids. Moreover, it may be speculated that a higher EPA-to-DHA ratio is needed for treating schoolchildren, consistent with the findings of a recent meta-analysis suggesting that higher EPA is associated with better clinical efficacy in improving symptoms of ADHD-type behavior.[122] More research is needed to answer these basic questions about dose and formulation in child populations.

SAFETY AND ADVERSE EFFECTS

Omega-3 supplementation is considered to be a safe intervention by the FDA, which currently advises that dietary dosage of up to 3 g daily of omega-3 fatty acids from marine sources are "Generally Recognized as Safe" (GRAS). The European Food Safety Authority has set a safe upper limit of 5 g daily for total omega-3 fatty acids, including DHA, EPA, and docosapentaenoic acid. These standards are set for adults, with no separate designations for children or adolescents.

At present, there is no established procedural system for reporting adverse events of food supplements, so systematically collected information is not available on a national scale. Several omega-3 products have been approved by the FDA for marketing in the United States as medications rather than as food supplements, and the manufacturing companies have reported mostly minor but some severe side effects. In addition, there is some information about adverse effects from clinical research trials, some of which use relatively higher omega-3 dosing regimens. Given the lack of systematic data, the monitoring of adverse effects in research and clinical settings should receive higher prioritization. Nonetheless, some general observations on adverse effects can be made (**Table 1**).

Omega-3 fatty acids can increase the incidence of excessive bleeding, including gastrointestinal bleeding and even hemorrhagic stroke. For patients who are

Table 1 Potential adverse effects of omega-3 HUFA supplementation	
Common (1%–10%)	Dyspepsia, nausea, diarrhea, increased bleeding
Uncommon (0.1%–1%)	Gastrointestinal symptoms, upper abdominal pain, allergic hypersensitivity, dizziness, headache, increased low-density lipoprotein levels, increased alanine aminotransferase levels, mania, depression
Rare (1/1000 to 1/10,000)	Hyperglycemia, headache, gastrointestinal pain, hepatotoxicity, acne, pruritic rash, ventricular tachycardia
Very rare (<1/10,000)	Hypotension, urticaria, nasal dryness, gastrointestinal hemorrhage, hemorrhagic stroke, increased blood lactate dehydrogenase, hemolytic anemia

Frequency figures are estimates for the general population, and certain individuals may be especially vulnerable based on their medical status, concurrent medication usage, and other individual factors.

anticipating surgery, it is advisable to ensure that surgeons are aware of when their patients are consuming HUFAs, because many surgeons will want to discontinue their use 3 to 7 days before surgery, depending on the type of surgery.

Gastrointestinal effects of omega-3 fatty acids are common, and may include loose stools, diarrhea, nausea, vomiting, and reduced appetite; some of these adverse effects may be mitigated by administration with meals or more gradual dose elevation. Omega-3 HUFAs may have hepatoprotective properties, and have been used to treat nonalcoholic fatty liver disease; however, there have been reports of increased liver transaminases (mainly alanine aminotransferase).

Short-term memory loss and headache have been reported, although increasing the EPA-to-DHA ratio has been reported to be a possible treatment for headache.[165]

Chronic treatment with HUFAs can cause vitamin E deficiency, so many clinicians provide advice about concurrent supplementation with vitamin E, especially at higher HUFA doses. Moreover, many commercial HUFA products include vitamin E as a preservative to reduce oxidation.

Many patients object to the fishy odor of some products, a result of the vulnerability of fatty acids to oxidation, which is especially problematic when weak manufacturing processes are used. High-quality preparations are also recommended to reduce the risks of exposure to potential contaminants, including mercury, dioxins, and polychlorinated biphenyls, although many products are now manufactured in accordance with WHO standards, which call for methods to reduce contaminants.

It should be emphasized that most data on the adverse effects of omega-3 HUFAs are derived from observations on adults, and the side-effect profile might be somewhat different in children and adolescents.

SUMMARY

Western diets can lead to imbalances in HUFA metabolism and alter molecular substrates in the brain. Omega-3 insufficiency and omega-6 excess can have particularly important effects on brain development, structure, and functioning. Malnutrition and inadequate nutrient intakes are well-established risk factors for both impaired cognitive development and adverse behavioral outcomes.

The case for nutritional intervention to reduce the burden of ADHD, aggressive and delinquent behaviors, and, possibly, major depressive disorder in youth is promising, but the research data at present are mainly suggestive. In adults, omega-3 HUFA supplementation is an inexpensive and safe adjunctive treatment for reducing symptom severity in mood disorders[146,166] and depression.[147] The role of omega-3 in adults with ADHD has not yet been investigated, but current research efforts are being undertaken by the authors' research team in the Section of Nutritional Neurosciences at the National Institutes of Health.

In applying the early intervention research to clinical practice, it is notable that omega-3 HUFAs are considered GRAS by the FDA in doses up to 3 g daily for adults, with no added specifications concerning children. This designation does not indicate that higher levels are unsafe, but rather that most cardiovascular and other health benefits are likely to have been achieved by that level of intake.

The American Psychiatric Association has recommended at least 1 g daily of omega-3 fatty acids, based on likely benefits for patients with certain psychiatric conditions as well as its more general medical benefits, but it has offered no specific recommendations for youth.[148] International guidelines recommend the consumption of a minimum of dose of 200 mg of DHA daily for pregnant and lactating women[167] to support the developing nervous system, but the authors are not aware of similar recommendations for children and adolescents. The *Dietary Guidelines for Americans, 2010* recommend consumption of seafood 2 to 3 times per week for children.[1] For children who refuse to eat fish, dietary supplements, fortified foods, or smoothie drinks may be more feasible sources to ensure daily recommended allowances.

In selecting a particular formulation of omega-3 fatty acids, clinicians should be aware that there are marked differences in quality among manufacturers. Total concentrations and ratios of omega-3 HUFAs vary widely across commercially available products (**Table 2**). In old, spoiled, or poorly manufactured products, oxidized omega

Table 2
Contents and ratios of omega-3 HUFAs vary widely across commercially available products

Total Oils in Capsules/ Serving	Total Omega-3 HUFA (mg)	EPA (mg)	DHA (mg)	% of EPA in Total Omega-3 HUFA	No. of Capsules Needed to Deliver HUFA at 2 g Daily	Daily Cost
Unconcentrated fish oil (1000 mg capsules)	300	120	180	40	7 caps	$
Molecularly distilled (1000 mg capsules)	500	300	200	60	4 caps	$$
Highly purified (1100 mg capsules)	1000	600	400	60	2 caps	$$$
Algal oils (625 mg capsules)	500	180	320	36	4 caps	$$$
Algal oils (500 mg capsules)	200	0	200	~100	10 caps	$$$
Liquid oil (highly concentrated) (1 teaspoon = 5 mL)	2510	1450	1060	58	3/4 teaspoon	$$
Emulsion (highly concentrated) (15 mL serving)	1500	910	590	60	20 mL (1.25 tablespoons)	$$$
Sardines, canned in oil (3.75 oz [106.3 g])	921	435	486	47	2 cans	$
Salmon, Atlantic, farmed, broiled (3 oz [85 g])	1824	586	1238	32	3.3 oz (93.5 g)	$$
White tuna, canned (3 oz [85 g])	733	198	535	27	8 oz (227 g)	$
Omega-3 eggs (1 egg, 50 g)	130	5	125	4	15 eggs	$

Box 1
Explanation of modified US Preventive Services Task Force (USPSTF) grading system used in Tables 3 and 4

Tables 3 and 4 use a modified form of the USPSTF system

Each treatment is assigned a grade for "Quality of Evidence" and a grade for "Strength of Recommendations"

The Quality of Evidence grade is a qualitative ranking of the strength of the published evidence in the medical literature regarding a treatment:

- Good: Consistent benefit in well-conducted studies in different populations
- Fair: Data show positive effects, but weak, limited, or indirect evidence
- Poor: Cannot show benefit owing to data weakness

The Strength of Recommendations grade provides a qualitative ranking of the clinical recommendations that can be drawn from findings of the studies:

- Insufficient data
- Recommend against: Fair evidence of ineffectiveness or harm
- Neutral: Fair evidence for, but appears risky
- Recommend: Fair evidence of benefit and safety
- Recommend strongly: Good evidence of benefit and safety

Adapted from U.S. Preventive Services Task Force Grade Definitions. May 2008. Available at: http://www.uspreventiveservicestaskforce.org/uspstf/grades.htm. Accessed February 26, 2014.

fatty acid HUFAs smell strongly of adverse fish odors. Fresh preparations have a clean smell akin to fresh seafood, unless masked by other natural flavors such as lemon, lime, or strawberry, and are more desirable to consume. Naturally flavored emulsions or capsules may also be beneficial to children or adults with olfactory neurosensory issues. In addition, honey placed on broiled salmon (or any fish) may increase the likelihood of consumption by children.

Owing to the small number of well-powered trials in adults and youth, more research is needed to better determine the optimal ratios and doses of EPA and DHA. Most studies indicate that symptom improvement in adults with depression and youth with ADHD symptoms is more likely using preparations containing higher levels of

Table 3
Evidence-based treatment evaluations derived from the medical literature (quality of evidence/strength of recommendations for each treatment and indication)

	EPA Alone	DHA Alone	Fish Oil
ADHD	Good/Recommend	Insufficient data	Fair/Recommend
Depression	Fair/Recommend	Poor/Insufficient data	Fair/Recommend
Aggression/Defiance	Fair/Insufficient data	Insufficient data	Fair/Recommend
Cognitive parameters	Fair/Insufficient data	Insufficient data	Good/Recommend
Dyspraxia	Insufficient data	Insufficient data	Good/Recommend
Basis for ADHD in youth	Multiple RCTs	Multiple RCTs	Meta-analyses

Levels of evidence based on US Preventive Services Task Force: http://www.uspreventiveservicestask force.org.

Table 4
Expert clinical opinion regarding HUFA treatment of ADHD (quality of evidence/Strength of recommendations for each treatment and indication)

Treatment	ADHD	Opinion
EPA >60%	Good/Recommend	Effects are consistent, but not as large as stimulant medications
DHA >60%	Insufficient data	Case reports for decreased anxiety and disruptive behaviors are encouraging
Fish oil	Fair/Recommend	Effects may be larger for aggression and mood than for inattention

Levels of evidence based on US Preventive Services Task Force: http://www.uspreventiveservicestask force.org.

EPA than DHA. The mechanisms of action of this tentative clinical finding are not well understood.

Supplementation with omega-3 fatty acids has proved to be safe, easy to use, and relatively inexpensive and, despite open questions regarding mechanisms of action in different psychiatric disorders, these treatments have a clear biological rationale. Preparations that are EPA-rich (as opposed to DHA-rich) appear to be linked to improvement in symptoms of both affect and cognition. However, more well-powered studies are needed in youth with ADHD, conduct disorder, and mood disorders before clinical treatment recommendations can be made (**Box 1, Tables 3 and 4**).

REFERENCES

1. US Department of Agriculture, US Department of Health and Human Services. Dietary guidelines for Americans, 2010. 7th edition. Washington, DC: U.S. Government Printing Office; 2010.
2. Georgieff MK. Nutrition and the developing brain: nutrient priorities and measurement. Am J Clin Nutr 2007;85:614S–20S.
3. Rees GA, Doyle W, Srivastava A, et al. The nutrient intakes of mothers of low birth weight babies - a comparison of ethnic groups in East London, UK. Matern Child Nutr 2005;1:91–9.
4. Doyle W, Rees G. Maternal malnutrition in the UK and low birthweight. Nutr Health 2001;15:213–8.
5. UNICEF. Sustainable elimination of iodine deficiency. New York: UNICEF; 2008. Available at: www.unicef.org/publications/index_44271.html.
6. The iodine deficiency—way to go yet [editorial]. Lancet 2008;372:88.
7. Peirano PD, Algarin CR, Chamorro R, et al. Sleep and neurofunctions throughout child development: lasting effects of early iron deficiency. J Pediatr Gastroenterol Nutr 2009;48(Suppl 1):S8–15.
8. Grantham-McGregor S, Ani C. A review of studies on the effect of iron deficiency on cognitive development in children. J Nutr 2001;131:649S–66S [discussion: 666S–8S].
9. McCann JC, Ames BN. An overview of evidence for a causal relation between iron deficiency during development and deficits in cognitive or behavioral function. Am J Clin Nutr 2007;85:931–45.
10. Lozoff B. Iron deficiency and child development. Food Nutr Bull 2007;28: S560–71.

11. Sachdev H, Gera T, Nestel P. Effect of iron supplementation on mental and motor development in children: systematic review of randomised controlled trials. Public Health Nutr 2005;8:117–32.

12. Venturi S, Donati FM, Venturi A, et al. Environmental iodine deficiency: a challenge to the evolution of terrestrial life? Thyroid 2000;10:727–9.

13. Coe CL, Lubach GR, Bianco L, et al. A history of iron deficiency anemia during infancy alters brain monoamine activity later in juvenile monkeys. Dev Psychobiol 2009;51:301–9.

14. Lozoff B, Beard J, Connor J, et al. Long-lasting neural and behavioral effects of iron deficiency in infancy. Nutr Rev 2006;64:S34–43 [discussion: S72–91].

15. Georgieff MK. The role of iron in neurodevelopment: fetal iron deficiency and the developing hippocampus. Biochem Soc Trans 2008;36:1267–71.

16. Beard JL, Connor JR. Iron status and neural functioning. Annu Rev Nutr 2003; 23:41–58.

17. Marszalek JR, Lodish HF. Docosahexaenoic acid, fatty acid-interacting proteins, and neuronal function: breastmilk and fish are good for you. Annu Rev Cell Dev Biol 2005;21:633–57.

18. Karr JE, Alexander JE, Winningham RG. Omega-3 polyunsaturated fatty acids and cognition throughout the lifespan: a review. Nutr Neurosci 2011;14: 216–25.

19. Siegel G, Ermilov E. Omega-3 fatty acids: benefits for cardio-cerebro-vascular diseases. Atherosclerosis 2012;225:291–5.

20. Innis SM. Dietary omega 3 fatty acids and the developing brain. Brain Res 2008; 1237:35–43.

21. Haag M. Essential fatty acids and the brain. Can J Psychiatry 2003;48:195–203.

22. Elmadfa I, Kornsteiner M. Fats and fatty acid requirements for adults. Ann Nutr Metab 2009;55:56–75.

23. Brenna JT, Salem N Jr, Sinclair AJ, et al. [alpha]-Linolenic acid supplementation and conversion to n-3 long-chain polyunsaturated fatty acids in humans. Prostaglandins Leukot Essent Fatty Acids 2009;80:85–91.

24. Crawford MA, Bazinet RP, Sinclair AJ. Fat intake and CNS functioning: ageing and disease. Ann Nutr Metab 2009;55:202–28.

25. Blasbalg TL, Hibbeln JR, Ramsden CE, et al. Changes in consumption of omega-3 and omega-6 fatty acids in the United States during the 20th century. Am J Clin Nutr 2011;93:950–62.

26. Rett BS, Whelan J. Increasing dietary linoleic acid does not increase tissue arachidonic acid content in adults consuming Western-type diets: a systematic review. Nutr Metab (Lond) 2011;8:36.

27. Wood JD, Enser M, Fisher AV, et al. Fat deposition, fatty acid composition and meat quality: a review. Meat Sci 2008;78:343–58.

28. Lauritzen L, Hansen HS, Jorgensen MH, et al. The essentiality of long chain n-3 fatty acids in relation to development and function of the brain and retina. Prog Lipid Res 2001;40:1–94.

29. Brenna JT, Diau GY. The influence of dietary docosahexaenoic acid and arachidonic acid on central nervous system polyunsaturated fatty acid composition. Prostaglandins Leukot Essent Fatty Acids 2007;77:247–50.

30. Diau GY, Hsieh A, Sarkadi-Nagy E, et al. The influence of long chain polyunsaturate supplementation on docosahexaenoic acid and arachidonic acid in baboon neonate central nervous system. BMC Med 2005;3:11.

31. Mitchell DC, Gawrisch K, Litman BJ, et al. Why is docosahexaenoic acid essential for nervous system function? Biochem Soc Trans 1998;26:365–70.

32. Bourre JM, Bonneil M, Chaudiere J, et al. Structural and functional importance of dietary polyunsaturated fatty acids in the nervous system. Adv Exp Med Biol 1992;318:211–29.

33. Jones CR, Arai T, Rapoport SI. Evidence for the involvement of docosahexaenoic acid in cholinergic stimulated signal transduction at the synapse. Neurochem Res 1997;22:663–70.

34. Condray R, Yao JK, Steinhauer SR, et al. Semantic memory in schizophrenia: association with cell membrane essential fatty acids. Schizophr Res 2008;106:13–28.

35. Yehuda S, Rabinovitz S, Mostofsky DI. Essential fatty acids are mediators of brain biochemistry and cognitive functions. J Neurosci Res 1999;56:565–70.

36. Tassoni D, Kaur G, Weisinger RS, et al. The role of eicosanoids in the brain. Asia Pac J Clin Nutr 2008;17(Suppl 1):220–8.

37. Carlson SE. Docosahexaenoic acid and arachidonic acid in infant development. Semin Neonatol 2001;6:437–49.

38. Levant B, Radel JD, Carlson SE. Decreased brain docosahexaenoic acid during development alters dopamine-related behaviors in adult rats that are differentially affected by dietary remediation. Behav Brain Res 2004;152:49–57.

39. McNamara RK, Carlson SE. Role of omega-3 fatty acids in brain development and function: potential implications for the pathogenesis and prevention of psychopathology. Prostaglandins Leukot Essent Fatty Acids 2006;75:329–49.

40. Mostofsky DI, Yehuda S, Salem N. Fatty acids: physiological and behavioral functions. (NJ): Humana Press; 2001.

41. Lands B. A critique of paradoxes in current advice on dietary lipids. Prog Lipid Res 2008;47:77–106.

42. Horrobin DF. Essential fatty acids, prostaglandins, and alcoholism: an overview. Alcohol Clin Exp Res 1987;11:2–9.

43. Marangoni F, Colombo C, De Angelis L, et al. Cigarette smoke negatively and dose-dependently affects the biosynthetic pathway of the n-3 polyunsaturated fatty acid series in human mammary epithelial cells. Lipids 2004;39:633–7.

44. Agostoni C, Riva E, Giovannini M, et al. Maternal smoking habits are associated with differences in infants' long-chain polyunsaturated fatty acids in whole blood: a case-control study. Arch Dis Child 2008;93:414–8.

45. Pawlosky RJ, Salem N Jr. Perspectives on alcohol consumption: liver polyunsaturated fatty acids and essential fatty acid metabolism. Alcohol 2004;34: 27–33.

46. Nakamura MT, Nara TY. Structure, function, and dietary regulation of delta6, delta5, and delta9 desaturases. Annu Rev Nutr 2004;24:345–76.

47. Brookes KJ, Chen W, Xu X, et al. Association of fatty acid desaturase genes with attention-deficit/hyperactivity disorder. Biol Psychiatry 2006;60:1053–61.

48. Simopoulos AP. The importance of the ratio of omega-6/omega-3 essential fatty acids. Biomed Pharmacother 2002;56:365–79.

49. Hibbeln JR, Nieminen LR, Lands WE. Increasing homicide rates and linoleic acid consumption among five Western countries, 1961-2000. Lipids 2004;39: 1207–13.

50. Chalon S. The role of fatty acids in the treatment of ADHD. Neuropharmacology 2009;57:636–9.

51. Yavin E, Himovichi E, Eilam R. Delayed cell migration in the developing rat brain following maternal omega 3 alpha linolenic acid dietary deficiency. Neuroscience 2009;162:1011–22.

52. McNamara RK, Jandacek R, Rider T, et al. Omega-3 fatty acid deficiency increases constitutive pro-inflammatory cytokine production in rats: relationship

with central serotonin turnover. Prostaglandins Leukot Essent Fatty Acids 2010; 83:185–91.

53. Kuipers RS, Luxwolda MF, Dijck-Brouwer DA, et al. Estimated macronutrient and fatty acid intakes from an East African Paleolithic diet. Br J Nutr 2010;104: 1666–87.

54. Ramsden CE, Zamora D, Leelarthaepin B, et al. Use of dietary linoleic acid for secondary prevention of coronary heart disease and death: evaluation of recovered data from the Sydney Diet Heart Study and updated meta-analysis. BMJ 2013;346:e8707.

55. Salem N Jr, Moriguchi T, Greiner RS, et al. Alterations in brain function after loss of docosahexaenoate due to dietary restriction of n-3 fatty acids. J Mol Neurosci 2001;16:299–307 [discussion: 317–21].

56. Wainwright PE. Dietary essential fatty acids and brain function: a developmental perspective on mechanisms. Proc Nutr Soc 2002;61:61–9.

57. Garcia-Calatayud S, Redondo C, Martin E, et al. Brain docosahexaenoic acid status and learning in young rats submitted to dietary long-chain polyunsaturated fatty acid deficiency and supplementation limited to lactation. Pediatr Res 2005;57:719–23.

58. Al MD, van Houwelingen AC, Hornstra G. Long-chain polyunsaturated fatty acids, pregnancy, and pregnancy outcome. Am J Clin Nutr 2000;71:285S–91S.

59. Alessandri JM, Guesnet P, Vancassel S, et al. Polyunsaturated fatty acids in the central nervous system: evolution of concepts and nutritional implications throughout life. Reprod Nutr Dev 2004;44:509–38.

60. Chalon S. Omega-3 fatty acids and monoamine neurotransmission. Prostaglandins Leukot Essent Fatty Acids 2006;75:259–69.

61. Zimmer L, Delpal S, Guilloteau D, et al. Chronic n-3 polyunsaturated fatty acid deficiency alters dopamine vesicle density in the rat frontal cortex. Neurosci Lett 2000;284:25–8.

62. Hibbeln JR, Ferguson TA, Blasbalg TL. Omega-3 fatty acid deficiencies in neurodevelopment, aggression and autonomic dysregulation: opportunities for intervention. Int Rev Psychiatry 2006;18:107–18.

63. Fedorova I, Salem JN. Omega-3 fatty acids and rodent behavior. Prostaglandins Leukot Essent Fatty Acids 2006;75:271–89.

64. Mathieu G, Denis S, Lavialle M, et al. Synergistic effects of stress and omega-3 fatty acid deprivation on emotional response and brain lipid composition in adult rats. Prostaglandins Leukot Essent Fatty Acids 2008;78:391–401.

65. Stein J. The magnocellular theory of developmental dyslexia. Dyslexia 2001;7: 12–36.

66. Antalis CJ, Stevens LJ, Campbell M, et al. Omega-3 fatty acid status in attention-deficit/hyperactivity disorder. Prostaglandins Leukot Essent Fatty Acids 2006;75:299–308.

67. Ward PE. Potential diagnostic aids for abnormal fatty acid metabolism in a range of neurodevelopmental disorders. Prostaglandins Leukot Essent Fatty Acids 2000;63:65–8.

68. Stevens LJ, Zentall SS, Deck JL, et al. Essential fatty acid metabolism in boys with attention-deficit hyperactivity disorder. Am J Clin Nutr 1995;62:761–8.

69. Chen JR, Hsu SF, Hsu CD, et al. Dietary patterns and blood fatty acid composition in children with attention-deficit hyperactivity disorder in Taiwan. J Nutr Biochem 2004;15:467–72.

70. Mitchell EA, Aman MG, Turbott SH, et al. Clinical characteristics and serum essential fatty acid levels in hyperactive children. Clin Pediatr (Phila) 1987;26:406–11.

71. Mitchell EA, Lewis S, Cutler DR. Essential fatty acids and maladjusted behaviour in children. Prostaglandins Leukot Med 1983;12:281–7.
72. Germano M, Meleleo D, Montorfano G, et al. Plasma, red blood cells phospholipids and clinical evaluation after long chain omega-3 supplementation in children with attention deficit hyperactivity disorder (ADHD). Nutr Neurosci 2007;10: 1–9.
73. Colter AL, Cutler C, Meckling K. Fatty acid status and behavioural symptoms of Attention Deficit Hyperactivity Disorder in adolescents: a case-control study. Nutr J 2008;7:8.
74. Richardson AJ, Montgomery P. The Oxford-Durham study: a randomized, controlled trial of dietary supplementation with fatty acids in children with developmental coordination disorder. Pediatrics 2005;115:1360–6.
75. Sinn N, Bryan J, Wilson C. Cognitive effects of polyunsaturated fatty acids in children with attention deficit hyperactivity disorder symptoms: a randomised controlled trial. Prostaglandins Leukot Essent Fatty Acids 2008;78:311–26.
76. Sinn N, Bryan J. Effect of supplementation with polyunsaturated fatty acids and micronutrients on learning and behavior problems associated with child ADHD. J Dev Behav Pediatr 2007;28:82–91.
77. Nemets H, Nemets B, Apter A, et al. Omega-3 treatment of childhood depression: a controlled, double-blind pilot study. Am J Psychiatry 2006;163: 1098–100.
78. Richardson AJ, Puri BK. A randomized double-blind, placebo-controlled study of the effects of supplementation with highly unsaturated fatty acids on ADHD-related symptoms in children with specific learning difficulties. Prog Neuropsychopharmacol Biol Psychiatry 2002;26:233–9.
79. McNamara RK, Able J, Jandacek R, et al. Docosahexaenoic acid supplementation increases prefrontal cortex activation during sustained attention in healthy boys: a placebo-controlled, dose-ranging, functional magnetic resonance imaging study. Am J Clin Nutr 2010;91:1060–7.
80. Richardson AJ, Burton JR, Sewell RP, et al. Docosahexaenoic acid for reading, cognition and behavior in children aged 7-9 years: a randomized, controlled trial (The DOLAB Study). PLoS One 2012;7:e43909.
81. Kirby A, Woodward A, Jackson S, et al. A double-blind, placebo-controlled study investigating the effects of omega-3 supplementation in children aged 8-10 years from a mainstream school population. Res Dev Disabil 2010;31: 718–30.
82. McNamara RK. The emerging role of omega-3 fatty acids in psychiatry. Prostaglandins Leukot Essent Fatty Acids 2006;75:223–5.
83. McNamara RK, Able J, Liu Y, et al. Omega-3 fatty acid deficiency during perinatal development increases serotonin turnover in the prefrontal cortex and decreases midbrain tryptophan hydroxylase-2 expression in adult female rats: dissociation from estrogenic effects. J Psychiatr Res 2009;43:656–63.
84. Cunnane SC, Plourde M, Kathy Stewart K, et al. Docosahexaenoic acid and shore-based diets in hominin encephalization: a rebuttal. Am J Human Biol 2007;19:578–81.
85. Cunnane SC, Stewart KM. Human brain evolution: the influence of freshwater and marine food resources. Hoboken (NJ): Wiley-Blackwell; 2010.
86. Crawford MA, Hassam AG, Williams G. Essential fatty acids and fetal brain growth. Lancet 1976;1:452–3.
87. Fiennes RN, Sinclair AJ, Crawford MA. Essential fatty acid studies in primates linolenic acid requirements of capuchins. J Med Primatol 1973;2:155–69.

88. Crawford MA, Leigh Broadhurst C, Guest M, et al. A quantum theory for the irreplaceable role of docosahexaenoic acid in neural cell signalling throughout evolution. Prostaglandins Leukot Essent Fatty Acids 2013;88:5–13.

89. Cordain L, Eaton SB, Sebastian A, et al. Origins and evolution of the Western diet: health implications for the 21st century. Am J Clin Nutr 2005;81:341–54.

90. Eaton SB, Eaton SB 3rd, Sinclair AJ, et al. Dietary intake of long-chain polyunsaturated fatty acids during the paleolithic. World Rev Nutr Diet 1998;83:12–23.

91. Eaton SB, Eaton SB 3rd, Konner MJ. Paleolithic nutrition revisited: a twelve-year retrospective on its nature and implications. Eur J Clin Nutr 1997;51:207–16.

92. Crawford M, Crawford S. What we eat today. New York: Stein and Day; 1972.

93. Wang Y, Lehane C, Ghebremeskel K, et al. Modern organic and broiler chickens sold for human consumption provide more energy from fat than protein. Public Health Nutr 2010;13:400–8.

94. Alvheim AR, Malde MK, Osei-Hyiaman D, et al. Dietary linoleic acid elevates endogenous 2-AG and anandamide and induces obesity. Obesity (Silver Spring) 2012;20:1984–94.

95. Mathers CD, Loncar D. Projections of global mortality and burden of disease from 2002 to 2030. PLoS Med 2006;3:e442.

96. Hibbeln JR, Davis JM, Steer C, et al. Maternal seafood consumption in pregnancy and neurodevelopmental outcomes in childhood (ALSPAC study): an observational cohort study. Lancet 2007;369:578–85.

97. US Food and Drug Administration and the Environmental Protection Agency. What you need to know about mercury in fish and shellfish: EPA and FDA advice for women who might become pregnant, women who are pregnant, nursing mothers, and young children. EPA-823-R-04-00 March 2004.

98. Moriguchi T, Greiner RS, Salem N Jr. Behavioral deficits associated with dietary induction of decreased brain docosahexaenoic acid concentration. J Neurochem 2000;75:2563–73.

99. FDA. Draft risk and benefit assessment report and draft summary of published research report of quantitative risk and benefit assessment of commercial fish consumption, focusing on fetal neurodevelopmental effects (measured by verbal development in children) and on coronary heart disease and stroke in the general population, and summary of published research on the beneficial effects of fish consumption and omega-3 fatty acids for certain neurodevelopmental and cardiovascular endpoints. Federal Register—74 FR 3615. Notice of Availability January 21 (Ed.), 2009.

100. Freeman MP, Mischoulon D, Tedeschini E, et al. Complementary and alternative medicine for major depressive disorder: a meta-analysis of patient characteristics, placebo-response rates, and treatment outcomes relative to standard antidepressants. J Clin Psychiatry 2010;71:682–8.

101. SanGiovanni JP, Parra-Cabrera S, Colditz GA, et al. Meta-analysis of dietary essential fatty acids and long-chain polyunsaturated fatty acids as they relate to visual resolution acuity in healthy preterm infants. Pediatrics 2000;105:1292–8.

102. Birch EE, Carlson SE, Hoffman DR, et al. The DIAMOND (DHA Intake and Measurement of Neural Development) Study: a double-masked, randomized controlled clinical trial of the maturation of infant visual acuity as a function of the dietary level of docosahexaenoic acid. Am J Clin Nutr 2010;91:848–59.

103. Forsyth JS, Willatts P, DiModogno MK, et al. Do long-chain polyunsaturated fatty acids influence infant cognitive behaviour? Biochem Soc Trans 1998;26:252–7.

104. Osendarp SJ, Baghurst KI, Bryan J, et al. Effect of a 12-mo micronutrient intervention on learning and memory in well-nourished and marginally nourished

school-aged children: 2 parallel, randomized, placebo-controlled studies in Australia and Indonesia. Am J Clin Nutr 2007;86:1082–93.

105. Stevens LJ, Zentall SS, Abate ML, et al. Omega-3 fatty acids in boys with behavior, learning, and health problems. Physiol Behav 1996;59:915–20.

106. Pawlosky R, Hibbeln J, Lin Y, et al. n-3 fatty acid metabolism in women. Br J Nutr 2003;90:993–4 [discussion: 994–5].

107. Voigt RG, Llorente AM, Jensen CL, et al. A randomized, double-blind, placebo-controlled trial of docosahexaenoic acid supplementation in children with attention-deficit/hyperactivity disorder. J Pediatr 2001;139:189–96.

108. Hirayama S, Hamazaki T, Terasawa K. Effect of docosahexaenoic acid-containing food administration on symptoms of attention-deficit/hyperactivity disorder—a placebo-controlled double-blind study. Eur J Clin Nutr 2004;58(3): 467–73.

109. Arnold LE, Kleykamp D, Votolato NA, et al. Gamma-linolenic acid for attention-deficit hyperactivity disorder: placebo-controlled comparison to D-amphetamine. Biol Psychiatry 1989;25:222–8.

110. Belanger SA, Vanasse M, Spahis S, et al. Omega-3 fatty acid treatment of children with attention-deficit hyperactivity disorder: a randomized, double-blind, placebo-controlled study. Paediatr Child Health 2009;14:89–98.

111. Raz R, Carasso RL, Yehuda S. The influence of short-chain essential fatty acids on children with attention-deficit/hyperactivity disorder: a double-blind placebo-controlled study. J Child Adolesc Psychopharmacol 2009;19:167–77.

112. Sumich A, Matsudaira T, Gow RV, et al. Resting state electroencephalographic correlates with red cell long-chain fatty acids, memory performance and age in adolescent boys with attention deficit hyperactivity disorder. Neuropharmacology 2009;57:708–14.

113. Gow RV, Matsudaira T, Taylor E, et al. Total red blood cell concentrations of omega-3 fatty acids are associated with emotion-elicited neural activity in adolescent boys with attention-deficit hyperactivity disorder. Prostaglandins Leukot Essent Fatty Acids 2009;80:151–6.

114. Singh SD, Ellis CR, Winton AS, et al. Recognition of facial expressions of emotion by children with attention-deficit hyperactivity disorder. Behav Modif 1998;22:128–42.

115. Boucher O, Burden MJ, Muckle G, et al. Neurophysiologic and neurobehavioral evidence of beneficial effects of prenatal omega-3 fatty acid intake on memory function at school age. Am J Clin Nutr 2011;93:1025–37.

116. Milte CM, Sinn N, Buckley JD, et al. Polyunsaturated fatty acids, cognition and literacy in children with ADHD with and without learning difficulties. J Child Health Care 2011;15(4):299–311.

117. Richardson AJ. Clinical trials of fatty acid treatment in ADHD, dyslexia, dyspraxia and the autistic spectrum. Prostaglandins Leukot Essent Fatty Acids 2004;70:383–90.

118. Johnson M, Ostlund S, Fransson G, et al. Omega-3/omega-6 fatty acids for attention deficit hyperactivity disorder: a randomized placebo-controlled trial in children and adolescents. J Atten Disord 2009;12:394–401.

119. Stevens L, Zhang W, Peck L, et al. EFA supplementation in children with inattention, hyperactivity, and other disruptive behaviors. Lipids 2003;38:1007–21.

120. Perera H, Jeewandara KC, Seneviratne S, et al. Combined ω3 and ω6 supplementation in children with attention-deficit hyperactivity disorder (ADHD) refractory to methylphenidate treatment: a double-blind, placebo-controlled study. J Child Neurol 2012;27(6):747–53.

121. Harding KL, Judah RD, Gant C. Outcome-based comparison of ritalin versus food-supplement treated children with AD/HD. Altern Med Rev 2003;8: 319–30.
122. Bloch MH, Qawasmi A. Omega-3 fatty acid supplementation for the treatment of children with attention-deficit/hyperactivity disorder symptomatology: systematic review and meta-analysis. J Am Acad Child Adolesc Psychiatry 2011;50: 991–1000.
123. Swan GE, Carmelli D, Rosenman RH. Psychological characteristics in twins discordant for smoking behavior: a matched-twin-pair analysis. Addict Behav 1988;13:51–60.
124. Gesch CB, Hammond SM, Hampson SE, et al. Influence of supplementary vitamins, minerals and essential fatty acids on the antisocial behaviour of young adult prisoners. Randomised, placebo-controlled trial. Br J Psychiatry 2002; 181:22–8.
125. Corrigan F, Gray R, Strathdee A, et al. Fatty acid analysis of blood from violent offenders. J Forensic Psychiatr Psychol 1994;5:83–92.
126. Schoenthaler SJ. Diet and criminal behavior: a criminological evaluation of the Arlington, Virginia proceedings. Pers Individ Dif 1991;12:339–40.
127. Schoenthaler SJ. The Alabama diet-behavior program: an evaluation at the Coosa Valley regional detention center. Pers Individ Dif 1991;12:336.
128. Schoenthaler SJ, Bier ID. The effect of vitamin-mineral supplementation on juvenile delinquency among American schoolchildren: a randomized, double-blind placebo-controlled trial. J Altern Complement Med 2000;6:7–17.
129. Weller EB, Weller RA, Rooney MT, et al. Children's interview for psychiatric syndromes (ChIPS). Arlington (VA): American Psychiatric Press, Inc; 1999.
130. Gow RV, Vallee-Tourangeau F, Crawford MA, et al. Omega-3 fatty acids are inversely related to callous and unemotional traits in adolescent boys with attention deficit hyperactivity disorder. Prostaglandins Leukot Essent Fatty Acids 2013;88(6):411–8.
131. Frick PJ, Stickle TR, Dandreaux DM, et al. Callous-unemotional traits in predicting the severity and stability of conduct problems and delinquency. J Abnorm Child Psychol 2005;33:471–87.
132. Frick PJ, White SF. Research review: the importance of callous-unemotional traits for developmental models of aggressive and antisocial behavior. J Child Psychol Psychiatry 2008;49:359–75.
133. Viding E. Annotation: understanding the development of psychopathy. J Child Psychol Psychiatry 2004;45:1329–37.
134. Viding E, Jones AP, Frick PJ, et al. Heritability of antisocial behaviour at 9: do callous-unemotional traits matter? Dev Sci 2008;11:17–22.
135. Zaalberg A, Nijman H, Bulten E, et al. Effects of nutritional supplements on aggression, rule-breaking, and psychopathology among young adult prisoners. Aggress Behav 2010;36:117–26.
136. Edwards R, Peet M, Shay J, et al. Omega-3 polyunsaturated fatty acid levels in the diet and in red blood cell membranes of depressed patients. J Affect Disord 1998;48:149–55.
137. Peet M, Murphy B, Shay J, et al. Depletion of omega-3 fatty acid levels in red blood cell membranes of depressive patients. Biol Psychiatry 1998;43: 315–9.
138. Conklin SM, Harris JI, Manuck SB, et al. Serum omega-3 fatty acids are associated with variation in mood, personality and behavior in hypercholesterolemic community volunteers. Psychiatry Res 2007;152:1–10.

139. Conklin SM, Manuck SB, Yao JK, et al. High omega-6 and low omega-3 fatty acids are associated with depressive symptoms and neuroticism. Psychosom Med 2007;69:932–4.
140. Hibbeln JR. Seafood consumption, the DHA content of mothers' milk and prevalence rates of postpartum depression: a cross-national, ecological analysis. J Affect Disord 2002;69:15–29.
141. Hibbeln JR. Fish consumption and major depression. Lancet 1998;351:1213.
142. Noaghiul S, Hibbeln JR. Cross-national comparisons of seafood consumption and rates of bipolar disorders. Am J Psychiatry 2003;160:2222–7.
143. Hibbeln JR. Seafood consumption and homicide mortality. A cross-national ecological analysis. World Rev Nutr Diet 2001;88:41–6.
144. McNamara RK, editor. Omega-3 fatty acid deficiency syndrome: opportunities for disease prevention. Hauppauge (NY): Nova Science Pub Incorporated; 2013.
145. Ginsberg Y, Lindefors N. Methylphenidate treatment of adult male prison inmates with attention-deficit hyperactivity disorder: randomised double-blind placebo-controlled trial with open-label extension. Br J Psychiatry 2012;200:68–73.
146. Jazayeri S, Tehrani-Doost M, Keshavarz SA, et al. Comparison of therapeutic effects of omega-3 fatty acid eicosapentaenoic acid and fluoxetine, separately and in combination, in major depressive disorder. Aust N Z J Psychiatry 2008;42:192–8.
147. Peet M, Horrobin DF. A dose-ranging study of the effects of ethyl-eicosapentaenoate in patients with ongoing depression despite apparently adequate treatment with standard drugs. Arch Gen Psychiatry 2002;59:913–9.
148. Freeman MP, Hibbeln JR, Wisner KL, et al. Omega-3 fatty acids: evidence basis for treatment and future research in psychiatry. J Clin Psychiatry 2006;67: 1954–67.
149. Appleton KM, Rogers PJ, Ness AR. Updated systematic review and meta-analysis of the effects of n-3 long-chain polyunsaturated fatty acids on depressed mood. Am J Clin Nutr 2010;91:757–70.
150. Kraguljac NV, Montori VM, Pavuluri M, et al. Efficacy of omega-3 fatty acids in mood disorders - a systematic review and metaanalysis. Psychopharmacol Bull 2009;42:39–54.
151. Martins JG. EPA but not DHA appears to be responsible for the efficacy of omega-3 long chain polyunsaturated fatty acid supplementation in depression: evidence from a meta-analysis of randomized controlled trials. J Am Coll Nutr 2009;28:525–42.
152. Martins JG, Bentsen H, Puri BK. Eicosapentaenoic acid appears to be the key omega-3 fatty acid component associated with efficacy in major depressive disorder: a critique of Bloch and Hannestad and updated meta-analysis. Mol Psychiatry 2012;17:1144–9 [discussion: 1163–7].
153. Sublette ME, Ellis SP, Geant AL, et al. Meta-analysis of the effects of eicosapentaenoic acid (EPA) in clinical trials in depression. J Clin Psychiatry 2011;72: 1577–84.
154. Lin PY, Mischoulon D, Freeman MP, et al. Are omega-3 fatty acids antidepressants or just mood-improving agents? The effect depends upon diagnosis, supplement preparation, and severity of depression. Mol Psychiatry 2012;17: 1161–3 [author reply: 1163–7].
155. Bloch MH, Hannestad J. Omega-3 fatty acids for the treatment of depression: systematic review and meta-analysis. Mol Psychiatry 2012;17:1272–82.
156. Kirsch I, Deacon BJ, Huedo-Medina TB, et al. Initial severity and antidepressant benefits: a meta-analysis of data submitted to the Food and Drug Administration. PLoS Med 2008;5:e45.

157. Hibbeln JR. Depression, suicide and deficiencies of omega-3 essential fatty acids in modern diets. World Rev Nutr Diet 2009;99:17–30.

158. Lewis MD, Hibbeln JR, Johnson JE, et al. Suicide deaths of active-duty US military and omega-3 fatty-acid status: a case-control comparison. J Clin Psychiatry 2011;72:1585–90.

159. Sublette ME, Hibbeln JR, Galfalvy H, et al. Omega-3 polyunsaturated essential fatty acid status as a predictor of future suicide risk. Am J Psychiatry 2006;163:1100–2.

160. Levin ED, McClernon FJ, Rezvani AH. Nicotinic effects on cognitive function: behavioral characterization, pharmacological specification, and anatomic localization. Psychopharmacology 2006;184:523–39.

161. Huan M, Hamazaki K, Sun Y, et al. Suicide attempt and n-3 fatty acid levels in red blood cells: a case control study in China. Biol Psychiatry 2004;56:490–6.

162. Amminger GP, Schafer MR, Papageorgiou K, et al. Long-chain omega-3 fatty acids for indicated prevention of psychotic disorders: a randomized, placebo-controlled trial. Arch Gen Psychiatry 2010;67:146–54.

163. Itomura M, Hamazaki K, Sawazaki S, et al. The effect of fish oil on physical aggression in schoolchildren—a randomized, double-blind, placebo-controlled trial. J Nutr Biochem 2005;16:163–71.

164. Hamazaki K, Syafruddin D, Tunru IS, et al. The effects of docosahexaenoic acid-rich fish oil on behavior, school attendance rate and malaria infection in school children—a double-blind, randomized, placebo-controlled trial in Lampung, Indonesia. Asia Pac J Clin Nutr 2008;17:258–63.

165. Ramsden CE, Mann JD, Faurot KR, et al. Low omega-6 vs. low omega-6 plus high omega-3 dietary intervention for chronic daily headache: protocol for a randomized clinical trial. Trials 2011;12:97.

166. Freeman MP. Omega-3 fatty acids and perinatal depression: a review of the literature and recommendations for future research. Prostaglandins Leukot Essent Fatty Acids 2006;75:291–7.

167. Carmelli D, Swan GE, Robinette D, et al. Genetic influence on smoking—a study of male twins. N Engl J Med 1992;327:829–33.

Single-Micronutrient and Broad-Spectrum Micronutrient Approaches for Treating Mood Disorders in Youth and Adults

 CrossMark

Charles W. Popper, MD[a,b],*

KEYWORDS

- Vitamins • Minerals • Micronutrients • Children • Adolescents
- Psychopharmacology • Major depressive disorder • Bipolar disorder

KEY POINTS

- Vitamins and minerals are involved in virtually every biologic process, so micronutrient deficiencies have broad effects throughout the body and brain.
- Micronutrient insufficiencies affect most people, even in "well-fed" populations, especially patients with psychiatric disorders, including mood disorders in youth and adults.
- Folic acid, chromium, and perhaps zinc may be effective adjunctive treatments for depression in adults but are not powerful enough to be monotherapies.
- Broad-spectrum micronutrient treatments appear effective in early controlled trials as potent treatments of ADHD, aggressive and disordered conduct, and mood disorders in youth and adults.
- For bipolar depression and mania, the effectiveness of broad-spectrum micronutrients appears comparable to conventional medications, but with fewer adverse effects and possibly greater long-term stability.
- In healthy adults, broad-spectrum micronutrients may reduce posttraumatic symptoms, benefit memory, and increase mental energy and clarity.

Disclosures: Dr C. Popper is an unpaid consultant to Truehope Nutritional Support and to NutraTek Health Innovations.
None of the agents discussed in this article have marketing approval for psychiatric uses by the US Food and Drug Administration.
a Child and Adolescent Psychiatry, McLean Hospital, Belmont, MA, USA; b Harvard Medical School, Boston, MA, USA
* 385 Concord Avenue, Suite 204, Belmont, MA 02478-3037, USA.
E-mail address: Charles_Popper@harvard.edu

Child Adolesc Psychiatric Clin N Am 23 (2014) 591–672
http://dx.doi.org/10.1016/j.chc.2014.04.001
1056-4993/14/$ – see front matter © 2014 Elsevier Inc. All rights reserved.

Abbreviations	
BDI	Beck Depression Inventory
CAARS	Conners Adult ADHD Rating Scales
CBCL	Child Behavior Checklist
CGI	Clinical Global Impression
CNS	Central nervous system
DHA	Docosahexaenoic acid
EAR	Estimated Average Requirement
EPA	Eicosapentaenoic acid
GAF	Global Assessment of Functioning
HAM-D	Hamilton Depression Rating Scale
MDD	Major depressive disorder
NHANES	National Health and Nutrition Examination Survey
OCD	Obsessive-Compulsive Disorder
POMS	Profile of Mood States
RCTs	Randomized controlled trials
RDAs	Recommended Daily Allowances
RDBPCTs	Randomized double-blind placebo-controlled trials
SAMe	S-adenosyl-methionine
SSRIs	Serotonin reuptake inhibitors

VITAMINS AND MINERALS IN HEALTH AND DISEASE

The technical term "micronutrients" refers to all vitamins and biologically active minerals required in trace and ultratrace amounts to sustain health. The term is often used more broadly to describe a variably defined group of dietary substances, including other bioactive nutrients required in "micro" amounts for a wide range of biologic processes (**Box 1**). In contrast, larger dietary quantities are needed of the macronutrients, which include carbohydrates, proteins, fats, and the macro-minerals (sodium, potassium, calcium, magnesium, chloride, phosphorus, and sulfur). For the purposes of this article, the term "micronutrients" will be used to signify vitamins and microminerals collectively.

Dietary intake of micronutrients must be maintained at nutritionally adequate levels to sustain biologic functionality and general health, both physical and mental.[1,2] At the level of global public health, iodine, iron, and vitamin A are usually considered the most common micronutrient deficiencies worldwide, especially in developing countries; but even in developed countries, deficiencies in iron, folate, and zinc are common. Children and pregnant mothers are considered particularly vulnerable to micronutrient deficiencies, and micronutrient deficiencies can have profound effects on physical growth and brain development.[3,4]

Micronutrient Functions in Biology

Micronutrients play a role in virtually every biologic, chemical, and physiologic process. Minerals and vitamins serve as cofactors in enzymatic reactions. Virtually all enzymes require some form of cofactor, and many enzymes require several cofactors. Vitamins may be a cofactor (biotin) or a component of a cofactor (folate in tetrahydrofolate). Minerals, in addition to functioning as cofactors, are also a structural part of some enzymes (iodine in thyroid hormone, magnesium and zinc in DNA polymerase) or may activate enzymes or other proteins (allosteric regulation). Enzymes are involved in neurotransmitter metabolism and drug biotransformation, potentially increasing or decreasing effects of pharmaceutical agents, among innumerable other

| **Box 1** |
| **Micronutrients** |

Vitamins

  Vitamin A: Retinol, retinal, retinoic acid, and other retinoids

  Vitamin B complex

    B1: Thiamine

    B2: Riboflavin

    B3: Niacin, nicotinic acid, niacinamide

    B5: Pantothenic acid

    B6: Pyridoxine, pyridoxal, pyridoxol, pyridoxamine

    B7: Biotin

    B9: Folic acid

    B12: Cobalamins

  Vitamin C: Ascorbic acid

  Vitamin D: Calciferol, cholecalciferol, ergosterol, ergocalciferol

  Vitamin E: Tocopherol, d-alpha tocopheryl, tocotrienols

  Vitamin K: K1 (phytomenadione), K2 (menaquinones)

Minerals

  Trace and ultratrace minerals, including zinc, iron, iodine, copper, selenium, chromium, manganese, molybdenum, boron, silicon, nickel, vanadium; cobalt, fluorine, aluminum (arguably, lithium and strontium).

  Macrominerals include sodium, potassium, calcium, magnesium, chloride, phosphorus, and sulfur.

Other compounds sometimes considered micronutrients

  Vitaminlike substances, including alpha-lipoic acid, coenzyme Q10 (ubiquinol, ubiquinone), L-carnitine, acetyl-L-carnitine, N-acetylcysteine, choline, inositol, phospholipids (phosphatidylcholine, phosphatidylserine)

  Essential fatty acids

    Alpha-linolenic acid, the omega-3 precursor for eicosapentaenoic acid (EPA), and docosahexaenoic acid (DHA)

    Linoleic acid, the omega-6 precursor for gamma-linolenic acid and arachidonic acid

  Amino acids, being constituents of protein, are technically macronutrients, but free amino acids are sometimes considered micronutrients.

  Other organic acids, including citric acid, acetic acid, lactic acid, taurine (2-aminoethanesulfonic acid), para-aminobenzoic acid, and orotic acid.

  Phytochemicals, including polyphenols (flavonoids) and carotenoids (alpha- and beta-carotene, lutein, lycopene, beta-cryptoxanthin, zeaxanthin).

roles. Transcription factors also require cofactors, and so micronutrients have an essential role in gene expression and epigenetic modification. With numerous and overlapping roles for vitamins and minerals, micronutrients are fundamental to biology (**Box 2**).

Box 2
A selection of (partially overlapping) mechanisms of micronutrient action

Modulation of enzyme activities (eg, cofactors "tune up" enzyme activity)

Regulation of the activity of transcription factors, so altering gene expression (eg, cofactors for transcription factors, changing DNA or histone methylation)

Transformation of receptors, transporters, ion channels, and pump mechanisms.

Alterations of membrane fluidity.

Varied effects on second and third messenger systems.

Modification of gastrointestinal absorption, the activity of vitamin-metabolizing enzymes, and the physiologic effects of other micronutrients.

Essential roles in neuron growth and brain development, neuronal repair, and the slowing of neuronal deterioration.

The nutrient requirements of an individual undergo continuous change, even though the establishment of Recommended Daily Allowances (RDAs) as fixed goals for nutrient intake may create the illusion that nutrient requirements are constant. The micronutrient status of an individual is governed by many factors that are related to both micronutrient utilization and micronutrient supply. Optimal dietary micronutrient intake is determined by these various factors. Some of these factors are relatively stable (genetics), some change over time and vary with development or physiologic state, and some are environmentally influenced (**Box 3**).

Physical activity and stress increase micronutrient utilization and needs. Micronutrient requirements are particularly high during pregnancy and early development, largely to optimize brain development.

Micronutrient bioavailability and absorption may be altered by changes in the intestinal flora. Gut flora help release micronutrients from partially metabolized food (digesting cellulose, releasing micronutrients from bound sites) and actively participate in vitamin synthesis and the conversion of minerals into more organically usable forms. Antibiotics, which diminish the gut flora, reduce micronutrient bioavailability and absorption. The nutrient supply is also reduced in advanced age, when senescent changes in the villae reduce intestinal absorption. Through these mechanisms, changes in the intestinal flora and aging gastrointestinal structures can affect brain function.[5]

Medical illnesses can alter micronutrient requirements in numerous ways. Intestinal and liver diseases affecting absorption degrade micronutrient supply. Hypermetabolic conditions (such as hyperthyroidism, infections, proliferative disorders) and conditions involving accelerated cell destruction (sickle cell anemia) increase nutrient requirements. Surgery and radiation treatment place a strain on micronutrient stores. Medications can modify nutrient intake, absorption, and bioavailability in complex ways.

Environmental factors influencing nutrient supply include the micronutrient content of local soil, which governs the nutritional value of foods grown from it; inhabitants may need increased oral supplementation in locales where the food supply comes from nutrient-poor soil. Sun exposure is critical for vitamin D synthesis, so indoor work, lack of outdoor recreation, illness, and bedridden status will reduce endogenous synthesis and increase dietary requirements. Cultural factors affecting nutrient supply include cuisine, cooking methods, and local food patterns[6]; for example, vegetarians are advised to take oral micronutrient supplementation. Inadequate food intake,

---

Box 3
Factors affecting dietary micronutrient requirements in an individual (most of which vary over time)

Age

Physical growth

Physical activity

Stress

Pregnancy and lactation

Geography (local micronutrient content of soil, sun exposure)

Cuisine and cooking methods

Food patterns (eg, Mediterranean, Western, vegetarianism, veganism, Norwegian, Chinese)

Inadequate intake (poverty, dieting)

Gastrointestinal flora (microbiome) alter micronutrient absorption

Antibiotic usage

Diseases

   Reduced gastrointestinal absorption, including gastrointestinal disease.

   Changes in metabolic requirements (eg, thyroid disease, infections, burns)

   Chronic liver or kidney disease

   Hematological conditions involving increased cell destruction (sickle cell anemia, hemolytic anemias)

   Certain brain disorders or injuries may lead to increasing or decreasing requirements.

Treatments of diseases

   Long-term use of certain medications alters micronutrient absorption, serum levels, and effects

   Surgery and radiation

Tobacco, alcohol, recreational drugs, and candy

Obesity

Aging

Genetics

---

whether due to poverty or dieting, will obviously alter the micronutrient status of an individual, and replenishment of depleted micronutrient stores requires more nutrient intake than normal health maintenance. Smoking, alcohol, and recreational drugs, as well as candy and processed foods with low nutrient density (ie, junk food) will increase utilization and reduce nutrient absorption.[7,8]

The micronutrient content of soil is an interesting factor. In developed countries, there is a dramatic depletion of many essential micronutrients in crops, largely caused by modern agricultural methods, which replenish soil with nitrogen and phosphorus, but generally fail to resupply the trace minerals and vitamins that are essential in the human diet. As a result, our soil has gradually become depleted of many essential nutrients, affecting the entire plant and animal food chain that comprises the bulk of human diets. In addition to overly selective soil replenishment and fertilization techniques, other factors contributing to reduced nutrient density in foods include overgrazing, overirrigation, soil aging (organic decomposition, acidification, or alkalinity buildup), loss of organic acids in the humus that helpfully chelate nutrients and enhance nutrient uptake and erosion. Another factor is the use of herbicides, which often contain glyphosates that bind certain minerals and substantially reduce their bioavailability in the soil.[9,10]

The effect of modern agricultural methods has been identified as a factor contributing to the progressive and marked reduction in the nutritional content of the plants and animals that comprise human sustenance. For example, in England, the micronutrient contents of fruits and vegetables grown in the 1930s and in the 1980s were quantitatively compared.[11] Significant reductions were found over those 50 years in the micronutrient content of both vegetables (copper by 81%, sodium by 43%, magnesium by 35%, and calcium by 19%) and fruits (copper by 36%, iron by 32%, potassium by 20%, and magnesium by 11%). Only phosphorus, which is routinely replenished in modern farming techniques, showed no appreciable change over the 50 years. Similar types of changes have been observed in vegetables and fruits grown on soil in the United States.[12] Although doubts have been raised about these figures based on a variety of technical grounds, including cultivars (varietal changes) that reflect trade-offs between market demands (such as productivity) and nutrient content, it seems likely that the micromineral content of the human diet has reduced in agriculturally advanced countries.[13]

Perhaps the most important of all factors affecting micronutrient requirements in an individual is genetics (including epigenetics). An individual's genetic polymorphisms or haplotypes affect genetic differences in all aspects of physiologic functioning. This factor, called "biochemical individuality" in some nutritional circles, is critical, but just one of many factors governing the micronutrient requirements of an individual.

Micronutrient Mechanisms Leading to Disease and Dysfunction

A large variety of diseases and subclinical dysfunctions can result from an inadequate availability of micronutrients. Apart from the frank deficiency diseases, suboptimal micronutrient status can increase the severity of many disorders and, more subtly, contribute to subclinical syndromes related to physiologic underperformance. Diverse mechanisms underlie these conditions, but several specific mechanisms are worth highlighting (**Box 4**).

Bruce Ames, one of the leading authorities on micronutrient medicine, estimates that one-third of single-gene enzyme mutations result in an enzyme with a decreased binding affinity for its cofactor, leading to a slower enzymatic reaction speed (and a higher cofactor concentration required to drive the reaction). He describes about 50 human genetic disorders that are likely to be at least partially ameliorated merely by increasing the dose of an orally administered vitamin cofactor.[15] In effect, the slightly deformed enzymes that characterize some genetic diseases can be made more functional by just increasing the cofactor supply. In this way, Ames suggests that a properly adjusted diet of micronutrients can in itself constitute effective treatment for a variety of genetic disorders.

Ames and colleagues[16] also provide evidence that micronutrient deficiencies can cause oxidative damage to nuclear DNA and to mitochondria, leading to metabolic changes, endothelial disruption, aggravated inflammatory processes, systemic diseases in various organs, neuronal decay, and accelerated aging.[17] These deteriorative processes can be slowed in rats by administration of alpha-lipoic acid and acetyl-L-carnitine.[18,19] Similarly, supplementation with a broad spectrum of micronutrients reduces the oxidative changes and DNA damage associated with chronic stress in

---

Box 4
Selected potential disease mechanisms related to micronutrient deficiencies

Inborn errors of metabolism: Genetic polymorphisms may cause reduced binding affinity (Km) of an enzyme for its micronutrient cofactor, leading to genetic disease.

Micronutrient deficiencies can increase oxidative damage to nuclear DNA (B12, folic acid, B6, C, E, iron, selenium, zinc), leading to numerous metabolic dysfunctions and increased risk for cancer.

Micronutrient deficiencies aggravate mitochondrial oxidative decay (iron, biotin), leading to inflammation-related diseases in multiple organ systems, neuronal deterioration, and accelerated aging.

Micronutrient deficiencies can lead to a temporary constriction of less essential biologic functions in order to preserve functions related to short-term survival (triage theory), but at the long-term cost of increased disease and aging.[14]

Adapted from Ames BN. Optimal micronutrients delay mitochondrial decay and age-associated diseases. Mech Ageing Dev 2010;131(7–8):473–9.

---

mice.[20] Ames[21,22] hypothesizes that physiologic functioning can be pervasively optimized by supplementation with a broad variety of micronutrients, a process he calls a "metabolic tune-up."

Need for a Full and Balanced Range of Micronutrients for Optimal Functioning

In considering the many biologic roles of micronutrients, it should be evident that optimal functioning requires fully adequate levels of all micronutrients, not just some or many. Given that depletion of specific micronutrients can result from a variety of physiologic stressors, it is especially critical that micronutrient supplies be well maintained during periods of stress. To that end, maintenance micronutrient stores in the body should be large enough to achieve and maintain adequate levels even during periods of stress.

With vitamins and minerals involved in virtually every biologic, chemical, and physiologic process, it should not be surprising that health effects of micronutrient inadequacies are abundant.

Micronutrient deficiencies in the general population

Most epidemiologic studies agree that most of the population in the developed world does not suffer from significant micronutrient deficiencies, if "deficiency" is defined as a severely compromised nutrient status. Nonetheless, there is substantive reason to believe that a broad array of specific micronutrient "insufficiencies" are common in the general population, even among the presumably well-fed.

According to data collected for the 2003 to 2006 National Health and Nutrition Examination Survey (NHANES), "10% or less" of the American population has nutritional deficiencies.[23,24] These data are largely based on biochemical indicators present in blood or urine, such as actual micronutrient concentrations or the activity of micronutrient-dependent enzymes. Wide age variations in specific micronutrient deficiencies are observed. For example, vitamin B12 deficiency is rare in children and adolescents (<1%) and more common in older adults (4%), whereas children are susceptible to iron deficiency (7%).[23] These estimates are based on a limited selection of biochemical indicators and so probably underestimate the true prevalence of deficiency.

Although the Centers for Disease Control and Prevention Executive Summary reports the deficiency prevalence as "10% or less," the NHANES data show a greater than 10% deficiency prevalence of vitamin B6 alone (**Fig. 1**). An individual may have one or several specific deficiencies. These studies examine micronutrient deficiencies one by one, not collectively across the range of possible deficiencies. The various micronutrient deficiencies are not all concentrated in the same "10%" of the population. Instead, different specific deficiencies are scattered sporadically across a larger segment of the population. There have been few attempts to estimate the prevalence of individuals who have one or more of the many possible micronutrient deficiencies, but it is apparent from these data that more than 10% of the population must have at least one micronutrient deficiency.

An alternative to selected biochemical assays are attempts to estimate deficiency in a population based on "food memory" questionnaires or food diaries, but these and other methods of measuring nutrient intake to assess nutrient status are fraught with problems.[27] If this approach were pursued anyway, it might seem reasonable to ask what percentage of the population fails to meet the RDA for a micronutrient, as the RDA is often interpreted by the public as a nutritional goal for individual intake. However, the RDA is defined as the intake level required by 97% of the healthy population (it is not possible to set a requirement that is generally applicable to unhealthy individuals), so attempting to aim the average intake standard at the 97% level would overestimate the prevalence of deficiencies.[28]

Instead of using RDAs, the preferred approach is to use the Estimated Average Requirement (EAR), which is the average daily intake that meets the nutrient requirements of 50% of the healthy population. Using this statistic, one can compare *average* intake to *average* requirement, which is a more meaningful way to estimate nutritional adequacy (**Fig. 2**). Approached this way, a similar picture emerges: Large segments of the population are not meeting intake standards for a variety of micronutrients. A variety of micronutrients are found to be ingested below intake standards.

All of these types of approaches to estimating nutritional deficiency in the population have limitations. Nonetheless, in looking at these types of data across the

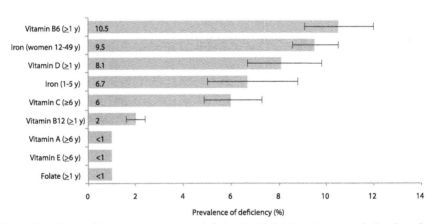

Fig. 1. Prevalence of single micronutrient deficiencies in the American population based on biochemical indicators of nutritional status. Prevalence estimates of nutritional deficiency based on data from the 2003–2006 NHANES in different age segments of the population. Error bars are 95% CIs. Similar profiles have been found in other databases in Canada[25] and England.[26] (*From* Centers for Disease Control and Prevention. Second national report on biochemical indicators of diet and nutrition in the US population. 2012 Executive Summary. Atlanta: Centers for Disease Control and Prevention; 2012. Available at: http://www.cdc.gov/nutritionreport/pdf/ExeSummary_Web_032612.pdf.)

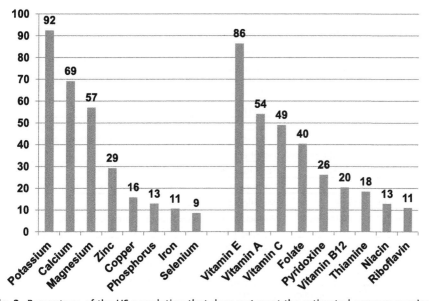

Fig. 2. Percentage of the US population that does **_not_** meet the estimated average requirements for specific nutrients. These figures do not include sources from vitamin supplements, so nutrient insufficiency may be overestimated. Also, not meeting the EAR (or the RDA) does not mean that an individual is nutrient insufficient. Food intake estimates are based on 1999–2004 data for the US population age 2 and older in "What We Eat in America," the dietary intake interview of NHANES. Food intake estimates are compared with EARs (or, if not available, Adequate Intakes), which is a component of the Dietary Reference Intake standards for nutritional recommendations set by the Institute of Medicine of the US National Academy of Sciences. (*Data from* United States Department of Agriculture (USDA), Agriculture Research Service (ARS). Community Nutrition Mapping Project. Available at: http://www.ars.usda.gov/Services/docs.htm?docid=15705. Accessed April 9, 2014. Data and figure assembled by Taron Fletcher.)

range of micronutrients, there is a consistent picture of gaps in nutrition in the general population, sporadic but not rare, varied and to some degree unpredictable, highly individual, and very hard to quantify. In view of the numerous nutritional insufficiencies in each individual micronutrient observed in parts of the population, it seems clear that a significant proportion of the population has suboptimal micronutrient status.[29] Despite their qualitative and quantitative vagueness, these data highlight the inadequacy of the common medical presumption that the American public has adequate micronutrient intake. To state the obvious, even a 10% prevalence of micronutrient deficiencies in a presumably well-fed or overfed nation is far from trivial and, based on NHANES data, this 10% figure appears to be a very significant underestimate. Even if these epidemiologic estimates do not and cannot describe them definitively, a priority goal for public health and a medical goal for individuals would be to address the sporadic micronutrient insufficiencies that these data imply.

Nutrient deficiencies and nutrient insufficiencies
The micronutrient intake standards, such as EAR and RDA, are generally established to help reduce the risk of deficiency states. Deficiency states were initially defined as the classic disorders associated with grossly inadequate nutrient intake (**Table 1**).

Table 1
Selected examples of vitamin deficiency diseases

Vitamin A	Retinol	Night blindness, corneal and conjunctival changes
Vitamin B1	Thiamine	Beriberi (including irritability, emotional lability) Wernicke encephalopathy (short-term memory loss, disorientation, confabulation, hallucinations)
Vitamin B2	Riboflavin	Seborrheic dermatitis
Vitamin B3	Niacin	Pellagra (including mental confusion, dementia, depression, anxiety, agitation, aggression, hallucinations, paranoia)
Vitamin B5	Pantothenic acid	Peripheral nerve damage
Vitamin B6	Pyridoxine	Seizures, amino acid metabolism disorders
Vitamin B7	Biotin	Carbohydrate and fat metabolic disorders, dermatitis
Vitamin B9	Folate	Megaloblastic anemia
Vitamin B12	Cobalamins	Pernicious anemia (including depression, mania, hallucinations, paranoia) with spinal cord degeneration
Vitamin C	Ascorbic acid	Scurvy (including depression, irritability)
Vitamin D	Calciferol	Rickets, osteomalacia, osteoporosis
Vitamin E	Tocopherol	Neurologic and muscular disorders
Vitamin K	Phytomenadione Menaquinone	Hemorrhagic diseases —

These disorders are not subtle, and they tend to be associated with relatively extreme deficiencies of particular micronutrients. An individual might have "deficient" micronutrient levels even if they do not have signs of frank deficiency disorders. Failure to meet RDA or EAR intake levels does not imply that an individual has a deficiency, and adequacy of dietary micronutrient intake does not guarantee that an individual has adequate nutrient status, because of individual variations in micronutrient supply and utilization. As a result, deficiencies may be conceptualized in terms of overt disease states and functional underperformance, or, alternatively, in terms of inadequate nutritional levels regardless of symptom status.

Mild inadequacies, characterized by suboptimal status but not severe enough to cause overt disease, are called "insufficiencies." Insufficiency states tend to be less clinically obvious but are much more prevalent. Short of overt disease, micronutrient insufficiencies imply some degree, or at least a risk, of compromise in physiologic functioning.

Formal definitions of deficiency and insufficiency levels are described for many micronutrients, often expressed in terms of serum concentrations. For example, based on bone health, vitamin D deficiency has traditionally been defined as serum concentrations of 25-hydroxyvitamin D below 20 ng/mL (50 nmol/L), but the consensus now holds that levels below 30 ng/mL are indicative of vitamin D insufficiency for the many other functions of vitamin D beyond bone health.

In the NHANES, which surveyed 6275 American children and adolescents from 2001 to 2004, the prevalence of vitamin D deficiency (<15 ng/mL) was 9%, and the prevalence of 25-hydroxyvitamin D insufficiency (<30 ng/mL) was a remarkable 61%.[30] Such data demonstrate that epidemiologic studies of vitamin *insufficiency* are needed to better understand nutritional needs at the population level.

Large-scale data from the Canadian Community Health Survey 2.2 (n = 34,381) similarly suggest that children (1–13 years old) have a very low prevalence of nutritional adequacy. Fewer than 30% of children were found to have sufficient intake of most micronutrients based on their dietary intake alone.[25] For the population 14 years or older, there was a similarly low level of nutritional adequacy, even when oral micronutrient supplementation was taken into account.

It should be clear that current data based on micronutrient *deficiencies* are likely to significantly underrepresent the extent of the problem and lead to policies that do not effectively serve the health needs of the public. Even conservative estimates of vitamin insufficiency implicate most of the population of both children and adults.

The intake amounts needed to obtain genuinely "optimal" functioning are above the cutoffs for vitamin insufficiency. There is no requirement that all areas of the body require similar amounts of a micronutrient, so optimal levels might vary depending on whether the target is hematological health, cardiac health, or brain health. In general, as more becomes known about nutritional effects on physiologic functioning, the standards of recommended micronutrient intake have tended to increase over time.

Still more subtle than nutrient insufficiencies are "relative insufficiencies," in which the biologically available amount of a nutrient might be adequate, but it is out of balance with respect to the availability of other micronutrients. Such imbalances in the ratios among micronutrients can have significant health consequences. A well-known example is the calcium-magnesium-phosphorus balance, in which excessive calcium leads to constipation and excessive magnesium leads to diarrhea. In another example, both chromium and vanadium can increase insulin sensitivity. The fact that chromium can counter insulin resistance does not mean that there is a chromium deficiency, because the problem might be due to low vanadium levels. These balances among micronutrients can be quite complex: the zinc-copper balance is strongly influenced by iron, magnesium, and manganese. A relative insufficiency may cause physiologic difficulty even if there is no absolute insufficiency of a micronutrient. Maintaining a proper balance among the various micronutrients can be critical to proper health.

The American problem in nutrition is minimal compared with the challenges in the developing world, where food shortages are endemic and food quality is too often abysmal. There remain enormous obstacles to dealing with the nutritional requirements and energy (calorie) needs of the world's population,[31] although some progress is being made in dealing with vitamin and mineral deficiencies on a worldwide basis.[32,33] Sufficient intakes of vitamin A, iodine, and iron have long been recognized as critical for immunologic and reproductive health, as well as physical growth and cognitive functioning, especially for children.[34]

Regardless of whether the health goal is to avoid deficiency diseases, to minimize insufficiency states, or to optimize functioning in part of (or the whole) body, the standard recommended intake levels are not assumed to be sufficient to replenish nutrient adequacy in the medically ill or in the seriously undernourished. Recommended dietary intake can vary by region, depending on the nutritional requirements and the nutritional resources of the local population. In geographic regions where low zinc levels in the soil might require local adjustment of copper intake standards, American RDA or EAR standards may not be helpful. In any case, the American population as a whole does not set a high standard for dietary competence.

General correlations between diet and mental health
Several epidemiologic reports have been extensively publicized for suggesting a link between depressive mood (not major depressive disorder) in adults and unhealthy "Western" dietary patterns (sugar-laden products, refined grains, red and processed meats, fatty and fried foods; low intake of fiber, fruits, and vegetables), but 2 recent

systematic reviews of these data (mostly in adults) found conflicting and inconclusive evidence of this link.[35,36] The only study examining bipolar disorder[37] in adults found some initial evidence that "Mediterranean" dietary patterns may be more favorable than Western or modern ("foodie") dietary patterns. Overall, the data in adults are limited and do not allow any clear conclusions.

Looking specifically at studies of youth, there appears to be a stronger correlation between diet and mental health, with more evidence of a link between poor diet and depressed mood. Several large independent studies have provided cross-sectional or prospective data supporting a link between an unhealthy diet in childhood[38] or adolescence[38-43] and lower general mental health scores. The 3 studies that collected data on internalizing (withdrawn/depressed) behaviors found correlations with poor diet quality.[38,39,42] Similarly, a study of 7114 adolescents (ages 10–14) found that depressive mood scores (Short Mood and Feelings Questionnaire) correlated with low diet-quality scores, with an adjusted odds ratio of 1.8 (1.5–2.1) for having depressive mood scores, when comparing the lowest and the highest quintiles for unhealthy diet scores.[44] One prospective study of 3757 children (ages 10–11) did not find diet quality correlating with internalizing disorders, but did find that increased variety in diet foods was associated with a lower prevalence of internalizing disorders,[45] so even this study could be viewed as positive evidence of a link.

The only clearly negative finding involved a different kind of experimental design. A prospective study of 23,020 mothers and their children found that higher intake levels of unhealthy foods (sugary drinks, salty snacks, refined cereals, processed meats) during pregnancy were not correlated with the presence of internalizing behaviors in the children at ages 1.5 to 5.0 years, although it did find a correlation with externalizing symptoms in early childhood.[38]

Overall, these studies provide reasonably consistent evidence of associations between diet quality and mental health in youth, with poor diets generally linked to an increased risk of internalizing disorders or depressive moods. These studies do not provide evidence addressing a possible connection to actual mood disorders in youth.

In fact, there are no studies of a mood-diet link in youths with mood disorders, but there is a study by Davison and Kaplan[46] that examined the relationship between dietary components and general functioning in 97 community adults with mood disorders. Scores for Global Assessment of Functioning were found to correlate with dietary intake of energy (calories), carbohydrates, fiber, total fat, linoleic acid, and certain micronutrients: magnesium ($r = 0.41$, $P<.001$); zinc ($r = 0.35$, $P<.001$); calcium, phosphorus, potassium, iron, B3, B5, B6, B9, and B12 (all $P<.05$). With each of the nutrients, there was a consistent pattern of increased nutrient intake correlating with better global functioning. However, depression and mania scores did not correlate with total daily intake of most micronutrients, except for iron and zinc. There was a correlation between decreased depression (Hamilton Depression Rating Scale [HAM-D]) scores and increased iron levels ($r = -0.22$, $P<.05$), and also a correlation between decreased mania (Young Mania Rating Scale [YMRS]) scores and increased levels of zinc ($r = -0.25$, $P<.05$). These findings are interesting but have not yet been subjected to replication in other samples.

Overall, the data linking general diet and mood seem suggestive but inconclusive in adults, even in adults with mood disorder. In contrast, the data in youth seem more suggestive, although there are no data on a link to mood disorders. Even if there is an association, it is unclear from these findings whether depressed mood is a cause or a result of a low-quality diet, although some prospective data suggest that the dominant mechanism is poor diet leading to a depressive mood, at least in adolescents.[40] A more definitive answer to the question of causation could be provided by intervention studies showing nutrient-induced improvements in mood.

TREATMENT OF MOOD DISORDERS WITH SINGLE MICRONUTRIENTS

Kaplan and Shannon[47] conducted a review of the evidence linking specific micronutrients to mood symptoms in children and adults. Based on clinical trials, as well as biochemical correlational studies, significant mood effects in humans were identified for a large number of vitamins and minerals (**Box 5**), and beneficial therapeutic effects have been identified for a small number of single micronutrients.

The study of individual micronutrients for treating psychiatric disorders is an endeavor that goes back decades.[48] Overall, these studies have yielded relatively few consistent replicable findings.[49] Many reports on the efficacy of single micronutrients for treating mood in adults, conducted in healthy volunteers and in patients with mood disorders, have not stood up well on replication. Nonetheless, a small number of micronutrients have shown consistent evidence of some degree of antidepressant effectiveness in adults as single micronutrient treatments,

---

Box 5
Single micronutrients associated with mood alterations in adults

Vitamins

    Vitamin B1: Thiamine

    Vitamin B3: Niacin

    Vitamin B6: Pyridoxine

    Vitamin B7: Biotin

    Vitamin B9: Folate

    Vitamin B12: Cobalamin

    Vitamin C: Ascorbic acid

    Vitamin D: Cholecalciferol

    Vitamin E: D-alpha tocopheryl

Minerals

    Lithium

    Magnesium

    Calcium

    Iron

    Copper

    Zinc

    Chromium

    Selenium

Data from Kaplan BJ, Crawford SG, Field CJ, et al. Vitamins, minerals, and mood. Psychol Bull 2007;133(5):747–60.

including folic acid and vitamin D for major depressive disorder (MDD), vitamin B12 for MDD in the elderly, and, more speculatively, chromium for atypical depression with carbohydrate craving and selenium for prevention of postpartum depression.

This is a large and largely unsatisfying literature, involving a huge number of methodologically unsound studies, which will not be reviewed here. Instead, we will focus mainly on the relatively small number of randomized double-blind placebo-controlled trials (RDBPCTs), with emphasis on the few single-micronutrient treatments whose findings in adults offer some plausible hope that they may someday prove to have value in youth.

Folic Acid (Vitamin B9)

Folic acid is involved in many biologic processes. In its active forms, tetrahydrofolates participate in single-carbon transfers, methylation (including the rate-limiting step in DNA synthesis), cell replication, brain development, and red blood cell formation, among many others. It is a cofactor in the biosynthesis of S-adenosyl-methionine (SAMe) and choline, 2 small molecules that have well demonstrated effects on mood, as well as on the synthesis of serotonin, dopamine, and norepinephrine, which are neurotransmitters implicated in mood disorders.[50–53]

Folate deficiencies have been implicated in diverse disease states and abnormalities, including depression in adults. Low serum folate levels are associated with lower levels of serotonin and dopamine metabolites in cerebrospinal fluid. Clinically, lower folate levels are correlated with greater severity of depression, weaker response to serotonin reuptake inhibitors (SSRIs), more rapid relapse after effective treatment, and perhaps to weaker responses to lithium augmentation and to electroconvulsive therapy.[54] Some preliminary data suggest a specific association between low folate status and the melancholic symptoms of depression.[55,56]

The Complementary and Alternative Medicine Task Force of the American Psychiatric Association[57] found that the data on folic acid were inadequate to draw any conclusions regarding its value as a monotherapy, but concluded that folic acid was a "reasonable" adjunctive treatment for MDD in adults.

Four RDBPCTs have examined antidepressant-treated adults (ages 21–65) who received augmentation with either folic acid[58,59] or L-methylfolate[51,60] or instead received augmentation with placebo. An additional randomized controlled trial (RCT) of antidepressant augmentation compared higher and lower doses of folic acid.[61] In these studies, antidepressant treatment usually consisted of an SSRI, typically fluoxetine 20 mg daily. All 5 RCTs showed that folic acid or L-methylfolate augmentation of antidepressants was effective (in comparison with placebo or a lower dose), with an effect size of 0.35 to 0.4.[62,63] In addition to folic acid and L-methylfolate, an open-label trial suggests that folinic acid also may effectively augment SSRI treatment.[64] One study showed that L-methylfolate augmentation was effective after patients had not responded to 8 weeks of treatment with fluoxetine 20 mg,[51] and that this clinical response appeared linked to obesity and to specific genetic and biologic markers related to inflammation and folate metabolism.[62]

The only negative study on folic acid augmentation was a naturalistic RCT that examined a low dose of folic acid (in combination with vitamin B12) in 209 elderly subjects (ages 60–74), but this unblinded study was conducted on a community sample that was not systematically diagnosed, entry into the study was based on patients attesting that they were taking antidepressants, and details of the antidepressant treatments were not specified.[65] Although a naturalistic study of folic acid augmentation would be useful, this study does not provide strong evidence against the treatment, especially in the face of 5 positive RDBPCTs. It might be noted, though, that 2 of the 5 RCTs were funded by pharmaceutical manufacturers.[51,58]

The available monotherapy studies of folic acid in MDD are methodologically limited. In fact, there are no RDBPCTs of folic acid monotherapy in MDD. In view of its relatively modest effect as an adjunctive therapy, folic acid seems unlikely to become a clinically relevant antidepressant monotherapy.

Several RCTs have examined the mood effects of folic acid in the general population. An RDBPCT of folic acid monotherapy, examining 211 women (ages 20–92) in a nonclinical sample, found positive effects after 35 days on cognition (including processing speed, recall, and recognition memory), but not on mood.[66] Three RCTs in the general population explored the effects of folic acid combined with other B vitamins, typically B12 and B6, and also found no beneficial effects on mood[67–69]; however, these samples consisted largely of elderly subjects, so it is unclear whether the B vitamin intervention did not have mood effects because the subjects were not depressed or because the sample was geriatric. In general, the effect of folic acid in nonpsychiatric and/or geriatric populations is unclear, but studies have generally been negative. However, one RDBPCT of 273 stroke survivors showed a reduced risk of developing MDD (18% vs 23%, adjusted hazard ratio 0.48) in subjects who were followed for a mean of 7 years after their stroke while taking folic acid combined with vitamins B12 and B6, although the effect did not reach significance in the intent-to-treat analysis.[70]

In youth, a cross-sectional study[71] conducted in 6517 community adolescents (ages 12–15) found that higher dietary folate intake was correlated with fewer depressive symptoms (adjusted odds ratio [OR] 0.6, $P<.002$). The same study found lower depression scores in youth correlated with low vitamin B6 (pyridoxine) intake (OR 0.73, $P<.02$) and (for girls only) low vitamin B2 (riboflavin) intake (OR 0.85, $P = .03$), but not with vitamin B12 (cobalamin) intake. No studies of folic acid are available in youth with depressive disorders, either as adjunctive treatment or as monotherapy.

Folic acid is generally well tolerated, but it is associated with a variety of adverse effects (**Box 6**). Central nervous system (CNS) reactions have included symptoms suggestive of depression[72] or mania,[73] although the mania has been questioned.[74] Rare allergic reactions[75–78] have been described with folic acid, even when used within moderate dose ranges. Folic acid treatment can lead to delayed recognition and treatment of vitamin B12 deficiency, because folic acid corrects the megaloblastic anemia that often heralds B12 deficiency (macrocytosis results from the inhibition of DNA synthesis caused by B12 or folate deficiency; B12 deficiency does not cause macrocytosis in the presence of adequate folate). There are also well-established nutrient-drug interactions involving folic acid with anticonvulsants, oral contraceptives, and alcohol.[79] Some epidemiologic data on folic acid raise the question of a possible increase in risk for cancer or cardiac events with chronic use,[80,81] a suggestive finding that underscores the need for safety testing, even for compounds as seemingly innocuous as folic acid.

Several versions of folic acid, L-methylfolate, and folinic acid are commercially available, but their clinical differences in treating depression are poorly defined. L-methylfolate is available by prescription at higher doses (7.5 or 15 mg) or over the counter at lower doses (0.8–1.0 mg). Although L-methylfolate was initially marketed for people who had difficulty in converting folate to its active form, some data suggest that methylfolate may help adults with depression who do not have the enzyme defect, consistent with the broader hypothesis that folic acid itself can contribute adjunctively to the treatment of MDD in adults.

Box 6
Clinical points on folic acid

Adverse Effects

Gastrointestinal effects, including nausea, anorexia, bloating, and flatulence.

Bitter or unpleasant taste.

Alterations in sleep (insomnia, vivid anxiety dreams), concentration, mood (depression and possibly mania), irritability, activity level, or mental clarity.

Seizures in patients receiving anticonvulsants, possibly due to lowered plasma anticonvulsant levels.

Question of increased risk of cancer and cardiac events.

Delayed recognition and treatment of vitamin B12 deficiency.

Allergic reactions, including erythema, rash, pruritis, urticaria, malaise, fever, and bronchospasm.

Nutrient-Drug Interactions

Folate absorption, blood levels, or effects are reduced by alcohol, nicotine (smoking), estrogens (oral contraceptives), nonsteroidal anti-inflammatory drugs (ibuprofen, naproxen, aspirin), H2 receptor antagonist antacids (ranitidine, famotidine), anticonvulsants (valproate, carbamazepine, lamotrigine, phenytoin, primidone), antibiotics (tetracycline), isotretinoin, metformin, diuretics (thiazides, furosemide), isoniazid.

Folic acid reduces levels or effects of anticonvulsants (phenytoin).

There is an RDBPCT describing folic acid as an effective augmentation agent for valproate treatment of acute mania in adults.[82] In an RDBPCT of 88 adults with mania treated with valproate, a 30% reduction in YMRS scores was apparent after 3 weeks of add-on folic acid (3 mg daily) compared with placebo augmentation ($P<.005$), with an effect size of 0.4. An early RDBPCT also suggests that folic acid (0.2 mg daily) may be effective for augmentation of lithium maintenance treatment in preventing relapse in adults with unipolar and bipolar depression, with the strength of the prophylactic effects correlating to plasma folate concentrations.[83] Neither of these studies has been replicated.

Overall, folic acid, L-methylfolate, and perhaps folinic acid appear to be modestly but clearly effective for augmentation of SSRI treatment of MDD in adults, with generally minimal adverse effects. It is unclear whether folic acid has value as a monotherapy of depression, whether its effectiveness for augmentation might be weaker in geriatric depression, and whether it alters mood in nonclinical samples. Based on findings in adults, folic acid appears to be the most likely of the single micronutrient treatments to have some potential role in treating depression in youth, albeit as an adjunctive option. However, there have been no trials of folic acid in youth with MDD.

Cobalamins (Vitamin B12)

The biologically active coenzyme forms of vitamin B12 are methylcobalamin (in intracellular fluids) and adenosylcobalamin (in mitochondria). Vitamin B12 is commercially available in oral supplements as cyanocobalamin, a synthetic but biologically inactive form, or in injectable depot form as hydroxocobalamin. Like folate, it participates in many biologic reactions, including methylation, DNA synthesis, hematopoiesis, and numerous metabolic processes, including synthesis of SAMe, conversion of folate to its active form as tetrahydrofolic acid, and myelin formation.

Its value in treating depression appears to be mainly in elderly patients. Elderly people are more susceptible to B12 deficiency because of declining absorption associated with senescence (about 30% of people older than 60 have atrophic gastritis), but patients of any age with inflammatory bowel disease or other gastrointestinal absorption impairments can be at risk.

B12 supplementation may have a role in treating certain older patients, but it is unlikely to be relevant for treating depressive disorders in otherwise healthy youth. Arguably, screening for serum B12 (or methylmalonic acid) levels might be considered for youths with chronic malabsorption, but it is not relevant for typical cases of depression in children or adolescents. Youths with very severe B12 deficiency may present with depressive and psychotic symptoms in association with obvious neurologic symptoms; their mental symptoms respond to B12 injections within 1 to 2 weeks.[84,85]

Although there are several trials of B12 combined with folic acid (and sometimes other vitamins) in treating depression, the 2 trials in adults of vitamin B12 monotherapy[86,87] were negative. The only trial of B12 as augmentation to an antidepressant[88] showed a positive effect, but was methodologically weak.

There are no studies of vitamin B12 for treating major depression in youth, and it does not appear to be a promising area for research, except speculatively in youth with chronic gastrointestinal absorption impairments. Folic acid would be a better candidate for a trial for treating depressed youth.

Calciferols (Vitamin D)

Vitamin D has received much less attention than the B vitamins in psychiatry, and so this micronutrient is covered in more detail.

Vitamin D is traditionally viewed as crucial for calcium and phosphate absorption, calcium homeostasis, and bone health, including its role in preventing rickets (childhood osteomalacia), osteomalacia in adults, and osteoporosis. More current understanding recognizes vitamin D as a series of steroid hormones that are relevant in a broad range of physiologic processes. Low vitamin D status has been implicated in apoptosis, immunologic regulation (increased proinflammatory cytokines and inflammation), insulin resistance, aberrant cell proliferation and differentiation, and neuronal connectivity.[89–91]

Hypovitaminosis D has been implicated in the pathophysiology of hypertension; cardiovascular disease (eg, left ventricular hypertrophy); type 2 diabetes; infectious, inflammatory, and autoimmune disorders (including asthma); and certain cancers (colorectal and possibly breast, prostate, and pancreatic). During pregnancy, low levels are associated with preeclampsia, infections, premature birth, and low birth weight.[92] Early evidence suggests that vitamin D supplementation may exert a therapeutic influence in all of these conditions.[90,93,94]

Similar to other steroid hormones and to thyroid hormones, vitamin D isomers may be viewed as neurohormones that are essential to brain development and functioning. Vitamin D (calcitriol) receptors are distributed diffusely in the brain, including in the hypothalamus, basal ganglia, hippocampus, cerebellum, and thalamus.[95] In the CNS, hypovitaminosis D has been linked to Alzheimer disease and other forms of cognitive dysfunction, epilepsy, Parkinson disease, multiple sclerosis, and chronic pain, as well as depression, bipolar disorder, schizophrenia, and autism.

The 2 main forms of vitamin D are cholecalciferol (vitamin D3) and ergocalciferol (vitamin D2). Vitamin D3 is synthesized in the skin after exposure to sunlight (ultraviolet

B radiation) or ingested in animal-derived foods. Vitamin D2 is obtained through the diet (eg, dairy, fish, plants). Both are converted to the biologically active form, called calcitriol or 1,25-dihydroxyvitamin D. The form that is most evident in circulation is 25-hydroxyvitamin D, and that is the form that is usually assayed to assess nutritional adequacy of vitamin D.

Although vitamin D *deficiency* has been conventionally defined by 25-hydroxyvitamin D serum levels below 10 to 20 ng/mL and vitamin D *insufficiency* by levels below 30 ng/mL, more recent data suggest that higher blood levels are desirable. Insufficiency is now increasingly defined as physiologic abnormalities associated with levels below 35 to 40 ng/mL. Many specialists clinically advise a normal range of 50 to 80 ng/mL. Undesirable effects may emerge above 80 to 120 ng/mL.

Low vitamin D levels often result from inadequate dietary intake and lack of sunlight exposure (eg, northern latitudes), but they also have been associated with female gender, older age, obesity, dark skin tone, low milk consumption (less than once weekly), more than 4 hours daily of screen time (television, computer, or video), high altitudes, malabsorption, and nonuse of vitamin D supplementation.

As previously noted, in the NHANES of more than 6000 American children and adolescents in 2001 to 2004, the prevalence of vitamin D insufficiency was 61% and of vitamin D deficiency was 9%.[30] Only 4% had consumed a daily mean of 400 IU, where the RDA is 600 IU. Among these youth, vitamin D deficiency was associated with more diabetes (OR 1.9), hypertension (OR 2.5), low high-density lipoprotein (OR 3.0), elevated C-reactive protein (OR 0.7), low serum calcium (OR 0.09), and increased parathyroid hormone levels (OR 3.6) compared with youths with 25-hydroxyvitamin D levels 30 ng/mL or higher.

Several clinical studies suggest a wide range of potential influences of vitamin D in the CNS. In a study of 308 girls who were followed from a gestational age of 18 weeks until age 20 years, the mothers' vitamin D levels at 18 weeks of pregnancy were found to be a significant predictor of the children's risk of eating disorders during adolescence.[96] Other data suggest a relationship between prenatal vitamin D status and language impairment at ages 5 and 10 years, although these may be specific deficits that do not apply to all aspects of CNS functioning.[97]

Correlations between vitamin D levels and depression in adults

Two recent reviews and meta-analyses examined large cross-sectional and prospective cohort studies assessing the link between serum 25-hydroxyvitamin D levels and the risk for depression in adults. In one meta-analysis,[98] lower vitamin D levels were found in adults with depression than in controls (Standardized Mean Difference = 0.60, 95% Confidence Interval [CI] 0.23–0.97). The cross-sectional studies showed an increased odds ratio of 1.31 for depression in the lowest compared with the highest vitamin D quartiles (95% CI 1.0–1.71), and the cohort studies showed an increased hazard ratio for depression of 2.21 (95% CI 1.40–3.49). The other analysis found low 25-hydroxyvitamin D levels to be significantly associated with depression in only 5 of the 11 case-control studies (n>43,000) and in 2 of the 5 prospective cohort studies (n>12,000, mostly elderly), but the overall data supported a small but significant reduction in risk for depression (OR 0.92–0.96) for each 10 ng/mg increase in serum 25-dihydroxyvitamin D levels.[99] Subsequently, 5 additional cross-sectional studies have examined this association. Four of the 5 studies showed a statistically significant correlation of lower vitamin D levels with increased depression.[100–104] The fifth study showed only a statistical trend.[105]

Despite the differences across studies, the overall findings point to a correlation between depression and low vitamin D status. Several instructive reasons may explain the variability in the data:

1. A cross-sectional study of 12,594 adults found that patients with a prior history of depression were at greater risk of depression associated with a low vitamin D level, whereas patients with no history of depression showed no correlation of vitamin D levels and current depression.[106] This suggests that the association of hypovitaminosis D with depression may be stronger in patients with repeated depressive episodes, a factor that other cross-sectional studies did not examine.
2. Two studies found that the depression/hypovitaminosis D correlation is strongest during low vitamin D months (eg, winter in North America) and that the association persisted only weakly during the high vitamin D months.[107,108]
3. A cross-sectional study in adults found that the risk of depression only began to reduce once the serum 25-hydroxyvitamin D levels were higher than 42 ng/mL,[109] suggesting that the standard cutoff for vitamin D insufficiency at 30 ng/mL might need to be revised for studies of depression, consistent with recent claims that optimal serum vitamin D levels are 50 to 80 ng/mL.

Correlations between vitamin D levels and depression in youth

Several cross-sectional studies in youth have been published and, as in adults, the findings are conflicting. A study of 945 young adults at age 20 years[110] found a 10% increase in serum 25-hydroxyvitamin D concentrations was associated with a 9% reduction in depression ($P<.001$) in males but not in females. Two smaller studies also found correlations of vitamin D status in youth with mood[111] or well-being scores.[112] In contrast, 4 cross-sectional studies in adolescents and young adults did not find such a correlation,[113–116] including a rigorous study of 104 adolescents finding no significant elevation of vitamin D deficiency among 36 youths with major depression or among 52 youths with other mood disorders.[114]

A large prospective cohort study[117] assessed vitamin D status at a mean age of 9.8 years and then evaluated depressive symptoms (Mood and Feelings Questionnaire) in 2750 youths at ages 10.6 and 13.8 years. Higher concentrations of 25-hydroxyvitamin D at 9.8 years predicted fewer depressive symptoms at 13.8 years (adjusted risk ratio 0.90, 95% confidence interval [CI] 0.86–0.95), but not at age 10.6 years (risk ratio 0.98), suggesting that the association between vitamin D3 levels and depression may emerge during early adolescence, perhaps related to puberty.

Overall, the correlational studies showed associations between vitamin D levels and depression in 7 of the 16 adult studies and in 4 of the 8 youth studies, so no clear age effect emerges. Again, the conflicting findings are difficult to interpret but could reflect a genuine correlation that is diluted by uncontrolled factors, such as single versus repeated depressive episodes, geographic differences (less sunlight exposure in northern latitudes), sampling season (winter vs summer), and dietary intake levels.

Correlational findings do not speak to causality; even if there is an association, it is unclear whether hypovitaminosis D is a cause or result of depression. Another possibility is that low vitamin D is a marker of upstream illness; for example, if inflammatory processes were a cause of low circulating vitamin D levels, then a wide range of inflammation-related medical disorders might be associated with reduced vitamin D levels, and treatment with vitamin D might have little or no value in treating these disorders. This explanation has been proposed to explain why so many medical illnesses are associated with low vitamin D levels and why so little health benefit has been seen in clinical trials in a variety of medical fields.[118] Nonetheless, clinical trials may be helpful in assessing whether hypovitaminosis D is a causal factor in depression as well as to determine whether vitamin D supplementation has antidepressant effects.

Treatment of depression with vitamin D

Ten RCTs in adults have examined whether vitamin D supplementation can treat depressive moods, although only a small number examined patients with psychiatric disorders. Four of the 10 RCTs in adults have yielded negative results,[119–122] but only 1 used acceptable depression measures, and it found no benefit in 230 adults who received either oral 40,000 IU weekly or placebo for 6 months.[121]

Six randomized placebo-controlled treatment studies in adults were positive, but 4 provided only weak evidence. A study found statistically significant improvement after 1 year of vitamin D treatment in 441 overweight adults, but the change was not clinically significant, mainly because the subjects started with only very mild depressive symptoms (mean baseline Beck Depression Inventory [BDI] 4–5).[123] A study of a single administration of high-dose vitamin D (intramuscular 300,000 IU) in 120 depressive adults (BDI>17) found improvement 3 months after injections compared with placebo, but standardized psychiatric diagnostic evaluations were not used and the study was not double-blind.[124] A study of seasonal affective disorder found improvement compared with bright-light therapy, but the study was small (n = 15).[125] Two used inadequate methodology.[126,127] The best data come from an RDBPCT examining 42 adults with formally diagnosed MDD being treated with fluoxetine 20 mg. Compared with placebo augmentation, augmentation with vitamin D3 1500 IU daily for 8 weeks produced significant improvements (HAM-D, BDI-21) starting at treatment week 4.[128]

Overall, there were 6 positive and 4 negative vitamin D studies in adults, and the most methodologically reliable studies were split with 1 positive and 1 negative result. Two recent systematic reviews found that the studies in adults were inconclusive.[129,130]

Only 1 treatment study of vitamin D has been conducted in youth with depression.[112] In this open-label case series, 48 adolescents (ages 10–19) with clinically diagnosed depression (without standardized evaluations) and low vitamin D levels (<25 ng/mL) were treated with vitamin D3 for 3 months (4000 IU daily for a month, then 2000 IU). Improvements were shown on self-rated depression scores on the Mood and Feelings Questionnaire-Short Version (14.7 $\pm$ 3.7 to 7.1 $\pm$ 5.3, $P<.05$) and on the World Health Organization Well-Being Scale-5 (25 $\pm$ 18 to 43 $\pm$ 25, $P<.001$), and an unvalidated scale showed improvements in daytime tiredness, insomnia, somatic complaints, irritability, and concentration. The study was conducted in Sweden, 74% of cases were initiated in November through April, with no dark-toned youth in the sample, and again all subjects had low vitamin D levels. Although this is an uncontrolled study in a population characterized by factors that increase the likelihood of response, its findings justify an RCT in youth.

Clinical recommendations

Current evidence does not support vitamin D supplementation in the treatment or prevention of depression in adults or youth, but additional studies are clearly warranted. Especially in view of its relatively low toxicity, clinicians may consider its use in vulnerable populations or individuals with known risk factors, and especially if vitamin D insufficiency is documented by blood testing.

Clinicians might consider a variety of risk factors. Given the role of sunlight exposure, the risk of low vitamin D levels increases with higher northern latitudes, more use of sunscreens, more indoor work, little outdoor recreation, darker skin tone, obesity, advanced age, chronic illness, or bedridden status. Seasonal changes render lower vitamin D levels during the autumn and winter months in the northern hemisphere,[131–133] so clinical supplementation may be most relevant in the cold weather months. Adolescents may be at generally higher risk of low vitamin D levels than children,[131] perhaps because of their reduced milk intake.

Hypovitaminosis D appears more marked in patients with more severe depressions. Some data suggest that hypovitaminosis D is more likely in patients with psychosis, both in youth[114] and adults,[134–137] and in suicidal patients.[108,133,138,139]

Future RCTs should evaluate the clinical risk factors in individuals with and without low vitamin D levels, examining both the general population and patients with mood (and other psychiatric) disorders, with attention to possible differences in supplementation effectiveness in winter versus summer.

Although the Institute of Medicine has suggested that most Americans across the nation do not need high-dose D supplements,[140] the NHANES finding of a 61% prevalence of 25-hydroxyvitamin D insufficiency (<30 ng/mL) in children and adolescents remains noteworthy.[30] Supplementation might be more relevant in northern states and perhaps especially in psychiatric populations. A chart review found that 75% of 544 psychiatric adult inpatients in Chicago had vitamin D insufficiency (<30 ng/mL), with a mean level of 22.[141] Similarly, the vast majority of patients in my psychiatric practice in New England have levels below 25 ng/mL. On the other hand, I rarely see vitamin D supplementation produce a clinically noticeable mood improvement. Supplementation can still be justified for general health reasons in patients with demonstrated vitamin D insufficiency.

Consonant with growing evidence that higher serum vitamin D levels are more helpful than traditionally believed, the Institute of Medicine has recently announced a sharp increase in the Dietary Reference Intakes for vitamin D: the RDA was raised from 200 IU to 600 IU daily (for individuals aged 1–70 years).[140] The maximum daily intake that can be safely used chronically without medical supervision (the Upper Level Intake) is 4000 IU daily for individuals aged 9 years and older (3000 IU daily for 4–8-year-olds). Generally, supplementation with vitamin D3 seems more effective than D2 in maintaining nutrient adequacy.[142]

Clinicians who offer vitamin D supplementation should be aware of its potential adverse effects, which are mostly related to hypercalcemia (with chronic use or acute intoxication), and nutrient-drug interactions (**Box 7**). However, the documentation regarding the proposed interactions is not uniformly strong.[143,144]

The wide range of medical disorders associated with hypovitaminosis D highlights that numerous physiologic mechanisms can be affected, underscoring the multiple roles that vitamin D plays in biology. Once thought to be "the bone vitamin," the plethora of effects of vitamin D in body and brain emphasizes the complexity of the influence of micronutrients in health and disease.

Pyridoxine (Vitamin B6)

Like other micronutrients, pyridoxine is involved in a vast number of biologic processes. As a cofactor for decarboxylase enzymes, pyridoxine plays an essential role in the synthesis of neurotransmitters, including dopamine, norepinephrine, serotonin, and gamma-aminobutyric acid. Vitamin B6 also participates in the metabolism of nucleic acids, proteins, carbohydrates (gluconeogenesis), fats (myelin, phospholipids,

---

Box 7
Clinical points on vitamin D

Adverse effects: Mainly related to hypercalcemia (increased risk if given with calcium)

  Anorexia, nausea, vomiting, constipation, diarrhea, weight loss

  Muscle weakness or pain, bone pain

  Irritability, confusion, dizziness, headache, fatigue

  Diabetes insipidus (excessive thirst and urination, low urine specific gravity)

  Proteinuria, azotemia

  Nephrolithiasis (kidney stones)

  Hypercalcification of the bones, soft tissues, kidneys, and heart

  Hypertension

  Cardiac arrhythmias

Proposed nutrient-drug interactions

  Vitamin D can reduce the effects of statins, calcium channel blockers, and digoxin (but also increase the risk of digoxin-induced cardiac arrhythmias).

  Vitamin D levels or effects can be reduced by alcohol, cimetidine, magnesium-containing antacids, certain anticonvulsants (valproate, carbamazepine, phenytoin), corticosteroids, orlistat (Xenical for weight loss), ketoconazole, and heparin.

  Vitamin D levels or effects can be increased by statins and thiazide diuretics.

---

prostaglandins), steroids, collagen, heme, and homocysteine, among many other functions in the body and brain.

There are 3 RDBPCTs of pyridoxine monotherapy on mood in healthy adults. A 5-week trial in 211 healthy women (ages 20–92) found no effect on mood (Center for Epidemiological Studies-Depression Scale, Profile of Mood States Questionnaire [POMS]), relative to placebo, although some cognitive benefits were observed, mainly in memory performance tasks.[66] A 3-month trial in 76 healthy elderly (ages 70–77) community volunteers also showed no effects of pyridoxine on mood, but it was inadequately assessed through a list of mood adjectives[145]; again, some limited cognitive improvements were noted. A RDBPCT examined the effects of pyridoxine on the adverse effects of oral contraceptives in 124 women (ages 18–40); outcome assessment was not rigorous, and trial duration was only 4 weeks, but again no effect of pyridoxine relative to placebo was observed on mood or physical symptoms; cognition was not assessed.[146] So the 3 monotherapy trials in healthy adults were negative.

Perhaps the strongest available suggestion that pyridoxine may be relevant to mood is an RDBPCT of 129 young healthy adults who took a 9-ingredient multivitamin (at 10 times RDA levels) for 1 year, which found that the observed improvements in "agreeable" feelings (and, in women, "composure" and general well-being) were positively correlated with pyridoxine (and riboflavin) levels.[147] Perhaps an interaction of pyridoxine with other B vitamins might explain this finding in the absence of monotherapy effectiveness. On the other hand, a large cross-sectional study of 6517 community adolescents (ages 12–15) unexpectedly found lower depression scores with *low* dietary intake of pyridoxine (OR 0.73, $P<.02$).[71] This finding is difficult to interpret.

Pyridoxine monotherapy has been specifically examined for specific effects on premenstrual mood. Reviews[148] and meta-analyses[149,150] of the many early trials found mostly conflicting effects or weakly supported positive effects, and 3 of the 4 best studies on premenstrual symptoms found no effect on mood.[151–154] All of these studies were compromised by use of outcome instruments not validated for mood measurement, lack of standardized diagnostic assessments, small unpowered sample sizes, inadequately presented data or statistical analyses, and uneven management or control for concurrent use of oral contraceptives. Few of the studies included adolescents, and none examined age effects.

Early questionable claims of pyridoxine benefits for autism have been largely dismissed[155,156] and, in any case, mood effects were not evaluated in those studies.

To my knowledge, there are no adequate RCTs of pyridoxine monotherapy in adults or youth with mood disorders. The best available data are inconclusive but do not support effects on mood, although there is a signal of possible benefit for cognition. There are no strong grounds for prioritizing pyridoxine trials on mood at this time.

Other Single Micronutrients

Several other micronutrients have been examined for mood effects in randomized controlled trials in adults, mostly with conflicting effects (**Table 2**). None of them have been examined in child or adolescent samples.

Chromium

Chromium monotherapy has been examined in 3 RDBPCTs. Two of the studies were conducted in atypical depression; one was small,[158] but the other[157] was adequately powered (n = 113). No overall change on mood was observed, but a subgroup with carbohydrate craving showed improvement in both carbohydrate craving and mood.[157] An RDBPCT on binge-eating disorder found nonsignificant reductions in depression ratings, binge frequency, and body weight.[159]

Zinc

Zinc has been examined in 3 RDBPCTs as a potential augmentation (add-on) treatment. In 2 studies of unipolar MDD from the same group, the earlier study found zinc augmentation of antidepressant treatment to be effective.[162] The second study had a more nuanced finding[160]: that zinc augmentation of imipramine was not routinely beneficial, but did appear helpful for patients who were previously known to be treatment-resistant (**Fig. 3**). The benefit of zinc for treatment-resistant depression, but not for routine depression, suggests a zinc-related mechanism in antidepressant treatment resistance, possibly glutaminergic: Glutaminergic neurons are the only intraneuronal location of zinc, where it is involved in allosteric modulation of N-methyl-D-aspartate and other receptors.[175] In a related study, zinc levels were lower in MDD than in 25 healthy controls, and zinc levels increased during imipramine treatment with or without zinc supplementation.[161]

Zinc "augmentation" of multivitamin supplements was examined in 30 young healthy volunteers (mean age 19) in an RDBPCT.[163] Compared with youths receiving a multivitamin formulation without minerals, the addition of zinc produced small but significant ($P<.02$) reductions in scores for depression/dejection (23% vs 18% for multivitamins alone) and anger/hostility (29% vs 13% for multivitamins alone) on the POMS Questionnaire.

All 3 RDBPCTs showed zinc to be an effective augmentation agent for mood, with 2 studies in patients treated for MDD and 1 study in healthy subjects on multivitamins.

Table 2
Randomized double-blind placebo-controlled trials of other single micronutrients on mood (not including folic acid, vitamin D, and pyridoxine; see text)

Treatment	Concurrent Treatment	Design	Age (y)	Population	Outcome Measures	Outcome (Statistically Significant Changes Compared to Placebo)	Citation
Chromium	Monotherapy	RDBPCT 2 mo n = 113	Mean 46	Atypical depression outpatients	HAM-D, CGI-I	No overall improvement; but in subgroup with carbohydrate craving, mood and carbohydrate craving improved	157
Chromium	Monotherapy	RDBPCT 2 mo n = 15	Mean 46	Atypical depression	HAM-D, CGI-I	Nonsignificantly reduced depression, perhaps more in overeaters	158
Chromium	Monotherapy	RDBPCT 6 mo n = 24	Mean 36	Binge-eating disorder, overweight	QIDS-SR, EDE-Q	Nonsignificant reductions in depression, binge frequency, and weight	159
Zinc	Imipramine	RDBPCT 12 wk n = 60	18–55	DSM-IV MDE unipolar	CGI, BDI, HAM-D, and MADRS	Zinc add-on had no benefit in nonresistant patients, but reduced depression in previously treatment-resistant patients	160,161
Zinc	Tricyclic or SSRI	RDBPCT 12 wk n = 20	25–57	DSM-IV MDE unipolar	HAM-D, BDI	Zinc add-on reduced depression	162
Zinc	Multivitamins	RDBPCT 10 wk n = 30	Mean 19	Healthy volunteers	POMS, Cornell Medical Index	Zinc add-on reduced depression and anger	163

Thiamine	Monotherapy	RDBPCT 2 mo n = 120	Mean 20	Healthy students	POMS, GHQ	Better mood and trend toward more clear-headedness	164
Thiamine	Monotherapy	RDBPCT 6 wk n = 80	65–92	Healthy elderly in thiamine-deficient region (65% had baseline insufficiency)	Subjective assessment	More well-being, energy, and appetite	165
Selenium	Some subjects took folate or iron	RDBPCT 8 mo n = 166	16–35	Postpartum depression	EPDS	Prenatal (starting first trimester) treatment reduced symptoms of postpartum depression	166
Selenium	Monotherapy	RDBPCT 5 wk n = 50	14–74	Healthy volunteers	POMS	Improved mood. Reduced anxiety. More mood changes in subgroup with lower baseline selenium levels	167,168
Selenium	Monotherapy	RDB 4 mo n = 11 No placebo, but 2 doses of selenium were compared	20–45	Healthy volunteers	POMS-BI	No change in mood, but more change in patients with lower baseline selenium levels	169

(continued on next page)

Table 2
(continued)

Treatment	Concurrent Treatment	Design	Age (y)	Population	Outcome Measures	Outcome (Statistically Significant Changes Compared to Placebo)	Citation
Selenium	Monotherapy	R 14 wk n = 30 No placebo, but two doses of selenium were compared Blinding unstated	18–45	Healthy volunteers	POMS-BI	Better mood, more clear-headed with high-dose selenium	170
Selenium	Monotherapy	RDBPCT 6 mo n = 448	60–74	Volunteers	POMS-BI	No benefit	171
Selenium	Monotherapy	RDBPCT 12 mo n = 115	24–53	HIV-positive drug users 25% probable MDE	BDI, POMS, STAI	Increased vigor Reduced anxiety No change in mood	172
Magnesium	Monotherapy	RDBPCT 2 mo n = 32	24–39	PMS	Moos Questionnaire	Reduced mood changes	173
Magnesium	Monotherapy	RDBPCT 2 mo n = 38	18–50 (mostly 18–25)	PMS	Moos Questionnaire	No effect on mood	174
Magnesium	Monotherapy	RDBPCT 1 mo n = 44	Mean 32	PMS	Moos Questionnaire	No mood improvement (but reduced anxiety if combined with pyridoxine)	151

Abbreviations: BDI, Beck Depression Inventory; CGI, Clinical Global Impression; EPDS, Edinburgh Postnatal Depression Scale; GHQ, General Health Questionnaire; HADRS, Hospital Anxiety and Depression Rating Scale; HAM-D, Hamilton Depression Rating Scale; MADRS, Montgomery-Asberg Depression Rating Scale; MDE, Major depressive episode; MMSE, Mini-Mental State Examination; Moos, Moos Menstrual Distress Questionnaire; PMS, Premenstrual syndrome; POMS, Profile of Moods State (BI, Bipolar); QIDS-SR, Quick Inventory of Depressive Symptomatology-Self Report; RDBPCT, Randomized double-blind placebo-controlled trial; STAI, State-Trait Anxiety Inventory.

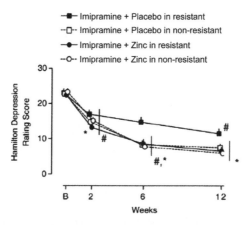

* *P*<.05 vs Imipramine + Placebo in resistant at a given time point
# *P*<.05 vs given groups' previous week score

Fig. 3. Zinc augmentation helps treatment-resistant adults with unipolar depression treated with imipramine, but does not help nonresistant patients. Adults (ages 18–55) with previously documented treatment-resistant unipolar major depression or with nonresistant depression were examined in an RDBPCT of zinc augmentation of antidepressant treatment. All subjects were treated with imipramine and improved significantly at week 2 compared with baseline on the HAM-D. By week 6, the treatment-resistant patients augmented with zinc continued to improve, comparably to the nonresistant patients, whereas the treatment-resistant patients augmented with placebo did not improve relative to week 2. This pattern persisted at week 12. n = 9–16 patients in each treatment group. (*From* Siwek M, Dudek D, Paul IA, et al. Zinc supplementation augments efficacy of imipramine in treatment resistant patients: a double blind, placebo-controlled study. J Affect Disord 2009;118(1–3):187–95; with permission.)

The finding of a selective effect of zinc augmentation in treatment-resistant depression has not been replicated. Zinc has not been examined as a monotherapy for depression.

Thiamine
Two RDBPCTs have examined thiamine as a monotherapy in community samples. Benton and colleagues[164] examined 120 healthy students (mean age 20) in a 2-month trial of thiamine monotherapy and found mood improvement (POMS, *P*<.05) and a trend toward more clear-headedness, a cognitive indicator. A trial in 80 healthy elderly (ages 65–92) subjects living in a region with endemic thiamine deficiency (65% of the sample had baseline insufficiency) showed subjective improvements in appetite, energy, and sense of well-being at 6 weeks.[165]

Although not a monotherapy trial, an RDBPCT of B vitamins examined a combination of thiamine (vitamin B1), riboflavin (B2), and pyridoxine (B6) as an augmentation strategy for antidepressant treatment.[176] Among 16 elderly (mean age 75) psychiatric inpatients with MDD, 4 weeks of augmentation of nortriptyline treatment yielded a trend toward less depression and toward better cognition. The interpretation of this study is complicated because there was also a trend suggesting that the B complex increased the plasma antidepressant levels, so the small clinical improvements might have been pharmacokinetically mediated rather than being a direct effect of B vitamins on mood or cognition.

Again, thiamine monotherapy trials for treating mood disorders are not available in adults or youth, but there is one good RDBPCT suggesting thiamine alone (50 mg mononitrate daily) may be effective for improving mood in college students.

Selenium

Low dietary intake of selenium has been associated with a tripling of the likelihood of developing new-onset MDD in adults.[177]

Selenium monotherapy has been examined in 6 RCTs. Four studies assessed selenium effects in healthy volunteers spanning the adult age range, using the POMS to assess mood. Two studies were placebo controlled, and 2 studies compared 2 doses of selenium. Treatment outcomes were mixed, with 2 positive[167,168,170] and 2 negative findings,[169,171] including a negative study with 448 subjects.[171] Another RCT conducted in HIV-positive drug users (about 25% with probable MDD) showed improvements in energy and anxiety, but no mood change.[172] An additional RCT of elderly subjects in a nursing home (mean age 82) found that selenium, combined with folic acid and vitamin C, improved mood at 8 weeks.[178]

Despite these mixed treatment findings (3 positive, 3 negative), 2 of the monotherapy studies reported more mood improvement in patients with lower baseline selenium levels,[167,169] so there might speculatively be some value of selenium supplementation for depressed patients with demonstrated selenium insufficiency. Although depression may be a symptom of selenium deficiency,[179] there is little to guide clinicians regarding which depressed patients might benefit from selenium blood sampling.

An additional noteworthy RDBPCT examined selenium for prevention of postpartum depression among 166 first-trimester mothers (ages 16–35) who were treated with selenium starting in the first trimester and continuing for 2 months after delivery.[166] It is unclear whether additional prenatal nutrients were used by this sample in Iran, but an unstated number of the mothers took folic acid or iron. Two months postpartum, Edinburgh Postnatal Depression Scale scores were 18% lower in the selenium-treated than the placebo-treated mothers ($P<.05$). This finding is consistent with the longitudinal Alberta Pregnancy Outcomes and Nutrition study showing that prenatal selenium supplementation was correlated with a reduced risk of postpartum depressive symptoms (OR 0.76 for each 10 μg of daily intake, $P = .0019$).[180] Although not a randomized or placebo-controlled study, the long-term follow-up data on the Alberta children will be interesting, especially regarding their CNS development.

Age effects of selenium interventions have not been examined, and no monotherapy trials of selenium for MDD are currently available.

Magnesium

All 3 RDBPCTs on magnesium examined its effects on premenstrual mood, with 2 negative findings[151,174] and 1 positive finding.[173] The quality of these studies was generally weak, with all relying on the Moos Menstrual Distress Questionnaire. Similar to the findings on pyridoxine for premenstrual mood, it is difficult to draw any conclusions regarding its effectiveness, but there is little to encourage further monotherapy studies. No studies of MDD have been conducted.

As an aside, magnesium also has been examined as an adjunctive treatment of mania. Magnesium or placebo was added to ongoing verapamil (calcium channel blocker) treatment of 20 subjects (ages 22–30) in a 4-month randomized single-blind trial. Mean changes were not reported, but Brief Psychiatric Rating Scale scores were stated to have improved ($P<.02$) in the magnesium augmentation group but not in the placebo subjects.[181]

Implications of the Single-Micronutrient Intervention Studies

At present, none of these single-nutrient monotherapies have been examined in RDBPCTs for treating mood disorders in youth. Based on findings from RDBPCTs in adults, only a few treatments seem promising as potential treatments for depression in youth:

1. Folic acid as an adjunctive treatment for MDD appears to be the most promising of the single-micronutrient treatments for further study in youth. Despite the absence of controlled trials in youth, but based on current adult findings and its minimal adverse effects, it may be justifiable to run empiric trials of adjunctive folic acid in youth with MDD, minding its interactions with alcohol, oral contraceptives, and anticonvulsants.
2. Vitamin B12 appears primarily useful for geriatric depression, probably due to senescent B12 absorption. Vitamin B12 appears particularly unpromising in youth, except speculatively for depressed youths with chronic gastrointestinal diseases and impaired absorption.
3. Vitamin D shows mixed findings in adults, but might still be found to have value in youth. Clinical trials and research studies should be tuned to high-risk indicators which, based on current data, might include recurrent depressions, northern climes, low sunlight exposure (seasonal effects, indoor work, bedridden status), darker skin tone, chronic illness, or obesity. In certain populations with these risk factors, and perhaps in psychiatric populations in general, treatment seems sensible in cases with documented vitamin D insufficiency. Controlled data in youth are not available.
4. Chromium might have a niche for treating atypical depression with carbohydrate craving, but additional studies are needed.
5. Zinc might have a role in antidepressant augmentation, perhaps especially for treatment-resistant MDD, and maybe not in routine cases, but again more study is needed.
6. Thiamine might have value for improving mood, energy, and possibly cognition in healthy students, according to a single study.
7. Selenium may have a role as a prenatal treatment to prevent postpartum depression, based on a single RDBPCT and some longitudinal correlational data.
8. Current data would put a low priority on studies of monotherapy with pyridoxine (vitamin B6) and magnesium, at least for premenstrual dysphoria, and there is little in the data to encourage trials in MDD.

Although we have emphasized only the RDBPCTs, there is an enormous literature examining single-nutrient treatments in psychiatry. In general, perhaps what is most striking about these single-micronutrient studies are the few positive findings and the mostly minor clinical improvements. Few if any of these treatments would stand up to conventional psychiatric medications as monotherapy treatments of depression. At best, some might serve as relatively weak adjunctive treatments. For this vast literature, there is surprisingly little to show.

Historically, treatments of disease states are examined one drug at a time, following the traditional medical model of investigating the effect of changing a single variable. This model has largely guided the exploration of micronutrient treatments of disease states, such as depression, with the vast majority of studies examining one micronutrient at a time.

This approach makes sense for drugs, but it is suspect for nutrients: micronutrients typically act in concert physiologically rather than as single actors. For example, B vitamins are known to work as a "complex," with different B vitamins working interactively.[1,2] Similarly, many enzymes have multiple co-factors, so trying to correct the activity of those enzymes by adjusting just a single micronutrient does not make much sense. In fact, treating with a single micronutrient is often disruptive, because it throws off the balance among the interacting micronutrients,[182,183] potentially creating relative micronutrient insufficiencies.

In view of such micronutrient interactions, it is not surprising that this decades-old endeavor of studying individual micronutrients in treating psychiatric disorders has yielded relatively few positive replicable findings. A more nutritionally and scientifically sensible approach would be to examine the effects of micronutrients acting in concert.

The standard term for these approaches is "multiple micronutrient supplementation." Although there is no formal definition, the term is often used to refer to formulations that contain 3 or more micronutrients, for example, by the World Health Organization.[184] However, to denote supplementation with a much broader and more complete array of micronutrients, we will use the term "broad-spectrum micronutrient supplementation" to refer to interventions that involve at least 10 different micronutrients.

BROAD-SPECTRUM MICRONUTRIENT INTERVENTIONS

Broad-spectrum micronutrient strategies supply a wide range of vitamins and minerals, an approach that is likely to provide more pervasive and significant physiologic changes than supplying just one or a few micronutrients at a time. Sometimes seen as an implicit challenge to the conventional model used in medical pharmacology conceptualizing 1 drug having 1 effect (eg, the standard dose-response curve), a "nutritional pharmacology" approach views a multi-ingredient supplement consisting of a broad spectrum of micronutrients as a single, although complex, intervention. For medical researchers who have traditionally investigated single-entity drugs as medical treatments and who have viewed 2-component products with some leeriness, the nutritional pharmacology model is a very different way of thinking.

At present, a complete assessment of the micronutrient status of an individual is not technically feasible. Certain micronutrients can be straightforwardly assessed by clinical blood tests, but blood levels are not indicative of nutritional adequacy for most micronutrients.[2,27] Blood assays are rough measures useful to estimate comparative micronutrient insufficiencies at the population level, but they do not provide a clinically accurate characterization of the nutritional status of an individual patient. (It might be mentioned that numerous commercial groups claim to offer such comprehensive nutritional evaluations, but they are largely based on scientifically unvalidated methodology and often based on scientifically disproven methodology.)

Until the development of comprehensive nutrient assessment methods for all micronutrients that could guide individualized nutritional supplementation for each patient, we have the practical and sensible alternative of providing broad-spectrum micronutrient supplementation with the aim of correcting the full range of potential nutritional deficiencies and insufficiencies. ("Full range" assumes that we have already identified all of the vitamins and essential minerals, which may not be the case; that is an important justification for the consumption of natural foods.) This population-based approach to individual care (supplying all the nutrients that an individual might need on the assumption that we do not know which single micronutrients might actually be needed) may seem unreasonable in the traditional medical model of treatment, but it is very sensible in a nutritional pharmacology model and a public health model.

The nutritional rationale for exploring broad-spectrum micronutrient interventions in medicine is based on several considerations:

1. The involvement of vitamins and minerals in virtually all biologic processes;
2. The requirement for completeness in the complement of vitamins and minerals to support the full range of biologic processes;
3. The complex interactions among micronutrients, requiring an appropriate balance in the ratios among the micronutrients;
4. Epidemiologic evidence confirming widespread micronutrient deficiencies in the general population, including among "well-fed" individuals in wealthy societies;
5. The progressive generalized depletion of various micronutrients in modern over-farmed soil, leading to the reduced availability of many nutrients in our food supply[11,12];
6. The increasing overconsumption of fats and refined sugars in the modern Western diet, resulting in the common intake of foods with low nutrient value[6];
7. Biochemical individuality (genetically determined variations in micronutrient requirements among individuals);
8. Individual variations in micronutrient requirements over time; and
9. The inability of current clinical methods to identify the full range of potential micronutrient deficiencies in an individual.

When considering all of these factors, the study of single micronutrient interventions can seem simplistic and a bit naïve. At the least, studies that examine the effects of broad-spectrum micronutrient interventions, aimed at correcting a diversity of micronutrient deficiencies, insufficiencies, and relative insufficiencies in the general population, have plausibility, practicality, and heuristic value, as well as making basic clinical sense, at least until an effective comprehensive nutritional evaluation can be developed to assess the profile of micronutrient insufficiencies in individual patients.

Broad-spectrum micronutrient interventions have been examined and found surprisingly effective for altering mood, cognition, and behavior. A recent comprehensive review by Rucklidge and Kaplan[185] of the psychiatric effects of micronutrient treatments involving 4 or more ingredients described beneficial effects on mood, anxiety and stress, aggressive and antisocial misconduct, substance abuse and dependence, attention-deficit/hyperactivity disorder (ADHD), and autism.

Although this article is primarily concerned with mood disorders, it is instructive to survey the effects of broad-spectrum micronutrient treatments on conditions that frequently appear comorbidly with mood disorders, as well as conditions that appear in healthy adults.

Violent and Antisocial Behavior in Youth and Adults

Broad-spectrum micronutrient interventions have been found to reduce violent and antisocial behavior in children and adolescents. A randomized double-blind placebo-controlled trial was conducted on 80 public school children (ages 6–12) with aggressive behaviors or disordered conduct.[186] A micronutrient formula (13 vitamins, 10 minerals, supplying about 50% of RDA) was administered for 4 months and resulted in a striking 47% reduction is disciplined violent and nonviolent misconduct, including threats, fights, vandalism, defiance, disrespect, and obscenities. In a similar 13-week study on 62 young delinquents (ages 13–17) in a maximum security hospital, treatment with micronutrients (12 vitamins at 3 times the RDA levels, 11 minerals at RDA level) led to an 83% reduction in the micronutrient group, compared with a 55% reduction in the control group, in both violent and nonviolent offenses ($P<.005$).[187] In the second study, improvement was noted predominantly in subjects whose blood samples showed evidence of improved nutritional status following supplementation, with little clinical improvement in subjects whose nutritional status remained unimproved by supplementation. These 2 RCTs demonstrated marked improvements in major conduct violations in American school children and delinquent adolescents following 3 to 4 months of broad-spectrum vitamin-mineral supplementation.

Two additional RDBPCTs conducted in young adults provide confirmation of these findings. In a very rigorous randomized multiply-blinded placebo-controlled study, Gesch and colleagues[188] examined the effects of nutritional supplementation with 13 vitamins and 12 minerals (all at or below RDA dosing), plus omega-3 and omega-6 fatty acids, on the disruptive behavior of 231 young prisoners (minimum age 18). The outcome measure was in-prison disciplinary offenses, consisting of violence or serious rule violations that required formal adjudication and were supported by "beyond reasonable doubt" evidence. Nutrient-supplemented prisoners committed a mean of 26% fewer offenses compared with the placebo group (95% CI 8.3%–44.3%, $P = .03$). Compared with baseline, nutritional supplementation (n = 90) for at least 2 weeks produced a mean 35% reduction in disciplinary offenses ($P = .001$), whereas placebo (n = 82) showed a nonsignificant 7% increase in offenses ($P > .1$). Both major and minor offenses showed a similar degree of improvement (**Table 3**). The period of supplementation was a mean of 142 days in both groups (range 2–9 months). No adverse responses to supplementation were reported. Compliance rates were high in both treatment groups, and the effectiveness of the placebo blinding was demonstrated. It is impressive that the improvements in antisocial behaviors were substantial (26%–36%), rapid (data based on prisoners who received nutrients for a minimum of 2 weeks), and observable across a range of severity of antisocial behaviors.

This rigorous study was replicated in detail by Zaalberg and colleagues[189] in 221 prisoners (mean age 21, range 18–25) who received nutritional supplementation that was virtually identical to Gesch and colleagues' formulation[188] (n = 115) or placebo (n = 106) for 1 to 3 months. Outcome findings based on incident reports were remarkably comparable to Gesch's, with a 34% decrease in staff-reported incidents of aggressive and rule-breaking behaviors (mainly alcohol or drug use), compared with

Table 3 Reduced frequency of major misconduct among incarcerated young adults who received nutrient intervention for at least 2 weeks		
	Broad-Spectrum Micronutrients with Omega-3 Fatty Acids	Placebo
	n = 82	n = 90
Total infringements before intervention (offenses per 1000 person-days)	16.0	16.0
Total infringements after intervention	10.4	14.9
Percent reduction in total infringements	35%, P<.001	6.7%, NS
Percent reduction in serious incidents, including violence	37%, P<.005	10.1%, NS
Percent reduction in minor incidents, mainly antisocial behaviors	33%, P<.025	6.5%, NS
Mean treatment compliance rate	91%	90%

Abbreviation: NS, not significant.
Data from Gesch CB, Hammond SM, Hampson SE, et al. Influence of supplementary vitamins, minerals and essential fatty acids on the antisocial behaviour of young adult prisoners. Randomised, placebo-controlled trial. Br J Psychiatry 2002;181:22–8.

a 14% increase in the placebo group ($P = .017$). Interestingly, no significant differences between the groups were observed when less concrete measures of behavior were used, such as several validated rating scales reflecting self-reported and staff-reported impressions of hostility feelings, disruptive behaviors, and (loosely assessed) psychiatric symptoms. This underscores a potential weakness of traditional rating scales, which remain somewhat subjective, and the value of using more concrete measures like incident reports.

These 3 RDBPCTs on adolescent and young adult prisoners, reasonably sized and independently conducted, show that supplementation with 23 to 25 vitamins and minerals at RDA doses induced 25% to 35% reductions in aggressive behavior and nonviolent misconduct.[187–189] The findings of these 3 studies are comparable to the RDBPCT in 6-year olds to 12-year-olds in public schools showing a 47% reduction in aggressive behaviors or conduct disorder symptoms among 80 children who received a 23-ingredient formulation of vitamins and minerals, administered at about 50% of RDA levels for 4 months, without fatty acid supplementation.[186]

The addition of omega fatty acid supplementation in 2 of the RDBPCTs[188,189] is sensible from a nutritional and public health perspective, in that it maximizes the likelihood of eliciting a positive response to nutritional intervention, but it has the unfortunate effect (from the point of view of this article) of obscuring how much of the observed behavioral improvements could be attributed to vitamins and minerals rather than to fatty acids. However, the 2 other RDBPCTs conducted in children and adolescents[186,187] showed that comparable results were obtained without fatty acids, supporting the notion that vitamins and minerals alone (without essential fatty acids) can be effective. These 4 RDBPCTs constitute replicated demonstrations that broad-spectrum micronutrient treatment, with or without essential fatty acids, can have marked clinical effects on major misconduct and aggressive behavior.

As an aside, an oft-cited, although flawed, study conducted at the Pfeiffer Treatment Center Health Research Institute in Illinois examined 207 patients (mean age 12, range 3–55 years) with ADHD, conduct disorder, or oppositional defiant disorder.[190] The protocol included a battery of 90 biochemical assays, standardized protocols to identify "chemical imbalances" to be treated, and individualized modular therapies consisting of micronutrients and amino acids, among other compounds. The targeted chemical imbalances were described as malabsorption, glucose dysregulation, elevated copper-to-zinc ratio, overmethylation or undermethylation, "pyrrole disorder," and heavy metal excesses. A 92% reduction in physical assaults and an 88% reduction in destructive episodes was reported. The individually varied treatments, open-label design, lack of a comparison group, unvalidated biochemical assay interpretations, and the lack of standardized outcome instruments make it difficult to interpret the findings.

In short, the 4 positive randomized double-blind placebo-controlled studies, with no negative studies, provide strong support for broad-spectrum micronutrients as a treatment for violence and major misconduct. Especially in view of the minimal side effects, the 3 RDBPCTs in young incarcerated offenders are sufficient grounds to proceed now with implementation in correctional facilities. The RDBPCT on public school children in the community needs replication before clinical recommendations can be made, but this should be an extremely high research priority.

None of these studies attempted to identify the diagnoses of the subjects, and so their implications regarding treatment of mood disorders (or ADHD) are speculative. These studies also leave open questions about which of the many micronutrients are the most crucial (or, instead, whether supplying a broad spectrum of nutrients is crucial), whether the effects are mainly seen in individuals with poor diets or low nutritional status, and whether higher micronutrient doses would be more effective than routine RDA dose levels.

ADHD

Open-label trials

Eight open-label studies on ADHD provide suggestive evidence that broad-spectrum micronutrient treatment may result in the improvement of both inattention and hyperactivity/impulsivity symptoms in youth[191–195] and adults.[196–198]

All but one of these studies[191] were conducted using a broad-spectrum micronutrient formulation, developed by David Hardy and Tony Stephan, consisting of relatively high but safe doses of about 36 ingredients, mainly vitamins, minerals, antioxidants, and a few amino acids. This type of formulation was originally developed as a nutritional intervention to reduce aggressive behavior among farm animals, but it was adapted for human use when it was observed to reduce symptoms of bipolar disorder. Several companies manufacture minor variations on this formulation (Daily Essentials Nutrients, manufactured by NutraTek Health Innovations, Raymond, Alberta, Canada; EMPowerPlus Advanced, manufactured by Truehope Nutritional Support, Raymond, Alberta, Canada; Equilib, manufactured by EvinceNaturals, Bountiful, Utah). These formulations contain more than 25 different vitamins and minerals. Most of the past research studies have used the EMPower version of the Hardy-Stephan formula. Possible differences among these minor variations of the formula have not been examined.

In a study of ADHD,[194] 11 youths (ages 8–15) with mood and behavior symptoms received open-label treatment with the Hardy-Stephan formula for 8 to 17 weeks and showed substantial improvement in Child Behavior CheckList (CBCL) scores for attention, as well as delinquent and aggressive behavior (all $P<.01$); 6 of the 11 children had ADHD, although their data were not analyzed separately because of sample size (**Fig. 4**).

A case series of 14 adults (ages 18–55) with ADHD and mood dysregulation reported that 8-week open-label treatment with the Hardy-Stephan formula led to significantly improved behavior and attention scores, as well as anxiety and quality of life ratings.[196] Hyperactivity/impulsivity and mood scores were normalized, but inattention ratings improved but remained within the clinically significant range (**Table 4**).

In a retrospective database analysis of 120 children (ages 7–18) with a parent-reported diagnosis of bipolar disorder, 24% of the subjects were also reported by the parents to have ADHD.[195] Open-label treatment with the Hardy-Stephan formula produced a 40% reduction in parent-reported ADHD symptoms, as well as a 43% reduction in parent-reported bipolar symptoms (**Fig. 5**). Also, the percentage of patients using conventional psychiatric medications declined from 79% to 38%, and the number of medications used decreased by 74%.

Most of the samples in these studies consisted of patients with presumptive ADHD and probable comorbid bipolar disorder. The morbidity makes it difficult to discern how much of the apparent micronutrient effect on ADHD symptoms might have been indirectly mediated by a micronutrient-induced reduction in bipolar symptoms (ie, without a direct micronutrient effect on ADHD itself). An additional study reportedly conducted on children with noncomorbid ADHD asserted the ADHD diagnosis without a standardized diagnostic evaluation (so comorbidity was not systematically assessed), and the treatment consisted of a complex chemical intervention including micronutrients as one component,[191] so it cannot help determine whether there is a direct micronutrient effect on ADHD. Perhaps more useful for this purpose was the subsample of 41 children from the database study whose parents reported their

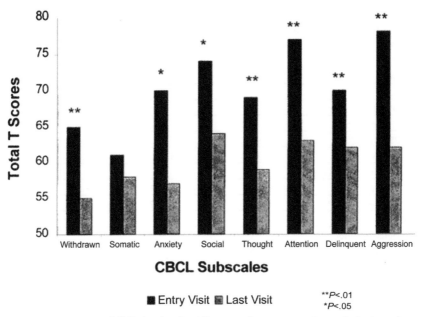

CBCL Subscales

■ Entry Visit ▦ Last Visit   ****P<.01**
                                   *P<.05

Fig. 4. Improvement on child behavior checklist scores in symptomatic youth during micronutrient treatment. Among 9 of 11 children with mixed mood and behavioral problems (mainly mood disorder and ADHD) who completed treatment with open-label EMPower for a mean of 14 weeks, Child Behavior Checklist scores improved significantly in all categories except somatic symptoms. (*From* Kaplan BJ, Fisher JE, Crawford SG, et al. Improved mood and behavior during treatment with a mineral-vitamin supplement: An open-label case series of children. J Child Adolesc Psychopharmacol 2004;14(1):115–22; with permission.)

diagnoses as ADHD without bipolar disorder.[195] In this subsample (in contrast to **Fig. 5**, which shows data from the entire sample predominated by ADHD-bipolar comorbidity), open-label treatment of ADHD (without bipolar disorder) for up to 6 months produced a 47% reduction in parent-reported ADHD symptoms from baseline to last observation (Cohen's d effect size [ES] 1.04). The response rates in this subsample of ADHD-only youths to micronutrient treatment are 63% to 76%, depending on the definition of clinical response (**Table 5**). These data suggest that micronutrient treatment can directly treat ADHD, but open-label data from a database that relies on parental reports of diagnosis and outcome leaves this question unsettled.

In most of the open-label reports examining the Hardy-Stephan formula as a broad-spectrum micronutrient treatment for ADHD, behavioral changes appeared stronger and sooner than attentional improvements, consistent with an indirectly mediated effect on attention or simply a weaker micronutrient effect on attention than behavior. For subjects who were using conventional psychiatric medications at baseline, the addition of micronutrient interventions appeared to reduce the dosage requirements for conventional medications or to allow their discontinuation in many cases.

Open-label reports are obviously limited by the lack of controls and blinding. Many reports lacked formally substantiated diagnoses, and the comorbidity obscured whether micronutrients directly reduced ADHD symptoms. In view of these limitations,

Table 4
EMPower treatment of 14 adults with "severe mood dysregulation" and ADHD: 8-week outcome of open-label treatment

Measure	Baseline Mean ± SD	8-wk Mean ± SD	P	ES
Mood				
MADRS (Depression)	22 ± 7.7	7.2 ± 3.4	<.001	1.96
DASS Depression	17 ± 9.3	7.1 ± 6.1	<.001	1.08
YMRS (Mania)	2.7 ± 3.7	0.7 ± 1.6	<.01	0.82
DASS Anxiety	12 ± 9.4	3.6 ± 2.6	<.01	0.88
CAARS Emotional Lability				
Self-Report[a]	68 ± 11	60 ± 11	<.001	1.29
Observer Report[a]	67 ± 11	56 ± 12	<.001	1.45
ADHD				
CAARS Self-Report				
DSM Inattention[a]	80 ± 8.9	70 ± 13	<.001	0.98
DSM Hyper/Imp[a]	67 ± 11	56 ± 13	<.001	1.88
DSM Combined[a]	78 ± 8.4	65 ± 13	<.001	1.58
CAARS Observer-Report				
DSM Inattention[a]	71 ± 8.4	65 ± 10	<.01	0.66
DSM Hyper/Imp[a]	65 ± 10	57 ± 12	<.01	0.70
DSM Combined[a]	70 ± 8.1	63 ± 11	<.01	0.70
GAF	54 ± 6.3	70 ± 6.5	<.001	2.44

[a] T scores.

P based on paired t tests (2-tailed).

Abbreviations: ADHD, attention-deficit/hyperactivity disorder; CAARS, Conners Adult ADHD Rating Scale; CGI-S, Clinical Global Impression-Severity; DASS, Depression, Anxiety, and Stress Scale; DSM, Diagnostic and Statistical Manual of Mental Disorders; ES, Cohen's d effect size; GAF, Global Assessment of Functioning; Hyper/Imp, Hyperactivity/Impulsivity; MADRS, Montgomery-Asberg Depression Rating Scale; YMRS, Young Mania Rating Scale.

Data from Rucklidge J, Taylor M, Whitehead K. Effect of micronutrients on behavior and mood in adults with ADHD: evidence from an 8-week open label trial with natural extension. J Atten Disord 2011;15(1):79–91.

the numerous open-label studies are only suggestive of a possible effect of micronutrients on ADHD.

Controlled trials on ADHD

There are 2 controlled studies of broad-spectrum micronutrients in treating ADHD or ADHD-like symptoms, 1 in children and 1 in adults. In the child RDBPCT,[199] broad-spectrum micronutrients at low doses (Multivitamins and Minerals for Kids; Blackmore, Warriewood, Australia) were administered in conjunction with omega-3 fatty acids to 132 children (ages 7–12) with ADHD-like symptoms, but not necessarily ADHD. Diagnostic interviews were not conducted, and the sample consisted of subjects who scored 2 SDs above the mean on the Conners ADHD Index. The children were randomized to 1 of 3 treatment arms: broad-spectrum micronutrients (at or below RDA levels) plus omega-3 fatty acids EPA 660 mg and DHA 175 mg (n = 41); omega-3 fatty acids alone (n = 36); or placebo (n = 27). The effects of micronutrients alone were not examined in this study. Randomized double-blind

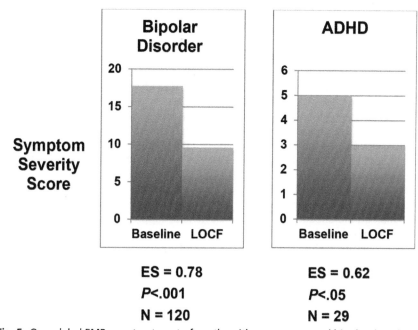

Fig. 5. Open-label EMPower treatment of youths with parent-reported bipolar disorder and ADHD comorbidity. Analysis of a database of open-label EMPower treatments of youths (ages 7–18) whose parents provided reports of clinical diagnoses of comorbid bipolar disorder and ADHD. Parents also provided daily symptom reports for 3 to 6 months using a Likert (0–3) scoring system for DSM-IV symptom clusters. Bipolar symptom severity scores range from 0 to 48. ADHD symptom severity scores range from 0 to 9. Mean ± SD. ES, Cohen's d effect size; LOCF, last observation carried forward. (*Data from* Rucklidge JJ, Gately D, Kaplan BJ. Database analysis of children and adolescents with bipolar disorder consuming a micronutrient formula. BMC Psychiatry 2010;10:74.)

Table 5
Response rates of youths treated with open-label EMPower: percentage of youths in database analysis showing improvement from baseline to last observation

	Bipolar (%)	ADHD (%)	Bipolar Disorder and Comorbid ADHD (%)
	n = 91	n = 41	n = 29
Response Criterion ≥30% Reduction in Symptom Severity			
Bipolar symptoms	68	—	55
ADHD symptoms	—	76	55
Response Criterion ≥50% Reduction in Symptom Severity			
Bipolar symptoms	45	—	48
ADHD symptoms	—	63	45

Response rates are expressed as the percentage of youths responding to treatment, based on 2 different definitions of response. Treatment reports were based on 3 to 6 months of treatment. Data from youths with comorbid bipolar disorder and ADHD are reported separately from youths with 1 primary diagnosis. Diagnoses and outcomes are based on parent report.
Abbreviation: ADHD, attention-deficit/hyperactivity disorder.
Data from Rucklidge JJ, Gately D, Kaplan BJ. Database analysis of children and adolescents with bipolar disorder consuming a micronutrient formula. BMC Psychiatry 2010;10:74.

treatments were administered for 15 weeks (104 completers), and there was a subsequent 15-week open-label extension. Both treatment groups did better than placebo on parent ratings of attention (ES 0.52–0.61) and behavior (ES 0.17–0.45), but teacher ratings showed no effects. The addition of broad-spectrum micronutrients did not improve on effect of omega-3 fatty acids alone, but the micronutrient doses were low in comparison with the previously mentioned studies on EMPower treatment, and the omega-3 fatty acid doses were low as well, so this study probably did not assess the full potential of the micronutrients or the fatty acids. The design also did not allow assessment of whether the effects of micronutrients would be improved by the addition of omega-3 fatty acids. In addition, despite the improvement in attentional measures, detailed neuropsychological testing showed few other areas of cognitive improvement.[200] The absence of significant effects on the teacher ratings, the lack of ADHD diagnoses, the low doses, and the lack of a micronutrients-only arm limit the value of these findings. This study does not provide information on the effectiveness of vitamin-mineral supplementation itself in treating ADHD in youth.

The best available study of micronutrient effects on ADHD was Rucklidge and colleagues' RDBPCT[201,202] conducted on 80 medication-free adults (age≥16) with formally diagnosed ADHD. Psychiatric comorbidity was intentionally retained in the sample to enhance generalizability. Subjects were randomized to receive the Hardy-Stephan formula (n = 42) or placebo (n = 38) for 8 weeks, without omega-3 fatty acids (**Table 6**). Dropout rate was 7.5%, and adherence rate was 95%. Compared with placebo, intent-to-treat analysis showed significant improvement on self-rated and observer-rated scores for hyperactivity/impulsivity (ES 0.46–0.67) and inattention (ES 0.33–0.62) on the Conners Adult ADHD Rating Scales (CAARS). Although changes were not significant on clinician-rated CAARS scores (ES 0.2), clinicians did report significant improvements on both Clinical Global Impression (CGI) for General Improvement and CGI for Improvement on ADHD symptoms (ES 0.53–0.57). At the end of 8 weeks, 64% of the micronutrient-treated and 37% of the controls

Table 6
Randomized double-blind placebo-controlled trial of the Hardy-Stephan formula in adults with ADHD

	Micronutrient-Treated, n = 42		Controls, n = 38			
	Baseline	8 wk	Baseline	8 wk	Treated vs Controls	Effect Size
CAARS DSM-IV ADHD Symptom Total						
Self-Report	80	67	75	70	$P = .009$	0.61
Observer	70	61	70	67	$P = .026$	0.59
Clinician	73	65	69	64	NS	0.23
MADRS	17	12	14	12	$P = .078$	0.41
GAF	59	64	62	64	$P = .045$	0.46

ADHD scores were reduced in self-report and observer (eg, a relative) reports, but not in clinician reports on CAARS. Mood (MADRS) and global functioning (GAF) also improved at 8 weeks.

Abbreviations: ADHD, attention-deficit/hyperactivity disorder; CAARS, Conners Adult ADHD Rating Scale; DSM-IV, *Diagnostic and Statistical Manual of Mental Disorders, Fourth Edition*; GAF, Global Assessment of Functioning; MADRS, Montgomery-Asberg Depression Rating Scale.

Adapted from Rucklidge JJ, Frampton CM, Gorman B, et al. Vitamin-mineral treatment of attention-deficit hyperactivity disorder in adults: double-blind randomised placebo-controlled trial. Br J Psychiatry 2014;204:306–15.

showed 30% or more reduction on at least one CAARS subscale, and 48% versus 21% showed much or very much improvement on the CGI-Improvement-ADHD scale. Approximately one-third of the micronutrient group appeared fully remitted at 8 weeks, compared with approximately one-sixth of the control group (Julia Rucklidge, personal communication, 2014).

One potential problem with this RDBPCT is that the micronutrient sample at baseline had more women (48% vs 18%) and more anxiety disorders (52% vs 29%) than the controls. However, the observed clinical effects of micronutrients relative to controls were not changed when gender and anxiety disorder diagnoses were entered as covariates. The baseline prevalence of mood disorders was comparable in both groups (past episodes 57%–60%, current episodes 21%–24%).

A 1-year follow-up study to this RDBPCT was conducted on 90% of the original sample.[203] After the 8-week RDBPCT, 51% of subjects stopped all medications, 24% switched to conventional psychiatric medications, and 19% continued on micronutrients. Participants who continued on micronutrients at the end of the study fared better than those who switched to conventional medications or to other natural treatments. Subjects who stayed on micronutrients throughout the follow-up year maintained their improvements or improved further, whereas subjects who discontinued micronutrients lost much of the treatment gains they had made while taking micronutrients. Even participants who switched to conventional psychiatric medications scored less well on ADHD and on depressive symptoms at 1-year follow-up than the micronutrient continuers. At 1 year, treatment response criteria (≥30% improvement from baseline on clinician CAARS) were met by 64% who stayed on the Hardy-Stephan formula, 35% on conventional medications, and 20% who discontinued treatment ($P = .009$). Remission criteria (within normal nonclinical range on the clinician CAARS) were met by 64% on the Hardy-Stephan formula, 29% on conventional medications, and 28% of those who stopped treatment ($P = .039$). The subjects who discontinued micronutrients primarily cited treatment cost as the reason, but some cited treatment inconvenience (15 pills daily) or nonresponse. The fact that those who discontinued micronutrients cited cost as the primary factor makes it unlikely that micronutrient nonresponders were overrepresented among the switchers. Interestingly, side effects were minimal and were not a significant factor contributing to treatment discontinuation.

The effect size of micronutrients on ADHD (ES 0.2–0.67) in this RDBPCT compares favorably to effects of omega-3 fatty acids (ES 0.2–0.3)[4] and of diets excluding artificial food colorings (ES 0.2–0.4),[204,205] but is lower than for psychostimulants (ES 0.6–0.8).[206] Despite some complications in this study, this RDBPCT gives strong evidence of a micronutrient effect on ADHD, at least in adults in a community sample with mixed comorbidity. Given its promising degree of effectiveness in this trial, the favorable side-effect profile, the possible reduction in dosage requirements for concurrently administered conventional medications, and the numerous open-label trials suggesting clinical value, additional controlled trials of micronutrient treatment of ADHD are warranted in youth and adults.

Compared with psychostimulants, micronutrients offer some significant advantages in terms of side effects: no rebound hyperactivity, abuse potential, daily on-off effects, appetite suppression, height or weight loss, blood pressure or pulse changes, or psychotic reactions.

Mood Disorders

There are 17 currently available studies of broad-spectrum micronutrient treatments for major mood disorders in youth and adults, including 1 RDBPCT. Some of the subjects had well-diagnosed bipolar disorder, and others had presumptive bipolar disorder by virtue of severe mood dysregulation, mood lability, and temper outbursts; some had major depression, and a few had dysthymia. Similar to the data available on ADHD, most of these reports are open-label studies, and most were conducted using the Hardy-Stephen formulation of broad-spectrum micronutrients (EMPower).

Open-label studies

In adults with bipolar disorder, several open-label case series[196,197,207–209] have suggested the effectiveness of broad-spectrum micronutrients for treating clinically diagnosed bipolar I or bipolar II disorder. In these reports, about 85% of the 40 adults (ages 18–68) showed improvement in mood and behavior over the course of 1 to 6 months of treatment, and most patients were treated successfully enough to be able to discontinue their previous conventional psychiatric medications entirely. For example, Kaplan and colleagues[207] noted reductions of 55% to 66% on depression (HAM-D) and mania (YMRS) scores in 11 adults over 6 months, with an effect size of about 0.80 for measures of depression and mania, and a reduction in the use of conventional medications of about 50%. Similarly, Rucklidge and colllegaues[196,197] described 14 adults with ADHD and severe mood dysregulation who were treated for 8 weeks with open-label EMPower, with 10 of 12 adults showing a 50% improvement in clinician-rated Montgomery-Asberg Depression Rating Scale (MADRS) scores. Mean MADRS scores reduced from 22 ± 7.7 to 7.2 ± 3.4 ($P<.001$; ES 1.96) and, although no subjects met criteria for mania, mean YRMS mania scores reduced from 2.7 ± 3.7 to 0.7 ± 1.6 ($P<.01$; ES 0.82).

In children and adolescents, several reports describe open-label treatments of presumptive bipolar disorder, mood lability and/or explosive rage. Some trials used multiple reversal designs (ABAB), meaning that treatment was applied, withdrawn, then reapplied. This approach allows open-label studies to provide evidence that the symptom change is actually linked to treatment rather than to incidental factors. The observation of several clinical changes (reversals) that are consistent and concurrent with dose changes increases the likelihood that the symptom change is, in fact, a result of the treatment.

Five reports used open-label ABAB designs in 6 youths. Kaplan and colleagues[193] described 2 children (ages 8 and 12) with mood lability and explosive rage whose symptom scores (Conners Parent Rating Scale, Child Behavior Checklist [CBCL]) improved with 3 weeks of broad-spectrum micronutrient treatment. In this naturalistic ABAB report, symptoms worsened when treatment was withdrawn, and improved again when treatment was reinstated. Both children then remained stable over 2 years of follow-up. In another report, a medication-naïve 10-year-old with clinically diagnosed *Diagnostic and Statistical Manual of Mental Disorders, Fourth Edition* (DSM-IV) bipolar disorder and major temper tantrums showed complete remission within 5 days of starting treatment,[208] followed by multiple naturalistic reversals (ABABA-BAB) over 3 years, confirming treatment effectiveness. Rucklidge[210] described an 18-year-old with major depression and obsessive-compulsive disorder (OCD) who showed improved mood (BDI), anxiety (Beck Anxiety Inventory), and obsessive symptoms (Yale-Brown Obsessive Compulsive Scale [YBOCS]) after 8 weeks of broad-spectrum micronutrient treatment; effectiveness was confirmed by subsequent treatment discontinuation and reinstatement (ABAB). Rucklidge and Harrison[198] also described a 21-year-old with bipolar disorder, ADHD, social anxiety, and panic disorder who had significantly improved depression (MADRS), mania (YMRS), hyperactivity/impulsivity (CAARS), processing speed (Wechsler Adult Intelligence Scale, WAIS-III), and verbal memory (Wide Range Assessment of Memory and Learning

[WRAML-II]) scores, with full remission at 1-year follow-up (**Fig. 6**). A 20-year-old with major depression had MADRS scores drop from 30 to 3 after 6 weeks of broad-spectrum micronutrient treatment, with confirmation in open-label ABAB reversals.[192]

Several additional open-label reports, although not using an ABAB design, suggest possible effectiveness of micronutrient treatment for treating mood disorders in 34 children and adolescents.[194,208,211–214] Frazier and colleagues[212] reported on 10 children (ages 6–12) with *Diagnostic and Statistical Manual of Mental Disorders, Fourth Edition, Text Revision* (DSM-IV-TR) bipolar disorder, 7 of whom completed a 6-month trial. The 3 dropouts had difficulty in swallowing the pills or adhering to the difficult regimen (5 pills, 3 times daily). Intent-to-treat analysis showed a statistically significant 45% decrease in YMRS mania scores ($P<.01$) and an almost-significant 37% reduction in depression scores ($P<.06$) from baseline to 6 months of treatment. For completers, statistically significant reductions were observed in both mania (58%) and depression (71%) scores.[213] Adverse effects consisted of transient mild dyspepsia and initial insomnia. Kaplan and colleagues[194] reported on 4 children (ages 8–15) with mood and behavioral problems whose YMRS scores reduced over 8 weeks of treatment ($P<.05$). One report described clinically significant improvement in 10 of 12 youths (9 adolescents, 3 preadolescents) with clinically diagnosed bipolar disorder,[208] with almost all able to completely discontinue their previous psychiatric medications. Two other reports describe complete resolution of psychotic symptoms and significant reductions in obsessive-compulsive symptoms associated with mood disorders in a 12-year-old[211] and an 11-year-old.[214]

In a retrospective database analysis on 358 adults with self-reported bipolar disorder,[215] mean symptom severity of self-reported symptoms of bipolar disorder reduced by 41% after 3 months and by 45% reduction at 6 months of treatment (ES 0.76, $P>.001$). At 6 months, 53% of patients reported greater than 50% symptom reduction, and improvements were found to be dose-dependent. This study is limited by the unverified diagnoses, self-reported outcome data, and open-label treatment, among other issues. In the absence of controlled data, these open-label studies on adults

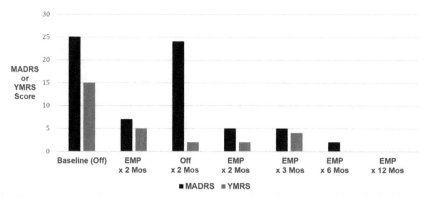

Fig. 6. Improvement in depression and mania scores in a 21-year-old with bipolar disorder and ADHD who was treated with open-label EMPower for one year. Starting medication-free at baseline, the patient was treated with EMPower for 2 months and then chose to discontinue treatment for 2 months. Follow-up data were available after 2, 3, 6, and 12 months of retreatment. MADRS and YMRS scores show treatment effects over time, including symptom-free status after 1 year. (*Data from* Rucklidge JJ, Harrison R. Successful treatment of bipolar disorder II and ADHD with a micronutrient formula: a case study. CNS Spectr 2010;15(5):289–95.)

with presumptive bipolar disorder suggest a clinically significant effect with a substantial effect size and apparent dose-dependent improvements in both depression and mania measures.

In the database analysis conducted on 120 youths (ages 7–18) with bipolar disorder, as reported by parents (not clinically verified by investigators), rage outbursts, or severe mood dysregulation, changes were quantitatively almost identical to findings in the adult database.[195] There was a 46% reduction in mean severity of bipolar symptoms at 6 months compared with baseline (ES 0.78), and 46% of the patients reported greater than 50% improvement in symptoms at 6 months (see **Fig. 5**). About 24% of this sample had ADHD (by parent report), and similar changes in bipolar symptoms were observed regardless of ADHD status. Similar to adult findings, the percentage of patients who needed to use conventional medications reduced from 79% to 38%, and mean doses reduced by 74%. Within the pediatric database, the observed improvements were found to be not age-dependent.

It is notable that the magnitude of outcome effects are so similar in the child and the adult databases, reinforcing the suggestion that the effect of broad-spectrum micronutrients on presumptive bipolar disorder is robust (ES 0.8) across the age spectrum.

Controlled studies of mood disorders

Beyond these open-label data, the one available RDBPCT provides better evidence for the effectiveness of broad-spectrum micronutrients for treating mood disorders.[201] As noted previously, in Rucklidge's RDBPCT on medication-free adults (ages>16) with ADHD, more than one-fifth of the patients had a current mood episode (21.4% in the micronutrient group, 23.7% in the control group), with mood disorder defined as dysthymia, MDD, or bipolar disorder, as assessed using the Structured Clinical Interview for DSM-IV-TR Axis I Disorders (SCID-I). The 8-week treatment produced only a trend ($P = .078$) toward improvement in clinician-rated MADRS depression scores in the overall ADHD sample, in which most of the 80 subjects had little or no depression (see **Table 6**).

However, there was a clear antidepressant effect of broad-spectrum micronutrients in the subsample of 21 patients with moderate or severe depression. Using a baseline MADRS score of 20 or more, which is a common cutoff score to qualify for entry into conventional antidepressant drug RCTs, there was a significant difference in depression outcome scores between patients treated with micronutrients (n = 11) and placebo (n = 10), with a moderate effect size (ES 0.64, $P<.04$) (**Fig. 7**). This compares favorably to a typical effect size of 0.3 to 0.6 for antidepressants in conventional registration RCTs, although the ES varies with baseline severity, among many other factors.[216–218] Most contemporary RCTs on conventional antidepressants purposively exclude patients with mild episodes of major depression, because their high placebo response rate makes it more difficult to demonstrate treatment effectiveness. So, as usual for antidepressant treatments, the effectiveness of micronutrients in this RDBPCT appeared to be more readily demonstrable for more moderate and severe depressive episodes. In this context, the micronutrient effect size of 0.64 appears comparable to the effectiveness of standard pharmaceutical antidepressants.

Other predictors in the Rucklidge and colleagues'[202] RDBPCT of a stronger antidepressant response to micronutrient treatment included lower baseline levels of vitamin D and copper, but not lower levels of folate, vitamin B12, iron, or ferritin. These predictor findings involved numerous comparisons and secondary exploratory analyses, so they require replication before being accepted at face value. This RDBPCT, which was designed for other purposes, does not allow an assessment of the effects of micronutrients in patients with bipolar disorder versus MDD versus dysthymia.

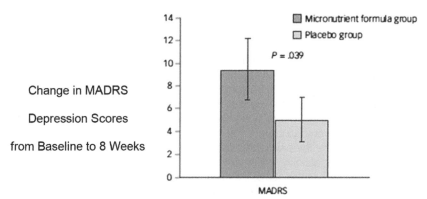

Fig. 7. Antidepressant effect of the Hardy-Stephan formula in a randomized double-blind placebo-controlled trial in adults with ADHD: effect size comparable to conventional antidepressant medications. In the RDBPCT of the Hardy-Stephan formula in adults, MADRS depression scores showed no significant change in the overall micronutrient-treated group compared with placebo (P = .078, ES 0.41, see **Table 6**). However, in this subsample of subjects with significant depression at baseline (MADRS$\geq$20), a clinically and statistically significant antidepressant effect of the Hardy-Stephan formula was demonstrated at 8 weeks (ES = 0.64). This subsample included 11 subjects treated with micronutrients and 10 subjects treated with placebo. (*From* Rucklidge JJ, Frampton CM, Gorman B, et al. Vitamin-mineral treatment of attention-deficit hyperactivity disorder in adults: double-blind randomised placebo-controlled trial. Br J Psychiatry 2014;204:306–15; with permission.)

Clinical caveats on the micronutrient treatment of mood disorders

Several observations, as yet undocumented in the literature, are commonly described by clinicians who are familiar with these micronutrient treatments. For example, once a patient with a mood disorder is stabilized on this treatment, the rate of symptom relapse is very low. Patients on micronutrients appear to have much fewer fluctuations in mood than patients on conventional medications, with fewer residual symptoms and fewer partial relapses into mild depressive or manic symptoms. This effect is apparent soon after stabilization, but it also increases over time. Whereas many patients treated with conventional medications require relatively frequent dose adjustments to manage the periodic variations in symptom control, physicians report a reduced frequency of necessary medication dose adjustments in patients receiving micronutrient treatment for mood disorders. (I would estimate that less than 1 yearly dose adjustment is required after a patient has been stabilized.) Some micronutrient-treated patients can be managed with much less than monthly medication check-ins. I have many patients who previously required close medication management on conventional drugs, but who now check in every 3 to 12 months with little symptomatology to report. Hospitalizations are rare. This "super stability" of micronutrient treatment relative to conventional psychiatric medication lowers the cost of medical care. Many of the open-label reports comment on this long-term stability, but it should be emphasized that these open clinical observations, although striking, are anecdotal opinion and have not been formally demonstrated in scientific studies.

One of the main disadvantages with this treatment is the dramatic interactions between micronutrients and psychiatric drugs. Drug-micronutrient interactions have been described with the Hardy-Stephan formula,[208] and several examples of effective micronutrient augmentation of psychiatric medications have been previously discussed involving folic acid,[54,58,82] vitamin B12,[88] a thiamine/riboflavin/pyridoxine combination,[176] vitamin D,[128] zinc,[160,162,163] and magnesium.[181] These drug-nutrient interactions become a problem when a patient who is receiving conventional medications is started on broad-spectrum micronutrient treatment. When the Hardy-Stephan formula is added to a regimen of psychiatric medications, it appears as if the micronutrients potentiate the effects of the psychiatric drugs, potentially flooding the patient with adverse effects unless the doses of the drugs are concurrently lowered. The potentiation is about threefold to fivefold, so psychiatric drug doses need to be gradually and carefully lowered to about 20% to 30% of the original level (although patients actually do better once the psychiatric medications are discontinued entirely). If drug doses are lowered too quickly, psychiatric symptoms may emerge; and if lowered too slowly, side effects characteristic of the psychiatric drug increase. Obviously, lowering doses or discontinuing psychiatric medications requires physician caution and patient cooperation. These transitions from conventional medications to the Hardy-Stephan formula are complex, especially when further complicated by withdrawal syndromes (from benzodiazepine or SSRI treatment), because the micronutrients appear to potentiate the withdrawal reactions as well. This transition process is not at all similar to transitioning from one psychiatric medication to another. It requires careful supervision by a clinician who is knowledgeable and experienced in the use of this micronutrient treatment.

For this reason, it is advised that any clinician who first begins to use broad-spectrum micronutrient treatment (1) obtain consultation with a clinician experienced with this particular treatment, both before and during the addition of micronutrient treatment to a psychiatric drug regimen, and (2) start first with a medication-naive patient. Treating a medication-naïve patient is much simpler and more straightforward, because of the absence of the drug-nutrient interactions. This allows the clinician to begin to get some experience with micronutrient treatment before adding the complexity of drug-nutrient interactions.

This micronutrient potentiation, which has been documented in several of the open-label reports, applies to all virtually drugs active in the CNS, including nonpsychiatric medications.

Lithium is a special case: this mineral has extremely strong interactions with micronutrients. Instead of the 3-fold to 5-fold potentiation seen with most CNS-active drugs, broad-spectrum micronutrients produce a 100-fold potentiation of lithium. When adding lithium to a broad-spectrum micronutrient treatment, I usually begin with a dosage of 1 mg 4 times daily, and gradually increase to up to 5 mg 4 times daily if tolerated. Most patients are treated with 10 to 20 mg total daily, with typical lithium side effects emerging at higher doses. The standard dosage range for lithium is approximately 1000 to 2000 mg daily in youth,[219] so this represents a 100-fold potentiation. Administration of these low dosages entails use of either the liquid lithium elixir (diluted with water) or compounded pills. In cases in which micronutrients are helpful but residual manic symptoms persist, the addition of these "micro doses" of lithium can, in my opinion, be very helpful. No studies of lithium combined with micronutrient treatment are available.

In other cases in which micronutrients appear effective but additional fine-tuning is needed, it is possible to combine broad-spectrum micronutrient treatment with certain other "natural" treatments without incurring drug-nutrient interactions. Options for such adjunctive treatments include SAMe or 5-hydroxytryptophan for residual depression, choline (or lecithin) for residual mania (although adjunctive lithium, which does interact with micronutrients, is more effective), inositol or L-theanine for anxiety, and inositol or melatonin for sleep.[52,63,130,220–222] Omega-3 fatty acids can be considered as well, although, based on anecdotal observation, it rarely seems to provide a significant benefit when added to the Hardy-Stephan formula.

Summary comment on mood disorders

The RDBPCT on adults with ADHD and the 16 open-label reports provide strong but early evidence that broad-spectrum micronutrient interventions can treat major symptoms of mood disorders, including depression and mania, in youth and adults. Virtually all of these studies conducted on youth and adults with mood disorders used the Hardy-Stephan formulation (eg, EMPower). In a recent systematic review, the Hardy-Stephan formulation was found to have substantial effect sizes for treating bipolar depression (Cohen d = 1.7) and bipolar mania (d = 0.83). By comparison, folic acid had a much lower effect size (d = 0.4) in bipolar depression.[63] Response rate (percentage of patients who improve significantly) appears to be about 80% for drug-naïve patients and about 50% for patients (as in the 2 database analyses) transitioning from previous psychiatric medications.

Particularly impressive in reviewing the reports on broad-spectrum micronutrient effects on mood disorders are (1) the virtual absence of significant adverse effects, (2) effectiveness for both manic and depressive symptoms, (3) the ability of most patients to discontinue their previous psychiatric medications entirely or at least reduce their doses, (4) the frequent reporting of remission rather than simple improvement of symptoms, (5) the low frequency of necessary medication dose adjustments, and (6) the anecdotal reports of long-term "super stability" in the treatment-responsive population, in which hospitalizations and even dose adjustments are rare.

Disadvantages of this treatment are significant. The lack of replicated RCTs assessing safety and efficacy remains a critical barrier at present. The cost of $150 monthly and the lack of insurance coverage puts these treatments out of consideration for many families, and cost (rather than adverse effects or ineffectiveness) is the most common reason for discontinuation by patients.[203] The treatment typically entails 8 to 15 pills daily for treating mood disorders, which is formidable for some patients, especially children. The drug-nutrient interactions are a challenge to patients when transitioning from conventional medications to the Hardy-Stephan formula (especially if withdrawal syndromes result from tapering of long-term treatments with benzodiazepines, SSRIs, or some antipsychotic agents) and to physicians (who need consultation or training when learning to conduct these transitions). Additional difficulties arise in the rare circumstance when a patient requires hospitalization, which is usually because of patient noncompliance or to unusually severe withdrawal syndromes from conventional medications. Most hospitals do not have these supplements in their formularies, and staff may decline to continue the treatments during hospitalization if they do not have access to a knowledgeable consultant.

The fact that there are so few reported negative open-label trials on broad-spectrum micronutrient treatment of mood disorders raises concern about publication bias. These concerns might be partially allayed by the 2 database analyses on several hundred youth and adults, which found that about half of patients show greater than 50% reduction in symptom scores. These estimates are based on a population in which 80% of patients were taking conventional medications at baseline, so this would underestimate the response rate that would be expected in a drug-naïve population. This substantial response rate in naturalistic data makes it unlikely that the highly favorable results in the open-label reports are due to publication bias alone.

It is evident that additional studies are needed before firm conclusions can be drawn. There are currently no RCTs examining broad-spectrum micronutrients in a population of youths or adults recruited for major depression or bipolar disorder. New studies should first examine patients who are drug-naïve or who have not recently used conventional psychiatric drugs to avoid drug-nutrient interactions that arise during treatment transitions. For the same reasons, patients should be excluded from initial studies if they regularly use CNS-active substances, such as alcohol, recreational drugs, nicotine, or significant amounts of caffeine. Recruitment of such adults with mood disorders might be difficult in some locations, so assembling this type of sample might be easiest in a child population.[212,213]

Micronutrients for Other Psychiatric Conditions

Preliminary data suggest that broad-spectrum micronutrient treatment may have some potential for treating OCD, autism, substance use, and other psychiatric conditions.

OCD

Positive effects of broad-spectrum micronutrient treatments have been reported on OCD in children[193,194,210–212,214] and adults.[196,207] Two of the case reports included multiple reversal (ABAB) confirmation of the treatment effect.[193,210,223] All of these reports were conducted using the Hardy-Stephen micronutrient formulation (EMPower). Because 63% of patients with OCD have a mood disorder,[224] OCD symptoms may be expected to improve, even if only mediated through improved mood symptoms.

Autism

Two RCTs examining broad-spectrum micronutrient formulations have been conducted in youths with autism, but both are methodologically limited. In an initial pilot RCT of treatment with a 34-ingredient micronutrient product (manufactured by Yasoo Health, Jonesborough, TN), 20 youths (ages 3–8) were studied without the use of outcome measures. Parents described improvements in sleep and gastrointestinal symptoms, but no behavior, language, or social changes.[225] This Yasoo micronutrient formulation was then examined in an RDBPCT involving 141 subjects with clinically diagnosed autism, mostly children and adolescents.[226] No change was noted on 3 standardized outcome instruments, but the report stated (without presenting full statistical analysis) that the micronutrient group showed improvements compared with placebo on unvalidated Parental Global Impression-R scales ($P = .008$), including tantrum ($P = .009$), hyperactivity ($P = .03$), and receptive language ($P = .03$) scores. Neither the pilot nor the RDBPCT used standardized diagnostic assessments, and comorbidity was not reported.

A well-conducted study in a clinical setting, although open-label, provided more interpretable data. A naturalistic open-label study of the Hardy-Stephan formula examined children and young adults (ages 2–28) with autism and a variety of forms of comorbidity.[227] The study compared 44 patients whose families preferred nonpharmaceutical treatment, and who received the Hardy-Stephan formula, with 44 participants who were treated with conventional psychiatric medications. Over the course of treatment (mean 15 months, range 3 months to 10 years), both treatment groups improved, but the micronutrient group showed significantly more improvement in scores for Aberrant Behavior Checklist ($P>.0001$), self-injurious behaviors ($P = .005$), and CGI ($P<.003$) than patients receiving conventional psychiatric medications. Micronutrients also appeared to be more effective in reducing social withdrawal, improving spontaneity, and reducing anger.

The possible mediating role of micronutrient-induced mood changes could not be clarified in these designs.

Substance use

A recent ABAB case report suggests a possible benefit of micronutrients in reducing marijuana and cigarette use in a 20-year-old, presumably mediated by reduced symptoms of depression and ADHD.[192] Several early reports suggest possible effects of micronutrient interventions, often in combination with amino acids, in reducing craving and relapse rates for abuse of alcohol[228–233] and cocaine,[228,231,234] but inadequate methodology or incomplete data presentation limits their value.

Broad-Spectrum Micronutrient Interventions in Healthy Populations

Broad-spectrum micronutrient treatments have been examined in healthy adults and youth for their effects on cognition, normal mood, sense of well-being, and response to stress. These RCTs used heterogeneous protocols (ingredient profiles, high-dose vs low-dose strategies, treatment durations, and outcome measures), and the findings are inconsistent and not robust, but still offer some perhaps unexpected intervention options.

Cognition in healthy adults

An extremely large number of studies have investigated micronutrient effects on cognition in adults. A meta-analysis of 10 selected quality RCTs in 3200 adults (age>18) concluded that broad-spectrum micronutrient interventions induce a small but consistent improvement in immediate free recall memory (ES 0.32, $P<.01$).[235] Among the studies examined, a large RDBPCT in 4447 middle-aged adults (ages 45–60) treated with broad-spectrum micronutrients for several years showed a slowing of age-related declines in executive functions and verbal memory.[236]

Later in life, in elderly populations with or without medical illness or dementia, micronutrient trials lasting 3 to 12 months do not show consistent effects on cognition. The RCTs have found either positive effects on cognition,[237–239] benefits only in subgroups on post hoc analysis,[240–244] or no benefits.[245–249] Senescent gastrointestinal absorption of nutrients and the many non-nutritional factors that interfere with brain function in the elderly[250–253] may contribute to these weak findings.

Berocca (Bayer Corporation, Pittsburgh, PA), a commercial formulation containing 12 micronutrients (mostly B vitamins) at RDA levels, has been examined in healthy adults (ages 18–65) in a series of RDBPCTs that show small but consistent improvements on a limited number of cognitive measures.[254–257] There are also some RCTs showing positive cognitive effects of other Berocca products that included caffeine-containing guaraná, which may have contributed to the observed changes.[258,259] It should be noted that these studies were funded by the manufacturer, and manufacturer representatives were coauthors on most of the Berocca studies. The Berocca studies comprised 4 of the 10 articles in the meta-analysis and so may have weighted its findings.

Cognition in healthy youth

A literature review by Benton[260] reported that 10 of 13 controlled and uncontrolled intervention studies provided evidence that micronutrients, either singly or in broad-spectrum, improved cognition in healthy school-age children, with selective increases in nonverbal intelligence (performance IQ) scores of 2 to 4 IQ points, and not in verbal intelligence. The changes were observed in only a subgroup of children, presumably with poor dietary status. A more recent meta-analysis of RCTs focused on micronutrient formulations containing 3 or more ingredients,[261] included newer rigorous studies, and analyzed 12 studies in healthy children (ages 5–16). No significant effects were found on cognitive processing speed, working memory, long-term memory, or sustained attention, and the effect on nonverbal intelligence was found to fall short of statistical significance (ES 0.14, P = .083). On the other hand, the 4 trials that examined academic performance collectively showed a cognitive benefit (ES 0.30, P = .44) in school-age children.[262–265]

It is not necessarily surprising that micronutrients could show a small or trending effect on nonverbal intelligence but no effect on verbal intelligence. Verbal intelligence can be viewed as more reliant on specific "crystallized" information, such as vocabulary and syntactic rules, and may depend more on education, environmental stimulation, interpersonal experience, and socioenvironmental influences. In contrast, nonverbal intelligence is more based on reasoning ability, problem-solving, reframing and set-shifting, and involves "fluid" or "organic" functioning that might be more reflective of biologic status. This division may be arbitrary to some extent, especially over time, as these types of intellectual functioning interact to promote individual development.[266]

An unexpected finding was raised by an RDBPCT of 81 healthy children (ages 8–14) using a commercial broad-spectrum micronutrient formulation (Pharmaton Kiddi, Boehringer Ingelheim GmbH, Ingelheim, Germany). It showed mixed effects on cognition, but included some improvements in selective attention that were apparent within 3 hours after the first dose administration.[267] The possibility that micronutrients might have rapid effects on cognition has not been well explored.

Surveying the cognitive effects of broad-spectrum micronutrients, healthy youths showed mild to moderate enhancement of academic performance (ES 0.44) and a trend toward a 2-point to 4-point improvement in performance IQ (ES 0.14). Adults showed some positive cognitive effects of micronutrients as well, including improved immediate free-recall memory (ES 0.32) and possibly a slowing of age-related declines in executive functioning and verbal memory. In the elderly, cognitive effects appeared mixed and inconclusive. These findings suggest that there are small but potentially clinically significant benefits of micronutrient interventions on cognition in youth and nonelderly adults.

Mood and well-being in healthy adults

Long and Benton[268] conducted a meta-analysis of RCTs examining mood and mood-related effects of broad-spectrum micronutrients in healthy adults. It found no overall effect on general mood in 8 RDBPCTs on 1292 healthy adults (ages 18–69) administered broad-spectrum micronutrients for 28 to 90 days. The 3 RDBPCTs examining subclinical depression in the general population also reported no effect (**Fig. 8**).[254,269,270]

Despite the absence of significant mood effects, the meta-analysis found that broad-spectrum micronutrients improved perceived stress (ES 0.35), anxiety (ES 0.32), fatigue (ES 0.27), mental fog (ES 0.23), and hostile mood (ES 0.23), all significantly ($P<.011$). Again, half of the 8 studies reviewed in the meta-analysis were manufacturer-sponsored reports on Berocca.[254–256,271] Two uncontrolled Berocca studies not included in the meta-analysis also found reductions in stress-related symptoms. The other four studies similarly showed positive effects on fatigue and mental clarity.[272–275]

Subsequent to the meta-analysis, an independent 4-month RDBPCT of a commercial formulation (Swisse Ultivite F1 Formula) in 138 healthy adults (ages 20–50) confirmed the meta-analysis findings of no change in mood measures, but some evidence of improved anxiety and physical fatigue scores,[276,277] including subjects' narrative reports describing an improved sense of well-being.[278]

As in the cognition studies, older adults ($\geq$50 years old) showed inconsistent results, with mood improvements in only 2[178,269] of 6 studies.[178,237,240,242,246,269]

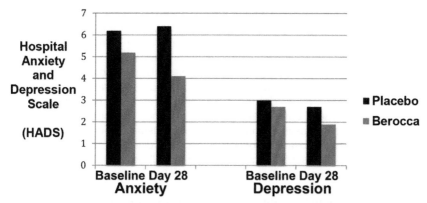

Fig. 8. Berocca, a commercial micronutrient supplement, reduced anxiety but not depression in healthy volunteers. A 4-week RDBPCT of Berocca in healthy male volunteers (ages 18–42, mean 25), with 40 subjects in each treatment group. The formulation of Berocca used in this study consisted several B vitamins, vitamin C, calcium, and magnesium, with no caffeine. At day 28, the effect on anxiety was significant ($P = .05$), but not on depression. (*Data from* Carroll D, Ring C, Suter M, et al. The effects of an oral multivitamin combination with calcium, magnesium, and zinc on psychological well-being in healthy young male volunteers: a double-blind placebo-controlled trial. Psychopharmacology (Berl) 2000;150(2):220–5.)

However, in contrast to the mixed results on mood and cognition, 2 studies in the elderly found positive micronutrient effects on measures of well-being and general functioning.[237,269]

In nongeriatric adults, 2 RDBPCTs again showed evidence of improved scores for feeling more "agreeable" ($P<.03$), and among women feeling more "composure" ($P<.01$).[147,279]

In youth, the only RDBPCT conducted on mood in children examined a commercial children's multivitamin/multimineral product (Pharmaton Kiddi) on 81 healthy children (8–14 years) in a 12-week study.[267] Mood data were collected via the Internet using only a visual analogue scale (faces) and a single number on a 7-point scale, so the findings are compromised by inadequate outcome measurement. The study found no effect on mood.

The meta-analysis found that micronutrient formulations with higher doses of B vitamins appeared to have more effect on actual mood ratings, especially if doses were well above RDA levels (5–10 times higher). This finding again challenges the validity of RDAs as reflecting optimal intake levels and instead suggests that supra-RDA levels may be needed to optimize brain function.

None of the studies conducted on cognition, mood, or well-being in healthy subjects have investigated the Hardy-Stephan formula. (It might be mentioned that none of the 28 reports on the Hardy-Stephan formula have been funded or coauthored by the manufacturers.)

Summing across these RCTs in healthy adults, broad-spectrum micronutrients appeared to have little effect on mood, but did improve sense of well-being, general energy, clear-headedness, and agreeable feelings and reduced anxiety and stress responses (ES 0.23–0.35). These statistically significant changes were not dramatic, but even these small changes should challenge some common preconceptions about nutrition and mental health. If judged by the standards of a therapeutic intervention for a medical disorder, this intervention might be viewed as worthwhile but not particularly strong. If judged by the standards of an inexpensive and easy life enhancement, these same findings might be viewed as dramatic. Who wouldn't want a consistent, albeit small, improvement in mental energy and clarity of mind? Who wouldn't want a subtle "tune-up" for anxiety and stress management?

Mental energy, clear-headedness, and agreeable feelings can be conceptualized as aspects of mood that are not tapped by the common psychiatric instruments for measuring outcome in mood disorders. These features could be "sub-subclinical" signs of mood disorders, but it is also possible that they are aspects of mood overlooked by psychiatric measures. Antidepressants are usually thought to contribute little to "normal" people who are free of subclinical mood disorders. These micronutrient data in healthy subjects suggest that the sense of well-being and clear-headedness may be valuable to conceptualize and target for intervention as aspects of "mood" that might not be affected by antidepressants.

These RCTs seem to highlight a possible value of micronutrients for the general population of nonelderly healthy adults. Micronutrients, unlike conventional antidepressants, may be a rational option for enhancing a quality of well-being, emotional reserve, clear-headedness, and freedom from stress and mental fatigue, even if the effects are subtle. At present, comparable data are not available for healthy youths.

Response to stress

Micronutrient effects on mood, anxiety, and well-being have been examined in highly stressful life circumstances. Three settings in which broad-spectrum micronutrient interventions have been studied in RCTs are stressful urban living, military training, and the aftermath of earthquakes.

A study of 300 community adults living in "2 centers with high stress levels" in South Africa, Durban and Johannesburg, were administered Berocca Calmag (not available in the United States) or placebo under RDBPC conditions.[271] Both groups improved between baseline and day 30, but the micronutrient group improved significantly more than the controls in anxiety or stress levels, as measured by the Hamilton Anxiety Rating Scale, the Psychological General Well-Being Index, and an unvalidated stress instrument. This study is compromised by the vague description of the population and recruitment procedures, and by the manufacturer's direct involvement. It is unclear whether the micronutrient-induced changes are due to treating stress responses or to correcting endemic nutritional deficiencies in these populations; however, stressful life circumstances increase micronutrient utilization and turnover, so these are not necessarily separable effects. Regardless of the conceptualization of the mechanism, it is interesting to see a micronutrient-induced reduction in stress response in an endemically stressful region.

Military training also can be viewed as a major life stressor. An RDBPC crossover study examined the effects of just a single week of micronutrient supplementation in 240 men who were subjected to physical "overtraining" in rigorous endurance military training.[280] Findings included a reduction in psychological stress responses (probably including anger, tension, somatization), compared with placebo, as well as in pituitary, adrenal, and thyroid changes. The Chinese government has made the abstract of this report available, but the article itself is officially unavailable because of its secret contents, so no further information can be described. Potential military applications of micronutrient treatments are plentiful.

A third example of micronutrient effects on extreme stress is evident in the open-label reports and an unblinded RCT suggesting that broad-spectrum micronutrients, even used on a short-term basis, can prevent or reduce posttraumatic stress symptoms following a natural disaster. An open-label study examined 33 adults with ADHD who had either been treated with the Hardy-Stephan formula or received no treatment for 2 weeks before a major earthquake.[281,282] The treatments were conducted in the context of research studies that were interrupted by the earthquake. These subjects were continued on open-label Hardy-Stephan formula or no treatment for 2 weeks after the earthquake and then assessed by using the Depression, Anxiety, and Stress Scale (DASS). Relative to baseline before the earthquake, the micronutrient-treated subjects at 2 weeks after the earthquake showed reductions in depression (ES 0.73, $P<.05$) as well as anxiety (ES 0.84, $P<.01$) and stress (ES 1.0, $P<.01$), with nonsignificant improvements in the untreated subjects. Two weeks after the earthquake, the micronutrient group showed lower anxiety and stress scores compared with controls (ES 0.69, $P<.05$). This study was conducted under extraordinary circumstances, involved nonrandom treatment assignments, an untreated control group, and differences in recruitment and treatment time, but nonetheless provides results suggesting that micronutrient treatment enhanced the resilience or recovery of adults with ADHD following a natural disaster.

A separate study was initiated as an RCT starting 2 to 3 months after a subsequent earthquake and conducted over a 4-week period while aftershocks were still occurring daily.[283] In this RCT, 91 healthy adults were randomized to 1 of 3 different micronutrient treatments: (1) EMPower administered at a moderate dose of 8 pills daily (the standard dose for treating mood disorders is 15 pills daily); (2) EMPower at a low dose of 4 pills daily; and (3) a once-daily dose of Berocca, which is the commercial RDA-level multivitamin/mineral formula that had been shown to have efficacy in reducing stress and anxiety (see **Fig. 8**),[254,255,271] with an effect size of 0.35.[268] A contrast group was separately recruited. All subjects had been selected for elevated baseline anxiety, depression, or stress scores. Although the study was randomized and different doses of micronutrients were compared with each other and with a separately recruited contrast group, this RCT was not blinded. One month later, all 3 micronutrient groups showed improvement ($P<.001$) on several scales (DASS; Impact of Event Scale; Perceived Stress Scale). The improvements in mood, anxiety, and energy were significant ($P<.03$) and appeared dose-dependent (**Fig. 9**). EMPower was more effective than Berocca in reducing intrusive thoughts ($P = .05$), and some other changes were significantly larger in the moderate-dose EMPower group than in the Berocca group. Over the 4-week trial, the prevalence of probable posttraumatic stress disorder (PTSD) reduced from 65% to 19% in the micronutrient groups, but increased from 44% to 48% in the control group ($P<.05$) (**Fig. 10**). In this postearthquake RCT, micronutrients appeared more effective than controls in diminishing anxiety, arousal, intrusive thoughts, and avoidance.

In a 1-year follow-up study to this RCT,[284] approximately 70% of the original subjects completed online questionnaires (Depression and Anxiety Stress Scale, Impact of Event Scale, CGI-I). Approximately 10% of the subjects still had PTSD symptoms at the 1-year point, but subjects treated with micronutrients soon after the earthquake had better DASS stress (ES 1.31), intrusions (ES 0.71), mood (ES 0.69), and energy (ES 0.71) scores, in comparison to controls after controlling for baseline values (**Table 7**). As in the ADHD RDBPCT, subjects who stayed on micronutrients for the entire year fared better than subjects who switched to conventional medications (**Fig. 11**).

These earthquake findings have potentially major implications, because they suggest that simple and inexpensive micronutrient supplementation may reduce acute

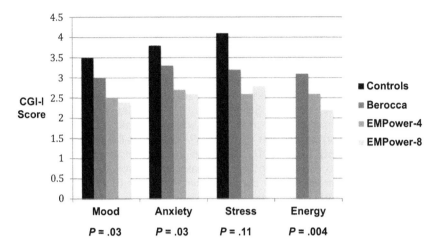

Fig. 9. Outcome after 4 weeks of micronutrient treatment following an earthquake. Two or 3 months after a catastrophic earthquake in New Zealand, 91 adults with elevated depression, anxiety, or stress scores were treated for 4 weeks with one of 3 micronutrient interventions: Berocca (1 pill daily), EMPower (4 pills daily), or EMPower (8 pills daily). A control group (n = 25) was separately assembled for comparison. All groups showed improvement in CGI scores for mood (DASS), anxiety (IES), and stress (Perceived Stress Scale) ratings. Clinical Global Impression-Improvement scores showed change from baseline to 4 weeks (1 = very much improved, 7 = very much worse, so lower score means better outcome). *P* values represent analysis of variance comparisons across treatments for each outcome measure. Comparison of combined micronutrient groups to controls was *P*<.001 for mood, anxiety, and stress (energy data for controls not available). (*Data from* Rucklidge JJ, Andridge R, Gorman B, et al. Shaken but unstirred? Effects of micronutrients on stress and trauma after an earthquake: RCT evidence comparing formulas and doses. Hum Psychopharmacol 2012;27(5):440–54.)

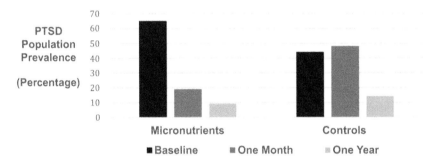

Fig. 10. Following a natural disaster, prevalence of probable PTSD was reduced after a 1-month RDBPC trial of EMPower, with follow-up at 1 year. Prevalence of probable PTSD was high in this population at baseline (2–3 months after earthquake). After a 1-month randomized double-blind placebo-controlled trial, probable PTSD was reduced in the micronutrient-treated subjects, but was unchanged in the separately recruited controls (comparison *P*<.05). After 1 year, part of the sample continued on micronutrients on an open-label basis, but by then, both groups had largely and equally improved. (*Data from* Rucklidge JJ, Andridge R, Gorman B, et al. Shaken but unstirred? Effects of micronutrients on stress and trauma after an earthquake: RCT evidence comparing formulas and doses. Hum Psychopharmacol 2012;27(5):440–54; and Rucklidge JJ, Blampied N, Gorman B, et al. Psychological functioning 1 year after a brief intervention using micronutrients to treat stress and anxiety related to the 2011 Christchurch earthquakes: A naturalistic follow-up. Hum Psychopharmacol 2014;29(3):230–43.)

Table 7
Earthquake victims treated for 1 month with the Hardy-Stephan formula in a randomized double-blind placebo-controlled trial showed better outcome 1 year later

	Micronutrient-Treated, n = 64			Control Group, n = 21			Effect Size for 4 vs 52 wk		
Months Treated	0	1	12	0	1	12	Treated	Controls	P
DASS									
Depression	16.0	8.2	7.2	12.0	8.5	8.1	0.13	0.10	NS
Anxiety	11.0	4.2	3.7	8.6	7.4	3.4	0.09	0.72	NS
Stress	22.0	11.0	3.7	17.0	15.0	9.9	0.80	1.12	<.001
Total	49.0	23.0	15.0	38.0	31.0	21.0	0.40	0.72	<.01
IES-R									
Avoidance	1.4	0.61	0.50	1.2	1.1	0.79	0.24	0.60	<.001
Arousal	2.1	1.2	0.82	1.6	1.8	1.1	0.39	0.62	<.001
Intrusion	1.9	1.1	0.76	1.7	1.5	1.1	0.44	0.77	NS
Total	39.0	21.0	15.0	33.0	32.0	22.0	0.44	0.74	<.001

Seventy percent of the original sample completed the 1-year followup evaluation, and all 3 randomized micronutrient-treated groups were merged for the 1-year follow-up data and compared with a separately recruited, nonrandomized control group.

All measures in both treatment groups showed improvement after 4 weeks and still more after 12 months (analysis of variance P<.001). Statistically significant improvements between 1 month and 1 year were observed for stress, avoidance, and arousal, but not for depression, anxiety, or intrusive thoughts. Given the large number of comparisons, change is considered significant only if P<.01.

Clinical Global Impression-Improvement (CGI-I) changes over time for mood, anxiety, and stress did not show statistically significant effects between treated and control groups.

Abbreviations: DASS, Depression, Anxiety, and Stress Scale; IES-R, Impact of Event Scale; NS, not significant.

Adapted from Rucklidge JJ, Blampied N, Gorman B, et al. Psychological functioning 1 year after a brief intervention using micronutrients to treat stress and anxiety related to the 2011 Christchurch earthquakes: A naturalistic follow-up. Hum Psychopharmacol 2014;29(3):230–43; with permission.

stress symptoms following natural disasters. These effects appear to be clinically significant, even with a brief 4-week intervention, similar to the improvement in anxiety and stress levels observed after a 4-week intervention in adults living in highly stressful urban centers in South Africa.[271] Although this earthquake study is limited by a lack of placebo controls, no blinding, and use of a nonrandomized control group, this RCT raises the possibility of an innovative and unique public health intervention for healthy populations following natural disasters.

Replicative studies are needed to assess micronutrients as an emergency intervention for treating and possibly preventing acute stress reactions in adults. Obviously, there are numerous potential applications for micronutrient interventions in response to major traumatic events in children and adolescents, but again, studies are needed.

Adverse Effects of Broad-Spectrum Micronutrient Interventions

The numerous open-label reports and controlled studies, both of the Hardy-Stephan formula and other broad-spectrum micronutrient formulations, have uniformly noted that broad-spectrum micronutrient treatments have a minimum of adverse effects in

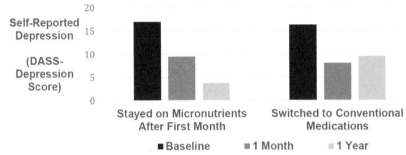

Fig. 11. After major stressor, staying on micronutrients for 1 year reduced depression scores more than switching to conventional medications. This is a reanalysis of the data, looking at outcomes (at 1 month and at 1 year) based on whether the subjects stayed on micronutrients for a full year or whether they switched to conventional medications after the 1-month RCT. Starting 2 to 3 months after the earthquake, all subjects in this subsample of the RDBPCT were treated with micronutrients for 1 month, and both groups responded about equally. After the first month, the 17 subjects who continued open-label micronutrients for 1 year had lower self-rated DASS depression scores than 12 subjects who switched to conventional medications after the first month (*P*<.05). The micronutrient continuers continued to improve between 1 month and 1 year, whereas the switchers did not. (*Data from* Rucklidge JJ, Blampied N, Gorman B, et al. Psychological functioning 1 year after a brief intervention using micronutrients to treat stress and anxiety related to the 2011 Christchurch earthquakes: A naturalistic follow-up. Hum Psychopharmacol 2014;29(3):230–43.)

children and adults. A naturalistic case-control study found markedly fewer adverse effects in 44 micronutrient-treated patients (ages 2–28) than in 44 medication-treated patients.[227] Two reports have given systematic descriptions of adverse effects in 151 children, adolescents, and adults,[213,285] including published and unpublished data.

The main adverse effects reported were mild nausea, dyspepsia, loose stools, initial insomnia, and headache (**Box 8**). In the ADHD RDBPCT, these symptoms appeared at similar frequency in the placebo-treated subjects, with no statistically significant differences between the 2 groups.[201] These adverse effects are typically mild and transient, and can be managed in the routine ways (taking capsules with food to reduce gastrointestinal symptoms, taking pills earlier to reduce insomnia, temporary dose reductions).

Anxiety, agitation, or impulsivity can appear if the broad-spectrum micronutrient dose is too high, but these exacerbations reliably resolve when the dose is lowered. Excessive dosing does not appear to trigger autonomous manic episodes. Another potential adverse effect is the aggravation of preexisting *Candida* (yeast) infections. In general, these infections can be adequately managed with antifungal medication, olive leaf extract, and probiotics.[286]

There was a report of a small asymptomatic increase in prolactin levels in micronutrient-treated patients (mean increased from 191 to 222 mIU/L, *P*<.006).[202] Two of 80 subjects had larger prolactin elevations, but no subject had levels rise beyond the normal range; it was unclear whether these changes were related to treatment. Two cases of mild blood sugar elevation also were described in that report, but they were judged not clinically significant, and again were not clearly related to treatment. No other changes have been observed in laboratory indices.

The systematic data and the numerous published descriptions document an absence of weight changes, sedation or fatigue, dry mouth, constipation, tremor,

---

Box 8
Clinical points on broad-spectrum micronutrient treatments

Adverse Effects

  Loose stools

  Nausea (rarely, vomiting)

  Dyspepsia

  Insomnia

  Headache

  "Neon" yellow urine (due to riboflavin excretion; not a medical problem)

  Flatulence

  Watery diarrhea

  Anxiety, agitation, or impulsivity if dose too high

  Aggravation of preexisting *Candida* (yeast) infections

  Slightly increased prolactin levels (reported in 1 study)[201]

Nutrient-drug interactions

  Critical: Interaction with virtually all psychiatric drugs and other medications with CNS effects, especially medications associated with discontinuation syndromes.

  Interaction with antibiotics (antibiotics reduce gastrointestinal absorption of nutrients, so micronutrient dosage needs to be increased during antibiotic treatment)

Strict contraindications

  Wilson disease (risk of copper overload)

  Hemochromatosis and hemosiderosis (risk of iron overload)

  Phenylketonuria (risk of phenylalanine overload)

  Trimethylaminuria (risk of choline overload)

Relative contraindications

  Recreational drug dependence, including caffeine, alcohol, and nicotine

  Recent use of medical drugs with withdrawal syndromes

  Necessary medical treatment with CNS-active agents

  Treatment-resistant *Candida*

  Autoimmune thyroid disease or nodular goiter (iodine)

  High alcohol intake, hyperlipidemia, or severe protein malnutrition (which are associated with increased susceptibility to vitamin A toxicity)

---

sexual side effects, blood pressure or pulse changes, seizures, thyroid changes, motor side effects, dependency, or discontinuation effects.[194,196,207,227] Electrocardiographic data have not been reported in the literature, but I have observed no micronutrient-related electrocardiogram abnormalities in several hundred youths and adults.

It is evident that the adverse effects of the broad-spectrum micronutrient treatments are mild in comparison with the side effects of most conventional psychopharmacological treatments.

SUMMARY

The main findings on micronutrient treatments provide some encouraging data (**Box 9**, **Tables 8** and **9**). Several single-nutrient interventions show promise as effective augmentation agents for antidepressant treatments, but not as monotherapies. In contrast, broad-spectrum micronutrient interventions appear to have the potential to become a genuine monotherapy for mood disorders whose effects may be comparable to conventional antidepressant and mood-stabilizing agents.

Main findings on broad-spectrum micronutrient treatments are as follows:

- Three RDBPCTs support the treatment of violence and major misconduct in adolescent and young adult incarcerated offenders.
- One RDBPCT shows a reduction in aggressive and disordered conduct in school children.
- One RDBPCT in adults with ADHD shows moderate effect sizes for changes in hyperactivity/impulsivity (ES 0.46–0.67), inattention (ES 0.33–0.62), and CGI (ES 0.53–0.57), with a response rate of 64%.
- In youth with ADHD, the best estimate of response rate is 63% to 76%.
- Treatment of probable MDD (MADRS≥20) in adults with comorbid ADHD has effect size comparable to antidepressants (ES 0.41) in the ADHD RCT.
- A sophisticated independent review gave higher estimates of the effect sizes for treating mood disorders: 1.7 for treating bipolar depression, and 0.83 for bipolar mania (Sarris 201).[63]
- Open-label data support possible effectiveness for OCD, autism, and substance abuse.
- Several RCTs suggest improved response to a diverse set of major stressors in healthy adults, including reduction in post-traumatic symptoms following a natural disaster.
- A meta-analysis finds improved academic performance in healthy school children (ES 0.44). (There is also a nonsignificant statistical trend suggesting a 2-point to 4-point improvement in performance IQ in healthy children.)
- A meta-analysis shows improved free-recall memory in healthy adults (ES 0.32), and a large multi-year RDBPCT showing a possible slowing of age-related decline in executive functioning and verbal memory.
- Subtle improvements in general energy, clear-headedness, and agreeable feelings in healthy adults (ES 0.2–0.3); no data in youth.

The main findings on single-micronutrient treatments provide some positive data as well:

- Folic acid is an effective, although not powerful, adjunctive treatment for MDD in adults (ES 0.4), but has not been evaluated in youth with MDD.
- Vitamin B12 appears useful in geriatric depression but is unlikely to be helpful for youth, except perhaps in depressed youth with chronic gastrointestinal malabsorption.
- Vitamin D might sometimes be useful in depressed patients with documented hypovitaminosis D, and several factors may help estimate level of risk in an individual.
- Chromium may prove to be useful for atypical depression with carbohydrate craving in adults, but has not been examined in youth.
- Zinc should be examined further for antidepressant augmentation, especially in treatment-resistant MDD.
- Thiamine needs further study for its potential to improve mood, energy, and cognition in psychiatrically healthy individuals.

Box 9
Explanation of modified US Preventive Services Task Force grading system used in Tables 8 and 9

Tables 8 and 9 use a modified form of the US Preventive Services Task Force (USPSTF) grading system for describing published evidence in the medical literature supporting a treatment intervention.

Each treatment is assigned a grade for "Quality of Evidence" and a grade for "Strength of Recommendations."

USPSTF Quality of Evidence grade is based on the strength of the published evidence:

- Good: Consistent effect in well-conducted studies in different populations.
- Fair: Data shows effects, but data are weak, limited, or indirect.
- Poor: Cannot determine effect due to data weakness.

USPSTF Strength of Recommendations grade provides a ranking of the clinical recommendations that can be drawn from data in the published studies:

- Insufficient Data
- Recommend Against: Fair evidence of ineffectiveness or harm.
- Neutral: Fair evidence for, but appears risky.
- Recommend: Fair evidence of benefit and of safety.
- Recommend Strongly: Good evidence of benefit and safety.

Adapted from U.S. Preventive Services Task Force Grade Definitions. May 2008. Available at: http://www.uspreventiveservicestaskforce.org/uspstf/grades.htm. Accessed February 26, 2014.

- Selenium may be useful as a prenatal measure to prevent postpartum depression, but more research is needed.

The fact that broad-spectrum micronutrient treatments are much more powerful than single-nutrient treatments is not surprising in view of the basics of nutrition. Indeed, one might question the general strategy of single-micronutrient interventions. The interactions among nutrients make their combined use much more potent (witness lithium), and the high rate of single nutrient insufficiencies in the population makes generalized supplementation sensible. In fact, the risks of creating micronutrient imbalances (relative insufficiencies) might serve as a warning against the introduction of just one or a few micronutrients, except in specific situations (eg, vitamin D for Northerners and for bedridden patients, iron for menstruating women).

The findings of widespread micronutrient deficiencies, even in presumably well-fed populations, should also serve as an alert that large sections of the general population might benefit from nutrient supplementation.[256] Judging by the early data, broad-spectrum micronutrient treatments seem to be helpful for several different psychiatric indications and in so-called "normal" people as well. This highlights the question of the specificity of broad-spectrum micronutrient treatments.

If broad-spectrum treatments are able to treat mood disorders and ADHD, as well as stress reactions in medical and nonmedical populations, could the effects of broad-spectrum micronutrient treatments operate through a promotion of general CNS functioning rather than through mechanisms specific to mood or mood disorders? A generalized improvement in CNS functioning would be consistent with Bruce Ames' concept[21,22] of a "metabolic tune-up," in which biologic functions are pervasively enhanced by broad-spectrum micronutrient supplementation.

Table 8
Evidence base in published medical literature for single-micronutrients and broad-spectrum micronutrients for treating major depression and bipolar disorder

Micronutrients	Major or Bipolar Depression		Bipolar Mania		Evidence Base for Recommendation
	Youth	Adults	Youth	Adults	
Folic acid adjunctive therapy					
Quality of evidence	No data	Good	No data	Poor	Multiple RCTs in adults
Clinical recommendation	Insufficient data	Recommend	Insufficient data	Insufficient data	
Vitamin B12 adjunctive therapy					
Quality of evidence	No data	Good in geriatrics Fair in adults	No data	No data	Multiple RCTs in geriatrics, 2 RCTs in adults
Clinical recommendation	Insufficient data	Recommend for geriatrics Recommend against in adults	Insufficient data	Insufficient data	
Vitamin D adjunctive therapy					
Quality of evidence	Poor	Fair	No data	No data	2 RCTs in adults
Clinical recommendation	Insufficient data	Neutral	Insufficient data	Insufficient data	One open-label in youth
Pyridoxine adjunctive therapy					
Quality of evidence	No data	Poor	No data	No data	4 RCTs in adults with premenstrual symptoms
Clinical recommendation	Insufficient data	Recommend against in adults	Insufficient data	Insufficient data	
Chromium monotherapy					
Quality of evidence	No data	Fair	No data	No data	2 RCTs in adults with atypical depression
Clinical recommendation	Insufficient data	Neutral	Insufficient data	Insufficient data	1 RCT in bulimia

					Evidence base
Zinc adjunctive therapy					
Quality of evidence	No data	Fair	No data	No data	
Clinical recommendation	Insufficient data	Neutral (to Recommend but weakly)	Insufficient data	Insufficient data	3 RCTs in adults
Thiamine monotherapy					
Quality of evidence	No data	No data	No data	No data	
Clinical recommendation	Insufficient data	Insufficient data	Insufficient data	Insufficient data	2 RCTs in nonclinical volunteers were positive
Selenium monotherapy					
Quality of evidence	No data	Poor	No data	No data	
Clinical recommendation	Insufficient data	Insufficient data	Insufficient data	Insufficient data	1 RCT for preventing postpartum depression; 3 of 5 positive RCTs in nonclinical adults
Magnesium monotherapy					
Quality of evidence	No data	Fair	No data	No data	
Clinical recommendation	Insufficient data	Recommend against	Insufficient data	Insufficient data	3 RCTs in adults with premenstrual symptoms
Broad-spectrum micronutrient monotherapy					
Quality of evidence	Poor	Fair	Poor	Fair	
Clinical recommendation	Neutral	Neutral	Neutral	Neutral	1 RCT in adults with MDD, 4 RCTs in nonclinical stressed adults

Abbreviations: MDD, major depressive disorder; RCT, randomized controlled trial.

Table 9
Author's personal opinion of single micronutrients and broad-spectrum micronutrients for treating mood disorders in youth and adults

Micronutrient	Treatment Evaluation	Author's Clinical Opinion
Folic acid	Good evidence as adjunctive treatment for major depression in adults; no data in youth.	Moderately useful in adults. Despite lack of data, reasonable to try in youth based on lack of risk.
Vitamin B12	Good evidence as adjunctive treatment for major depression in geriatrics, but not in other adults; no data in youth.	Unlikely to help youth, unless chronic gastrointestinal malabsorption.
Vitamin D	Little evidence to support use for major depression in adults, few data in youth.	May be useful in depressed youth and adults with documented low serum levels of vitamin D, but even in those cases, effects on mood appear small.
Pyridoxine	Mostly negative results as adjunctive treatment of premenstrual mood.	Overall, little evidence of benefit.
Chromium	Mixed results as monotherapy for atypical depression in adults, no data in youth.	Might be useful for subgroup of atypical depression with carbohydrate craving.
Zinc	Mostly positive effects as adjunctive treatment in 3 RCTs in adults, perhaps mainly in treatment-resistant depression.	Needs more data, but low risk of harm.
Thiamine	Few data on monotherapy for depression, but might brighten mood in nonclinical youth and adults.	Unclear implications for treating mental illness.
Selenium	One RCT suggests possible preventive intervention for postpartum depression; conflicting data on mood in nonclinical samples.	Unclear implications for treating mental illness.
Magnesium	Monotherapy mostly ineffective for premenstrual mood.	Little mood effect, but not examined in major depression.
Broad-spectrum micronutrients	In mostly open trials, appears effective as monotherapy for bipolar depression, unipolar depression, and mania in youth and adults; one RCT in adults with ADHD shows antidepressant benefit that is comparable in effect size to conventional medications.	May prove useful as monotherapy. Because of few adverse effects compared with standard treatment, can be considered for medication-free youth and adults with mood disorders, but drug-nutrient interactions make this unsuitable for currently medicated patients unless treated by clinician familiar with this approach.

Abbreviations: ADHD, attention-deficit/hyperactivity disorder; RCT, randomized controlled trial.

Such a "metabolic tune-up" also could explain why broad-spectrum micronutrient treatments can amplify the effects of virtually all CNS-active drugs. Perhaps most psychiatric patients, or most people, are underresponding to their conventional medications because their biologic responses are not generally optimized. Tuning up the nutritional status of patients might speculatively improve their response to psychiatric medications, or to medications in general, by enhancing overall biological functioning.

Until there is more substantial evidence of the efficacy of these broad-spectrum micronutrient treatments, discussion of mechanisms in treating diseases remains entirely speculative. Once there is strong scientific evidence that these treatments are effective, then it will make sense to ask questions about mechanism: How do micronutrients alter disease processes? Are there particular nutrients that are essential, or is a broad-spectrum approach required? Is the same approach needed for all patients with a particular disorder, or does the optimal intervention depend on the nutritional requirements of the particular individual? Are nutritional insufficiencies even relevant, or are other individual factors more decisive? Until more clinical efficacy data are available, such questions are premature. The model of a metabolic tune-up is appealing, but it is not the only possible model. Nonetheless, at this time, Ames' notion of a broad-spectrum micronutrient "tune-up" of a broad range of physiological functions is sensible, supported by diverse biologic examples, and highly applicable to the seemingly wide-ranging effects of micronutrients on brain functioning.

The notion that broad-spectrum micronutrient supplementation might have broad-ranging effects on brain function and brain development is supported by a series of experiments conducted in rats. Celeste Halliwell and Bryan Kolb[287,288] have examined the effects of EMPower on recovery from early brain injury. Rats lesioned on postnatal day 3 in the frontal cortex show drastic permanent reductions in cortical thickness and functional performance, including decrements on tasks that involve motor skills and spatial learning and memory. When tested as adults, lesioned rats administered EMPower in their chow throughout their lives showed, relative to rats fed standard chow, increased brain weight, increased cortical thickness, and restoration of normal functioning on both behavioral tasks, as well as evidence of enhanced new dendritic growth and increased spine density (**Figs. 12** and **13**). Rats with perinatal posterior parietal lesions, when fed EMPower, showed generally similar anatomic recovery (including reversal of decreased brain size, atrophy of dendritic arborizations, and reduced spine density in pyramidal cells in the cortex), as well as restoration of cognitive and motor capacity.

These studies suggest a powerful neurotrophic effect of broad-spectrum micronutrients on rat brain structure, function, and development following early perinatal cortical lesions. The potential clinical implications of these findings for children with prenatal or perinatal brain injury (for example, in response to intrauterine drug or nicotine exposure, or to perinatal anoxia) or with neurodevelopmental disorders (for example, learning disorders or schizophrenia) have not been investigated.[289,290]

In addition to such broad-spectrum approaches, more targeted interventions also might have generalized neurotrophic effects on cerebral plasticity, dendrite growth, spine density, brain development, and brain function.[291,292] Halliwell and Kolb,[287,288] as well as Richard Wurtman,[293] have provided evidence that choline can have similar effects. Wurtman[293,294] has noted that increasing the dietary intake of choline, the omega-3 fatty acid DHA, and the nucleoside uridine can improve synaptogenesis during early development and in senescence.

In this review, we have glossed over a variety of technical details in the clinical studies. Optimally, intervention studies would control for subjects' oral micronutrient intake obtained through foods and supplements. We have not discussed proper

Standard
Chow

Chow with
EMPower

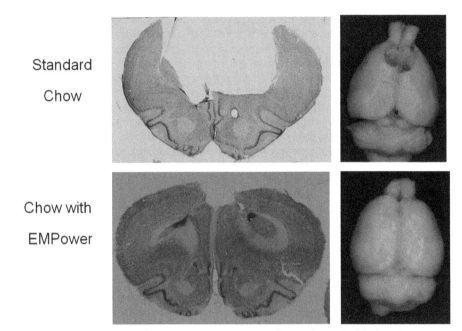

Fig. 12. Micronutrients enhance anatomic recovery after early cortical lesions in rats. Rats received aspiration lesions in the midline medial frontal cortex on postnatal day 3, and were then examined anatomically in adulthood. Animals receiving standard rat chow showed the expectable permanent damage resulting from early cortical lesions. Animals receiving EMPower in their rat chow showed significant restoration of brain tissue, although the cortical structures were not fully normal.[287] (*Courtesy of* Celeste Halliwell, PhD and Bryan Kolb, PhD, University of Lethbridge, Alberta, Canada.)

dose levels for the various micronutrient interventions or what goes into creating a well-balanced micronutrient supplement. We have not emphasized different responses in subgroups based on baseline micronutrient sufficiency status, or that data analyses could be stratified based on endogenous micronutrient deficiency markers. We have only glanced at the issue of micronutrient-micronutrient interactions. We have ignored the less popular minerals, such as molybdenum, which in deficiency can cause CNS symptoms ranging from fatigue to mental retardation[2] and which may be involved in the allosteric modulation of glutamate receptors.[295] Similar to pinning down mechanisms of micronutrient action, all of these questions will become more important once the basic principles and place of micronutrients in psychiatric care become better acknowledged.

One of the interesting findings embedded in this research is that therapeutic effects of broad-spectrum micronutrients have been reported with a diverse range of micronutrient formulations. It does not appear that any particular nutrients are required to produce improvements, although the effect sizes can vary, but a larger number of different micronutrients does appear to deliver more effectiveness. Most of the broad-spectrum micronutrient research on mood disorders and ADHD has been conducted using the Hardy-Stephan formulation (such as EMPower or Daily Essential Nutrients), so this broad-spectrum product containing vitamins, minerals, and antioxidants at relatively high doses has some data to support its use. There also has been a series of papers on Berocca, a formulation consisting mainly of several B vitamins, which appears effective for enhancing stress responses and perhaps a sense of

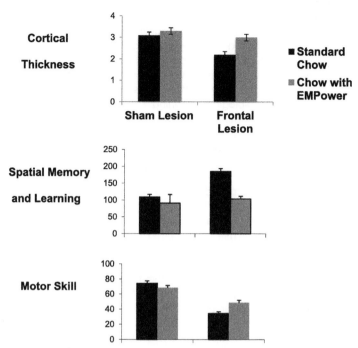

Fig. 13. Broad-spectrum micronutrients help restore structure and function in rats following early lesions of the frontal cortex. After receiving midline medial frontal lesions at postnatal day 3 (which cause permanent structural changes and chronic functional deficits), rats were fed either standard chow or chow fortified with EMPower throughout their lives, and then assessed as adults. In rats fed standard chow, cortical lesions produced a reduction in cortical thickness (measured in millimeters). The lesions also caused chronic deficits in spatial memory and learning, demonstrated on the Morris Water Navigation Task that requires rats to learn to swim to a safe zone (measured in the seconds it takes to reach the safe zone in several runs). In addition, the lesions produced decrements in motor skill performance, assessed by the Tray Reach Task that involves skilled forelimb movements, scored as percent success in obtaining food. The rats fed chow with broad-spectrum micronutrient showed a return to the normal range of cortical thickness and of performance on the spatial processing task, as well as a partial normalization on the motor skill task. Generally similar findings were observed following early lesions in the posterior parietal cortex. (*Adapted from* Halliwell C. Dietary choline and vitamin/mineral supplement for recovery from early cortical injury. Master of Science thesis, University of Lethbridge, Department of Psychology and Neuroscience; 2003.[287] Available at: https://www.uleth.ca/dspace/handle/10133/222; and Halliwell C, Kolb B. Diet can stimulate functional recovery and cerebral plasticity after perinatal cortical injury in rats. Soc Neuroscience Abstracts 2003;459:11.[288])

well-being. In a direct comparison, the Hardy-Stephan formula at 4 or 8 pills daily outperformed Berocca at 1 pill daily in enhancing stress responses in the post-earthquake RCT, but a head-to-head comparison using equivalent doses is not available. In general, it appears that stronger effects have been seen with formulations involving a more diverse range of micronutrients and higher doses, especially when aiming at optimal functioning. On the other hand, some studies have shown effectiveness at RDA levels, perhaps mostly in subgroups with low baseline nutritional status, when aiming at the correction of deficiencies.

Using high doses of micronutrients has the potential to induce vitamin or mineral toxicity. The Hardy-Stephan formulation has been well-researched for a vitamin-mineral product (although not by Food and Drug Administration standards for novel medications). It conforms to governmental guidelines for safety, and it appears safe in clinical trials at recommended doses. Using higher doses of other formulations should be approached with caution, although other formulations may work as well.

What constitutes optimal dosing remains an open issue. As discussed earlier, the doses of micronutrients required to avoid frank classical deficiency diseases is almost certainly too low to optimize biologic functioning. Optimization of biologic functioning is a complex concept. Should optimal functioning be defined based on cardiovascular indicators, mood or cognitive parameters, stress responses (capacity for higher than routine demands), or longevity goals? It is clear that RDAs were never aimed at optimizing brain functioning.[260]

Although the term "anti-aging" suffers from tremendous baggage, the findings that micronutrients can reduce oxidative damage to nuclear and mitochondrial DNA, and reduce chronic inflammation, raises the possibility micronutrients might slow age-related deterioration in multiple organ systems. This possibility is underscored by recent findings that multivitamin use is associated with longer telomere length[296]: daily multivitamin users were found to have 5% longer telomeres (leukocyte DNA) than non-users ($P = .002$).

To be sure, micronutrients do not help everything. Various studies examining micronutrient interventions have produced disappointing findings regarding their effects on cardiovascular functioning, cancer prevention, and all-cause mortality.[297,298] These findings may be criticized on various technical grounds,[299,300] and it is clear that multivitamins may be helpful for subpopulations and for other health goals.[301] It is also possible that multivitamin use could have negative effects.[302–305] Single-nutrient or narrow-spectrum interventions also could have adverse effects, including the induction of relative deficiencies in other micronutrients, and there are reports of deleterious effects at routine doses of beta-carotene, vitamin A, B vitamins, or vitamin E.[80,81,306–311] Most of these reviews of adverse micronutrient effects have generally examined formulations with 3 or more ingredients, and it appears that the findings become more favorable with formulations containing 10 or more micronutrients.[312] The benefits, risks, and scope of micronutrient interventions will be decided empirically in the future.

In the meantime, psychiatrists have an opportunity to explore a new set of tools and principles for treatment and prevention. This is a new approach to mental health care, and one that youths and families embrace as de-stigmatizing. Micronutrient treatments are acceptable to many individuals who hesitate to use conventional psychiatric medications. Some parents seek the opportunity to use micronutrients to forestall or prevent the initial appearance of psychiatric illness by introducing these treatments early, including to patients' troubled younger siblings.

It is advisable for clinicians to be prepared to deal with overly enthusiastic families (and colleagues) whose excitement about a "natural" treatment might cloud their thinking or disrupt their balance in assessing risks. It also is sensible to be ready to deal with excessive skeptics, especially colleagues (and some patients), whose doubts about "natural" treatment might lead them to disregard evidence of effectiveness because micronutrients do not fit the prevailing models of disease and pharmaceutical treatment.

Some clinicians have raised the question of whether the low risks involved in micronutrient treatments, compared with conventional treatments, might justify their use as first-line treatments in some cases. Normally, there would be a simple response based on the absence of controlled trials showing the efficacy and safety of these treatments. However, for a treatment whose safety appears significantly better than the standard of care, the answer could be more nuanced in some situations. In response to patient and family interest, I have chosen to offer broad-spectrum micronutrient treatments, despite the lack of RCTs, in cases in which (1) the symptoms are mild and nonacute, (2) there is low clinical risk in a temporary delay of established treatment, and (3) chart documentation outlines informed consent based on a discussion of the available established treatments, reasons for the patient and/or family preference to use a nonestablished treatment, an explicit statement of the lack of controlled trials regarding safety and efficacy, risks (including unknown risks), drug interactions with CNS-active medical drugs, and adverse effects (including aggravation of preexisting *Candida*). Needless to say, this option is restricted to families who are competent to make these judgments and who understand the financial burdens compared with insurance-covered conventional treatment.

Although emphasized previously, it is worth restating that clinicians are energetically advised to avoid using broad-spectrum micronutrient treatments for patients receiving psychopharmacotherapy without ongoing consultation with a specialist familiar with this treatment approach. Until a clinician is well informed about the techniques of managing nutrient-drug interactions and the pitfalls involved in transitioning a patient from psychiatric medications to micronutrient treatment, it is not sensible to attempt to reduce doses of prior psychiatric medications in a patient with active illness. Although treatment of drug-naïve patients is much more straightforward, clinicians are still advised to have an established connection to a consultant who can advise on technical details.

The hope generated by this line of inquiry is the possible development of a low-risk, low-stigma, health-promoting treatment for violence in prisons and conduct disorder in schools; a nonabusable treatment for ADHD that is more likely to enhance growth than to diminish it; a treatment for MDD and bipolar disorder with fewer side effects and seemingly greater long-term stability than current approaches; and the enhancement of stress response, cognition, and sense of well-being in healthy individuals. Obviously, additional research is needed. Interestingly, perhaps because of its low risks and adverse effects, broad-spectrum micronutrient intervention is one area of psychiatry in which treatment research to date has been generally well-balanced between studies in adults and youth.

The recent trends toward greater openness in general medicine to look at the role of nutrition and the health effects of micronutrients is commendable and exciting. Significant advances in the future may be attainable by a more focused consideration of the biology of micronutrients and their place in medical treatment, health promotion, and wellness.

ACKNOWLEDGMENTS

The author thanks Julia Rucklidge, Bonnie Kaplan, and Cathy Field for their contributions to this field and also for their comments on an earlier form of this article.

REFERENCES

1. Pizzorno JE, Murray MT. Textbook of natural medicine. 4th edition. St Louis (MO): Elsevier Churchill Livingstone; 2013.
2. Ross AC, Caballero B, Cousins RJ, et al, editors. Modern nutrition in health and disease. 11th edition. Philadelphia: Lippincott Williams & Wilkins; 2012.
3. Anjos T, Altmäe S, Emmett P, et al, NUTRIMENTHE Research Group. Nutrition and neurodevelopment in children: focus on NUTRIMENTHE project. Eur J Nutr 2013;52(8):1825–42.

4. Hibbeln JR, Gow RV. Omega-3 fatty acid and nutrient deficits in adverse neuro-development and childhood behaviors. In: Simkin D, Popper C, editors. Alternative and complementary therapies for children with psychiatric disorders, part 2. Child Adolesc Psychiatr Clin N Am 2014;23(3):555–90.

5. Diaz Heijtz R, Wang S, Anuar F, et al. Normal gut microbiota modulates brain development and behavior. Proc Natl Acad Sci U S A 2011;108(7):3047–52.

6. Davis DR. Declining fruit and vegetable nutrient composition: what is the evidence? Hort Science 2009;44:15–9.

7. Farris RP, Nicklas TA, Myers L, et al. Nutrient intake and food group consumption of 10-year-olds by sugar intake level: the Bogalusa Heart Study. J Am Coll Nutr 1998;17(6):579–85.

8. Kant AK. Reported consumption of low-nutrient-density foods by American children and adolescents: nutritional and health correlates, NHANES III, 1988 to 1994. Arch Pediatr Adolesc Med 2003;157(8):789–96.

9. Johal GS, Huber DM. Glyphosate effects on diseases of plants. Eur J Agron 2009;31:144–52.

10. Zobiole LH, Rubem S, Oliveira RS, et al. Glyphosate affects seed composition in glyphosate-resistant soybean. J Agric Food Chem 2010;58:4517–22.

11. Mayer AM. Historical changes in the mineral content of fruits and vegetables. Br Food J 1997;99:207–11.

12. White PJ, Broadley MR. Historical variation in the mineral composition of edible horticultural products. J Hort Sci Biotechnol 2005;80:660–7.

13. Davis DR, Epp MD, Riordan HD. Changes in USDA food composition data for 43 garden crops, 1950-1999. J Am Coll Nutr 2004;23:669–82.

14. McCann JC, Ames BN. Vitamin K, an example of triage theory: is micronutrient inadequacy linked to diseases of aging? Am J Clin Nutr 2009 Oct;90(4): 889–907.

15. Ames BN, Elson-Schwab I, Silver EA. High-dose vitamin therapy stimulates variant enzymes with decreased coenzyme binding affinity (increased K_m): relevance to genetic disease and polymorphisms. Am J Clin Nutr 2002;75(4): 616–58.

16. Ames BN, Atamna H, Killilea DW. Mineral and vitamin deficiencies can accelerate the mitochondrial decay of aging. Mol Aspects Med 2005;26(4–5):363–78.

17. Shigenaga MK, Hagen TM, Ames BN. Oxidative damage and mitochondrial decay in aging. Proc Natl Acad Sci U S A 1994;91(23):10771–8.

18. Aliev G, Liu J, Shenk JC, et al. Neuronal mitochondrial amelioration by feeding acetyl-L-carnitine and lipoic acid to aged rats. J Cell Mol Med 2009;13(2): 320–33.

19. Ames BN. Optimal micronutrients delay mitochondrial decay and age-associated diseases. Mech Ageing Dev 2010;131(7–8):473–9.

20. Hasan S, Fatima N, Bilal N, et al. Effect of chronic unpredictable stress on short term dietary restriction and its modulation by multivitamin-mineral supplementation. Appetite 2013;65:68–74.

21. Ames BN. A role for supplements in optimizing health: the metabolic tune-up. Arch Biochem Biophys 2004;423(1):227–34.

22. Ames BN. The metabolic tune-up: metabolic harmony and disease prevention. J Nutr 2003;133(5 Suppl 1):1544S–8S.

23. Centers for Disease Control and Prevention. Second national report on biochemical indicators of diet and nutrition in the US population. Atlanta (GA): Centers for Disease Control and Prevention; 2012. Available at: http://www.cdc.gov/nutritionreport/pdf/Nutrition_Book_complete508_final.pdf#zoom=100.

24. Centers for Disease Control and Prevention. Second national report on biochemical indicators of diet and nutrition in the US population 2012 executive summary. Atlanta (GA): Centers for Disease Control and Prevention; 2012. Available at: http://www.cdc.gov/nutritionreport/pdf/ExeSummary_Web_032612.pdf.

25. Shakur YA, Tarasuk V, Corey P, et al. A comparison of micronutrient inadequacy and risk of high micronutrient intakes among vitamin and mineral supplement users and nonusers in Canada. J Nutr 2012;142(3):534–40.

26. Ruston D, Hoare J, Henderson L, et al. The National Diet and Nutrition Survey: adults aged 19-64 years (volume 4): nutritional status (anthropometry and blood analytes), blood pressure and physical activity. London: The Stationery Office [formerly, Her Majesty's Stationery Office]; 2004.

27. Willett W, editor. Nutritional epidemiology. 3rd edition. New York: Oxford University Press; 2013.

28. Younger KM. Dietary reference standards. Chapter 7. In: Gibney MJ, Lanham-New SA, Cassidy A, et al, on behalf of The Nutrition Society, editors. Introduction to human nutrition. 2nd edition. West Sussex (England): Wiley-Blackwell; 2009. p. 122–31.

29. Kennedy DO, Haskell CF. Vitamins and cognition: what is the evidence? Drugs 2011;71(15):1957–71.

30. Kumar J, Muntner P, Kaskel FJ, et al. Prevalence and associations of 25-hydroxyvitamin D deficiency in US children: NHANES 2001-2004. Pediatrics 2009; 124(3):e362–70.

31. Boy E, Mannar V, Pandav C, et al. Achievements, challenges, and promising new approaches in vitamin and mineral deficiency control. Nutr Rev 2009; 67(Suppl 1):S24–30.

32. United Nations International Children's Emergency Fund (UNICEF), The Micronutrient Initiative, Adamson P. Vitamin and Mineral Deficiency: A Global Progress Report. Oxfordshire, England, P&LA, 2004. Available at: http://www.micronutrient.org/CMFiles/PubLib/VMd-GPR-English1KWW-3242008-4681.pdf.

33. United Call to Action. Investing in the future: a united call to action on vitamin and mineral deficiencies: global report 2009. Ottawa (Canada): United Call to Action; 2009. Available at: http://www.unitedcalltoaction.org/documents/Investing_in_the_future.pdf.

34. Kapil U, Bhavna A. Adverse effects of poor micronutrient status during childhood and adolescence. Nutr Rev 2002;60(5 Pt 2):S84–90.

35. Quirk SE, Williams LJ, O'Neil A, et al. The association between diet quality, dietary patterns and depression in adults: a systematic review. BMC Psychiatry 2013;13:175.

36. Rahe C, Unrath M, Berger K. Dietary patterns and the risk of depression in adults: a systematic review of observational studies. Eur J Nutr 2014. [Epub ahead of print].

37. Jacka FN, Pasco JA, Mykletun A, et al. Diet quality in bipolar disorder in a population-based sample of women. J Affect Disord 2011;129(1–3):332–7.

38. Jacka FN, Ystrom E, Brantsaeter AL, et al. Maternal and early postnatal nutrition and mental health of offspring by age 5 years: a prospective cohort study. J Am Acad Child Adolesc Psychiatry 2013;52(10):1038–47.

39. Herbison CE, Hickling S, Allen KL, et al. Low intake of B-vitamins is associated with poor adolescent mental health and behaviour. Prev Med 2012;55(6): 634–8.

40. Jacka FN, Kremer PJ, Berk M, et al. A prospective study of diet quality and mental health in adolescents. PLoS One 2011;6(9):e24805.

41. Jacka FN, Rothon C, Taylor S, et al. Diet quality and mental health problems in adolescents from East London: a prospective study. Soc Psychiatry Psychiatr Epidemiol 2013;48(8):1297–306.

42. Oddy WH, Robinson M, Ambrosini GL, et al. The association between dietary patterns and mental health in early adolescence. Prev Med 2009;49(1):39–44.

43. Oellingrath IM, Svendsen MV, Hestetun I. Eating patterns and mental health problems in early adolescence - a cross-sectional study of 12-13-year-old Norwegian schoolchildren. Public Health Nutr 2013;1–9. [Epub ahead of print].

44. Jacka FN, Kremer PJ, Leslie ER, et al. Associations between diet quality and depressed mood in adolescents: results from the Australian Healthy Neighbourhoods Study. Aust N Z J Psychiatry 2010;44(5):435–42.

45. McMartin SE, Kuhle S, Colman I, et al. Diet quality and mental health in subsequent years among Canadian youth. Public Health Nutr 2012;15(12):2253–8.

46. Davison KM, Kaplan BJ. Nutrient intakes are correlated with overall psychiatric functioning in adults with mood disorders. Can J Psychiatry 2012;57(2):85–92.

47. Kaplan BJ, Shannon S. Nutritional aspects of child and adolescent psychopharmacology. Pediatr Ann 2007;36(9):600–9. Reprinted in: Psychiatr Ann 2007;37(7):519–28.

48. Werbach MR. Nutritional influences on mental illness: a sourcebook of clinical research. Tarzana (CA): Third Line Press; 1999.

49. Kaplan BJ, Crawford SG, Field CJ, et al. Vitamins, minerals, and mood. Psychol Bull 2007;133(5):747–60.

50. Caverzasi E, Pichiecchio A, Poloni GU, et al. Magnetic resonance spectroscopy in the evaluation of treatment efficacy in unipolar major depressive disorder: a review of the literature. Funct Neurol 2012;27(1):13–22.

51. Papakostas GI, Shelton RC, Zajecka JM, et al. L-methylfolate as adjunctive therapy for SSRI-resistant major depression: results of two randomized, double-blind, parallel-sequential trials. Am J Psychiatry 2012;169(12):1267–74.

52. Popper CW. Mood disorders in youth: exercise, light therapy, and pharmacologic complementary and integrative approaches. In: Simkin D, Popper C, editors. Alternative and complementary therapies for children with psychiatric disorders, part 1. Child Adolesc Psychiatr Clin N Am 2013;22(3):403–41.

53. Sylvia LG, Peters AT, Deckersbach T, et al. Nutrient-based therapies for bipolar disorder: a systematic review. Psychother Psychosom 2013;82(1):10–9.

54. Mischoulon D, Rosenbaum JF. Natural medications for psychiatric disorders. 2nd edition. Philadelphia: Lippincott Williams & Wilkins; 2008.

55. Fava M, Borus JS, Alpert JE, et al. Folate, vitamin B12, and homocysteine in major depressive disorder. Am J Psychiatry 1997;154(3):426–8.

56. Seppälä J, Koponen H, Kautiainen H, et al. Association between folate intake and melancholic depressive symptoms. A Finnish population-based study. J Affect Disord 2012;138(3):473–8.

57. Freeman MP, Fava M, Lake J, et al. Complementary and alternative medicine in major depressive disorder: The American Psychiatric Association Task Force report. J Clin Psychiatry 2010;71(6):669–81.

58. Coppen A, Bailey J. Enhancement of the antidepressant action of fluoxetine by folic acid: a randomised, placebo controlled trial. J Affect Disord 2000;60(2):121–30.

59. Resler G, Lavie R, Campos J, et al. Effect of folic acid combined with fluoxetine in patients with major depression on plasma homocysteine and vitamin B12, and serotonin levels in lymphocytes. Neuroimmunomodulation 2008;15(3):145–52.

60. Godfrey PS, Toone BK, Carney MW, et al. Enhancement of recovery from psychiatric illness by methylfolate. Lancet 1990;336(8712):392–5.

61. Venkatasubramanian R, Kumar CN, Pandey RS. A randomized double-blind comparison of fluoxetine augmentation by high and low dosage folic acid in patients with depressive episodes. J Affect Disord 2013;150(2):644–8.

62. Papakostas GI, Shelton RC, Zajecka JM, et al. Effect of adjunctive L-methylfolate 15 mg among inadequate responders to SSRIs in depressed patients who were stratified by biomarker and genotype: results from a randomized clinical trial. J Clin Psychiatry 2014;75. [Epub ahead of print]. http://dx.doi.org/10.4088/JCP.13m08947.

63. Sarris J, Mischoulon D, Schweitzer I. Adjunctive nutraceuticals with standard pharmacotherapies in bipolar disorder: a systematic review of clinical trials. Bipolar Disord 2011;13(5–6):454–65.

64. Alpert JE, Mischoulon D, Rubenstein GE, et al. Folinic acid (Leucovorin) as an adjunctive treatment for SSRI-refractory depression. Ann Clin Psychiatry 2002; 14(1):33–8.

65. Christensen H, Aiken A, Batterham PJ, et al. No clear potentiation of antidepressant medication effects by folic acid+vitamin B12 in a large community sample. J Affect Disord 2011;130(1–2):37–45.

66. Bryan J, Calvaresi E, Hughes D. Short-term folate, vitamin B-12 or vitamin B-6 supplementation slightly affects memory performance but not mood in women of various ages. J Nutr 2002;132(6):1345–56.

67. Andreeva VA, Galan P, Torrès M, et al. Supplementation with B vitamins or n-3 fatty acids and depressive symptoms in cardiovascular disease survivors: ancillary findings from the Supplementation with FOLate, vitamins B-6 and B-12 and/ or OMega-3 fatty acids (SU.FOL.OM3) randomized trial. Am J Clin Nutr 2012; 96(1):208–14.

68. Ford AH, Flicker L, Thomas J, et al. Vitamins B12, B6, and folic acid for onset of depressive symptoms in older men: results from a 2-year placebo-controlled randomized trial. J Clin Psychiatry 2008;69(8):1203–9.

69. Walker JG, Mackinnon AJ, Batterham P, et al. Mental health literacy, folic acid and vitamin B12, and physical activity for the prevention of depression in older adults: randomised controlled trial. Br J Psychiatry 2010;197(1):45–54.

70. Almeida OP, Marsh K, Alfonso H, et al. B-vitamins reduce the long-term risk of depression after stroke: The VITATOPS-DEP trial. Ann Neurol 2010;68(4): 503–10.

71. Murakami K, Miyake Y, Sasaki S, et al. Dietary folate, riboflavin, vitamin B-6, and vitamin B-12 and depressive symptoms in early adolescence: the Ryukyus Child Health Study. Psychosom Med 2010;72(8):763–8.

72. Aisen PS, Schneider LS, Sano M, et al. High-dose B vitamin supplementation and cognitive decline in Alzheimer disease: a randomized controlled trial. JAMA 2008;300(15):1774–83.

73. Hunter R, Barnes J, Oakeley HF, et al. Toxicity of folic acid given in pharmacological doses to healthy volunteers. Lancet 1970;1(7637):61–3.

74. Hellström L. Lack of toxicity of folic acid given in pharmacological doses to healthy volunteers. Lancet 1971;1(7689):59–61.

75. Roy S, Roy M. A case of folic acid allergy in pregnancy. J Obstet Gynaecol India 2012;62(Suppl 1):33–4.

76. Sanders GM, Fritz SB. Allergy to natural and supplemental folic acid as a cause of chronic, intermittent urticaria and angioedema. Ann Allergy Asthma Immunol 2004;93(5 Suppl 3):S51–2.

77. Smith J, Empson M, Wall C. Recurrent anaphylaxis to synthetic folic acid. Lancet 2007;370(9588):652.
78. Valdivieso R, Cevallos F, Caballero MT, et al. Chronic urticaria caused by folic acid. Ann Allergy Asthma Immunol 2009;103(1):81–2.
79. Lambie DG, Johnson RH. Drugs and folate metabolism. Drugs 1985;30(2): 145–55.
80. Ebbing M, Bønaa KH, Nygård O, et al. Cancer incidence and mortality after treatment with folic acid and vitamin B12. JAMA 2009;302(19):2119–26.
81. Figueiredo JC, Grau MV, Haile RW, et al. Folic acid and risk of prostate cancer: results from a randomized clinical trial. J Natl Cancer Inst 2009;101(6):432–5.
82. Behzadi AH, Omrani Z, Chalian M, et al. Folic acid efficacy as an alternative drug added to sodium valproate in the treatment of acute phase of mania in bipolar disorder: a double-blind randomized controlled trial. Acta Psychiatr Scand 2009;120(6):441–5.
83. Coppen A, Chaudhry S, Swade C. Folic acid enhances lithium prophylaxis. J Affect Disord 1986;10(1):9–13.
84. Dogan M, Ariyuca S, Peker E, et al. Psychotic disorder, hypertension and seizures associated with vitamin B12 deficiency: a case report. Hum Exp Toxicol 2012;31(4):410–3.
85. Tufan AE, Bilici R, Usta G, et al. Mood disorder with mixed, psychotic features due to vitamin b12 deficiency in an adolescent: case report. Child Adolesc Psychiatry Ment Health 2012;6(1):25.
86. Hvas AM, Juul S, Lauritzen L, et al. No effect of vitamin B-12 treatment on cognitive function and depression: a randomized placebo controlled study. J Affect Disord 2004;81(3):269–73.
87. Oren DA, Teicher MH, Schwartz PJ, et al. A controlled trial of cyanocobalamin (vitamin B12) in the treatment of winter seasonal affective disorder. J Affect Disord 1994;32(3):197–200.
88. Syed EU, Wasay M, Awan S. Vitamin B12 supplementation in treating major depressive disorder: a randomized controlled trial. Open Neurol J 2013;7: 44–8.
89. Bell DS. Protean manifestations of vitamin D deficiency, part 2: deficiency and its association with autoimmune disease, cancer, infection, asthma, dermopathies, insulin resistance, and type 2 diabetes. South Med J 2011;104(5):335–9.
90. Bell DS. Protean manifestations of vitamin D deficiency, part 3: association with cardiovascular disease and disorders of the central and peripheral nervous systems. South Med J 2011;104(5):340–4.
91. McCann JC, Ames BN. Is there convincing biological or behavioral evidence linking vitamin D deficiency to brain dysfunction? FASEB J 2008;22(4):982–1001.
92. Bell DS. Protean manifestations of vitamin D deficiency, part 1: the epidemic of deficiency. South Med J 2011;104(5):331–4.
93. Eyles DW, Burne TH, McGrath JJ. Vitamin D, effects on brain development, adult brain function and the links between low levels of vitamin D and neuropsychiatric disease. Front Neuroendocrinol 2013;34(1):47–64.
94. Nimitphong H, Holick MF. Vitamin D, neurocognitive functioning and immunocompetence. Curr Opin Clin Nutr Metab Care 2011;14(1):7–14.
95. Harms LR, Burne TH, Eyles DW, et al. Vitamin D and the brain. Best Pract Res Clin Endocrinol Metab 2011;25(4):657–69.
96. Allen KL, Byrne SM, Kusel MM, et al. Maternal vitamin D levels during pregnancy and offspring eating disorder risk in adolescence. Int J Eat Disord 2013;46(7):669–76.

97. Whitehouse AJ, Holt BJ, Serralha M, et al. Maternal serum vitamin D levels during pregnancy and offspring neurocognitive development. Pediatrics 2012; 129(3):485–93.
98. Anglin RE, Samaan Z, Walter SD, et al. Vitamin D deficiency and depression in adults: systematic review and meta-analysis. Br J Psychiatry 2013;202:100–7.
99. Ju SY, Lee YJ, Jeong SN. Serum 25-hydroxyvitamin D levels and the risk of depression: a systematic review and meta-analysis. J Nutr Health Aging 2013; 17(5):447–55.
100. Brandenbarg J, Vrijkotte TG, Goedhart G, et al. Maternal early-pregnancy vitamin D status is associated with maternal depressive symptoms in the Amsterdam Born Children and Their Development cohort. Psychosom Med 2012;74(7):751–7.
101. Cizza G, Mistry S, Nguyen VT, et al, POWER Study Group. Do premenopausal women with major depression have low bone mineral density? A 36-month prospective study. PLoS One 2012;7(7):e40894.
102. Jamilian H, Bagherzadeh K, Nazeri Z, et al. Vitamin D, parathyroid hormone, serum calcium and phosphorus in patients with schizophrenia and major depression. Int J Psychiatry Clin Pract 2013;17(1):30–4.
103. Maddock J, Berry DJ, Geoffroy MC, et al. Vitamin D and common mental disorders in mid-life: cross-sectional and prospective findings. Clin Nutr 2013;32(5): 758–64.
104. Premkumar M, Sable T, Dhanwal D, et al. Vitamin D homeostasis, bone mineral metabolism, and seasonal affective disorder during 1 year of Antarctic residence. Arch Osteoporos 2013;8(1–2):129.
105. Brouwer-Brolsma EM, Feskens EJ, Steegenga WT, et al. Associations of 25-hydroxyvitamin D with fasting glucose, fasting insulin, dementia and depression in European elderly: the SENECA study. Eur J Nutr 2013;52(3):917–25.
106. Hoang MT, Defina LF, Willis BL, et al. Association between low serum 25-hydroxyvitamin D and depression in a large sample of healthy adults: the Cooper Center longitudinal study. Mayo Clin Proc 2011;86(11):1050–5.
107. Chan R, Chan D, Woo J, et al. Association between serum 25-hydroxyvitamin D and psychological health in older Chinese men in a cohort study. J Affect Disord 2011;130(1–2):251–9.
108. Nanri A, Mizoue T, Matsushita Y, et al. Association between serum 25-hydroxyvitamin D and depressive symptoms in Japanese: analysis by survey season. Eur J Clin Nutr 2009;63(12):1444–7.
109. Jaddou HY, Batieha AM, Khader YS, et al. Depression is associated with low levels of 25-hydroxyvitamin D among Jordanian adults: results from a national population survey. Eur Arch Psychiatry Clin Neurosci 2012;262(4):321–7.
110. Black LJ, Jacoby P, Allen KL, et al. Low vitamin D levels are associated with symptoms of depression in young adult males. Aust N Z J Psychiatry 2014; 48(5):464–71.
111. Smith BA, Cogswell A, Garcia G. Vitamin D and depressive symptoms in children with cystic fibrosis. Psychosomatics 2014;55(1):76–8.
112. Högberg G, Gustafsson SA, Hällström T, et al. Depressed adolescents in a case-series were low in vitamin D and depression was ameliorated by vitamin D supplementation. Acta Paediatr 2012;101(7):779–83.
113. Fazeli PK, Mendes N, Russell M, et al. Bone density characteristics and major depressive disorder in adolescents. Psychosom Med 2013;75(2):117–23.
114. Gracious BL, Finucane TL, Friedman-Campbell M, et al. Vitamin D deficiency and psychotic features in mentally ill adolescents: a cross-sectional study. BMC Psychiatry 2012;12:38.

115. Kwasky AN, Groh CJ. Vitamin D and depression: is there a relationship in young women? J Am Psychiatr Nurses Assoc 2012;18(4):236–43.

116. Obeidat BA, Alchalabi HA, Abdul-Razzak KK, et al. Premenstrual symptoms in dysmenorrheic college students: prevalence and relation to vitamin D and parathyroid hormone levels. Int J Environ Res Public Health 2012;9(11):4210–22.

117. Tolppanen AM, Sayers A, Fraser WD, et al. The association of serum 25-hydroxyvitamin D3 and D2 with depressive symptoms in childhood—a prospective cohort study. J Child Psychol Psychiatry 2012;53(7):757–66.

118. Autier P, Boniol M, Pizot C, et al. Vitamin D status and ill health: a systematic review. Lancet Diabetes Endocrinol 2014;2(1):76–89.

119. Arvold DS, Odean MJ, Dornfeld MP, et al. Correlation of symptoms with vitamin D deficiency and symptom response to cholecalciferol treatment: a randomized controlled trial. Endocr Pract 2009;15(3):203–12.

120. Bertone-Johnson ER, Powers SI, Spangler L, et al. Vitamin D supplementation and depression in the women's health initiative calcium and vitamin D trial. Am J Epidemiol 2012;176(1):1–13.

121. Kjærgaard M, Waterloo K, Wang CE, et al. Effect of vitamin D supplement on depression scores in people with low levels of serum 25-hydroxyvitamin D: nested case-control study and randomised clinical trial. Br J Psychiatry 2012; 201(5):360–8.

122. Sanders KM, Stuart AL, Williamson EJ, et al. Annual high-dose vitamin D3 and mental well-being: randomised controlled trial. Br J Psychiatry 2011;198(5): 357–64.

123. Jorde R, Sneve M, Figenschau Y, et al. Effects of vitamin D supplementation on symptoms of depression in overweight and obese subjects: randomized double blind trial. J Intern Med 2008;264(6):599–609.

124. Mozaffari-Khosravi H, Nabizade L, Yassini-Ardakani SM, et al. The effect of 2 different single injections of high dose of vitamin D on improving the depression in depressed patients with vitamin D deficiency: a randomized clinical trial. J Clin Psychopharmacol 2013;33(3):378–85.

125. Gloth FM, Alam W, Hollis B. Vitamin D vs broad spectrum phototherapy in the treatment of seasonal affective disorder. J Nutr Health Aging 1999; 3(1):5–7.

126. Lansdowne AT, Provost SC. Vitamin D3 enhances mood in healthy subjects during winter. Psychopharmacology (Berl) 1998;135(4):319–23.

127. Vieth R, Kimball S, Hu A, et al. Randomized comparison of the effects of the vitamin D3 adequate intake versus 100 mcg (4000 IU) per day on biochemical responses and the wellbeing of patients. Nutr J 2004;3:8.

128. Khoraminya N, Tehrani-Doost M, Jazayeri S, et al. Therapeutic effects of vitamin D as adjunctive therapy to fluoxetine in patients with major depressive disorder. Aust N Z J Psychiatry 2013;47(3):271–5.

129. Li G, Mbuagbaw L, Samaan Z, et al. Efficacy of vitamin D supplementation in depression in adults: a systematic review. J Clin Endocrinol Metab 2014 Mar;99(3):757–67.

130. Qureshi NA, Al-Bedah AM. Mood disorders and complementary and alternative medicine: a literature review. Neuropsychiatr Dis Treat 2013;9:639–58.

131. Holmlund-Suila E, Koskivirta P, Metso T, et al. Vitamin D deficiency in children with a chronic illness-seasonal and age-related variations in serum 25-hydroxy vitamin D concentrations. PLoS One 2013;8(4):e60856.

132. Kasahara AK, Singh RJ, Noymer A. Vitamin D (25OHD) serum seasonality in the United States. PLoS One 2013;8(6):e65785.

133. Melander KR, Justinussen K. Vitamin D plasma levels during summer in a psychiatric population are comparable to the winter levels of healthy individuals. Dan Med J 2013;60(3):A4598.

134. Belvederi Murri M, Respino M, Masotti M, et al. Vitamin D and psychosis: mini meta-analysis. Schizophr Res 2013;150(1):235–9.

135. Berg AO, Melle I, Torjesen PA, et al. A cross-sectional study of vitamin D deficiency among immigrants and Norwegians with psychosis compared to the general population. J Clin Psychiatry 2010;71(12):1598–604.

136. Crews M, Lally J, Gardner-Sood P, et al. Vitamin D deficiency in first episode psychosis: a case-control study. Schizophr Res 2013;150(2–3):533–7.

137. McGrath J, Saari K, Hakko H, et al. Vitamin D supplementation during the first year of life and risk of schizophrenia: a Finnish birth cohort study. Schizophr Res 2004;67(2–3):237–45.

138. Tariq MM, Streeten EA, Smith HA, et al. Vitamin D: a potential role in reducing suicide risk? Int J Adolesc Med Health 2011;23(3):157–65.

139. Umhau JC, George DT, Heaney RP, et al. Low vitamin D status and suicide: a case-control study of active duty military service members. PLoS One 2013;8(1):e51543.

140. Food and Nutrition Board, Institute of Medicine, National Academies of Science: Daily Reference Intakes (DRIs): Estimated Average Requirements 2010. Available at: http://www.iom.edu/Activities/Nutrition/SummaryDRIs/DRI-Tables.aspx. Accessed April 20, 2014.

141. Rylander M, Verhulst S. Vitamin D insufficiency in psychiatric inpatients. J Psychiatr Pract 2013;19(4):296–300.

142. Logan VF, Gray AR, Peddie MC, et al. Long-term vitamin D3 supplementation is more effective than vitamin D2 in maintaining serum 25-hydroxyvitamin D status over the winter months. Br J Nutr 2013;109(6):1082–8.

143. Robien K, Oppeneer SJ, Kelly JA, et al. Drug-vitamin D interactions: a systematic review of the literature. Nutr Clin Pract 2013;28(2):194–208.

144. Rogovik AL, Vohra S, Goldman RD. Safety considerations and potential interactions of vitamins: should vitamins be considered drugs? Ann Pharmacother 2010;44(2):311–24.

145. Deijen JB, van der Beek EJ, Orlebeke JF, et al. Vitamin B-6 supplementation in elderly men: effects on mood, memory, performance and mental effort. Psychopharmacology (Berl) 1992;109(4):489–96.

146. Villegas-Salas E, Ponce de León R, Juárez-Perez MA, et al. Effect of vitamin B6 on the side effects of a low-dose combined oral contraceptive. Contraception 1997;55(4):245–8.

147. Benton D, Haller J, Fordy J. Vitamin supplementation for 1 year improves mood. Neuropsychobiology 1995;32:98–105.

148. Kleijnen J, Ter Riet G, Knipschild P. Vitamin B6 in the treatment of the premenstrual syndrome—a review. Br J Obstet Gynaecol 1990;97(9):847–52.

149. Bendich A. The potential for dietary supplements to reduce premenstrual syndrome (PMS) symptoms. J Am Coll Nutr 2000;19(1):3–12.

150. Wyatt KM, Dimmock PW, Jones PW, et al. Efficacy of vitamin B-6 in the treatment of premenstrual syndrome: systematic review. BMJ 1999;318(7195):1375–81.

151. De Souza MC, Walker AF, Robinson PA, et al. A synergistic effect of a daily supplement for 1 month of 200 mg magnesium plus 50 mg vitamin B6 for the relief of anxiety-related premenstrual symptoms: a randomized, double-blind, crossover study. J Womens Health Gend Based Med 2000;9(2):131–9.

152. Doll H, Brown S, Thurston A, et al. Pyridoxine (vitamin B6) and the premenstrual syndrome: a randomized crossover trial. J R Coll Gen Pract 1989;39(326): 364–8.
153. Kendall KE, Schnurr PP. The effects of vitamin B6 supplementation on premenstrual symptoms. Obstet Gynecol 1987;70(2):145–9.
154. Williams MJ, Harris RI, Dean BC. Controlled trial of pyridoxine in the premenstrual syndrome. J Int Med Res 1985;13(3):174–9.
155. Findling RL, Maxwell K, Scotese-Wojtila L, et al. High-dose pyridoxine and magnesium administration in children with autistic disorder: an absence of salutary effects in a double-blind, placebo-controlled study. J Autism Dev Disord 1997; 27(4):467–78.
156. Pfeiffer SI, Norton J, Nelson L, et al. Efficacy of vitamin B6 and magnesium in the treatment of autism: a methodology review and summary of outcomes. J Autism Dev Disord 1995;25(5):481–93.
157. Docherty JP, Sack DA, Roffman M, et al. A double-blind, placebo-controlled, exploratory trial of chromium picolinate in atypical depression: effect on carbohydrate craving. J Psychiatr Pract 2005;11(5):302–14.
158. Davidson JR, Abraham K, Connor KM, et al. Effectiveness of chromium in atypical depression: a placebo-controlled trial. Biol Psychiatry 2003;53(3): 261–4.
159. Brownley KA, Von Holle A, Hamer RM, et al. A double-blind, randomized pilot trial of chromium picolinate for binge eating disorder: results of the Binge Eating and Chromium (BEACh) study. J Psychosom Res 2013;75(1):36–42.
160. Siwek M, Dudek D, Paul IA, et al. Zinc supplementation augments efficacy of imipramine in treatment resistant patients: a double blind, placebo-controlled study. J Affect Disord 2009;118(1–3):187–95.
161. Siwek M, Dudek D, Schlegel-Zawadzka M, et al. Serum zinc level in depressed patients during zinc supplementation of imipramine treatment. J Affect Disord 2010;126(3):447–52.
162. Nowak G, Siwek M, Dudek D, et al. Effect of zinc supplementation on antidepressant therapy in unipolar depression: a preliminary placebo-controlled study. Pol J Pharmacol 2003;55(6):1143–7.
163. Sawada T, Yokoi K. Effect of zinc supplementation on mood states in young women: a pilot study. Eur J Clin Nutr 2010;64(3):331–3.
164. Benton D, Griffiths R, Haller J. Thiamine supplementation mood and cognitive functioning. Psychopharmacology (Berl) 1997;129(1):66–71.
165. Smidt LJ, Cremin FM, Grivetti LE, et al. Influence of thiamin supplementation on the health and general well-being of an elderly Irish population with marginal thiamin deficiency. J Gerontol 1991;46(1):M16–22.
166. Mokhber N, Namjoo M, Tara F, et al. Effect of supplementation with selenium on postpartum depression: a randomized double-blind placebo-controlled trial. J Matern Fetal Neonatal Med 2011;24(1):104–8.
167. Benton D, Cook R. The impact of selenium supplementation on mood. Biol Psychiatry 1991;29(11):1092–8.
168. Benton D, Cook R. Selenium supplementation improves mood in a double-blind crossover trial. Psychopharmacology (Berl) 1990;102(4):549–50.
169. Hawkes WC, Hornbostel L. Effects of dietary selenium on mood in healthy men living in a metabolic research unit. Biol Psychiatry 1996;39(2):121–8.
170. Finley JS, Penland JG. Adequacy or deprivation of dietary selenium in healthy men: clinical and psychological findings. J Trace Elem Exp Med 1998;11(1): 11–27.

171. Rayman M, Thompson A, Warren-Perry M, et al. Impact of selenium on mood and quality of life: a randomized, controlled trial. Biol Psychiatry 2006;59(2): 147–54.
172. Shor-Posner G, Lecusay R, Miguez MJ, et al. Psychological burden in the era of HAART: impact of selenium therapy. Int J Psychiatry Med 2003;33(1):55–69.
173. Facchinetti F, Borella P, Sances G, et al. Oral magnesium successfully relieves premenstrual mood changes. Obstet Gynecol 1991;78(2):177–81.
174. Walker AF, De Souza MC, Vickers MF, et al. Magnesium supplementation alleviates premenstrual symptoms of fluid retention. J Womens Health 1998;7(9): 1157–65.
175. Swardfager W, Herrmann N, McIntyre RS, et al. Potential roles of zinc in the pathophysiology and treatment of major depressive disorder. Neurosci Biobehav Rev 2013;37(5):911–29.
176. Bell IR, Edman JS, Morrow FD, et al. Brief communication. Vitamin B1, B2, and B6 augmentation of tricyclic antidepressant treatment in geriatric depression with cognitive dysfunction. J Am Coll Nutr 1992;11(2):159–63.
177. Pasco JA, Jacka FN, Williams LJ, et al. Dietary selenium and major depression: a nested case-control study. Complement Ther Med 2012;20(3):119–23.
178. Gosney MA, Hammond MF, Shenkin A, et al. Effect of micronutrient supplementation on mood in nursing home residents. Gerontology 2008;54(5):292–9.
179. Sher L. Depression and suicidal behavior in alcohol abusing adolescents: possible role of selenium deficiency. Minerva Pediatr 2008;60(2):201–9.
180. Leung BM, Kaplan BJ, Field CJ, et al, APrON Study Team. Prenatal micronutrient supplementation and postpartum depressive symptoms in a pregnancy cohort. BMC Pregnancy Childbirth 2013;13:2.
181. Giannini AJ, Nakoneczie AM, Melemis SM, et al. Magnesium oxide augmentation of verapamil maintenance therapy in mania. Psychiatry Res 2000;93(1):83–7.
182. Mertz W. A balanced approach to nutrition for health: the need for biologically essential minerals and vitamins. J Am Diet Assoc 1994;94(11):1259–62.
183. Mertz W. Mineral elements: new perspectives. J Am Diet Assoc 1980;77(3): 258–63.
184. Kawai K, Spiegelman D, Shankar AH, et al. Maternal multiple micronutrient supplementation and pregnancy outcomes in developing countries: meta-analysis and meta-regression. Bull World Health Organ 2011;89:402–411B. Available at: http://www.who.int/bulletin/volumes/89/6/10-083758/en/.
185. Rucklidge JJ, Kaplan BJ. Broad-spectrum micronutrient formulas for the treatment of psychiatric symptoms: a systematic review. Expert Rev Neurother 2013;13(1):49–73.
186. Schoenthaler SJ, Bier ID. The effect of vitamin-mineral supplementation on juvenile delinquency among American schoolchildren: a randomized, double-blind placebo-controlled trial. J Altern Complement Med 2000;6(1):7–17.
187. Schoenthaler SJ, Amos S, Doraz W, et al. The effect of randomized vitamin-mineral supplementation on violent and non-violent antisocial behavior among incarcerated juveniles. J Nutr Environ Med 1997;7:343–52.
188. Gesch CB, Hammond SM, Hampson SE, et al. Influence of supplementary vitamins, minerals and essential fatty acids on the antisocial behaviour of young adult prisoners. Randomised, placebo-controlled trial. Br J Psychiatry 2002; 181:22–8.
189. Zaalberg A, Nijman H, Bulten E, et al. Effects of nutritional supplements on aggression, rule-breaking, and psychopathology among young adult prisoners. Aggress Behav 2010;36(2):117–26.

190. Walsh WJ, Glab LB, Haakenson ML. Reduced violent behavior following biochemical therapy. Physiol Behav 2004;82(5):835–9.

191. Harding KL, Judah RD, Gant C. Outcome-based comparison of Ritalin versus food-supplement treated children with AD/HD. Altern Med Rev 2003;8(3): 319–30.

192. Harrison R, Rucklidge JJ, Blampied N. Use of micronutrients attenuates cannabis and nicotine abuse as evidenced from a reversal design: a case study. J Psychoactive Drugs 2013;45(2):168–78.

193. Kaplan BJ, Crawford SG, Gardner B, et al. Treatment of mood lability and explosive rage with minerals and vitamins: two case studies in children. J Child Adolesc Psychopharmacol 2002;12(3):205–19.

194. Kaplan BJ, Fisher JE, Crawford SG, et al. Improved mood and behavior during treatment with a mineral-vitamin supplement: an open-label case series of children. J Child Adolesc Psychopharmacol 2004;14(1):115–22.

195. Rucklidge JJ, Gately D, Kaplan BJ. Database analysis of children and adolescents with bipolar disorder consuming a micronutrient formula. BMC Psychiatry 2010;10:74.

196. Rucklidge J, Taylor M, Whitehead K. Effect of micronutrients on behavior and mood in adults with ADHD: evidence from an 8-week open label trial with natural extension. J Atten Disord 2011;15(1):79–91.

197. Rucklidge JJ, Harrison R, Johnstone J. Can micronutrients improve neurocognitive functioning in adults with ADHD and severe mood dysregulation? A pilot study. J Altern Complement Med 2011;17(12):1125–31.

198. Rucklidge JJ, Harrison R. Successful treatment of bipolar disorder II and ADHD with a micronutrient formula: a case study. CNS Spectr 2010;15(5):289–95.

199. Sinn N, Bryan J. Effect of supplementation with polyunsaturated fatty acids and micronutrients on learning and behavior problems associated with child ADHD. J Dev Behav Pediatr 2007;28(2):82–91.

200. Sinn N, Bryan J, Wilson C. Cognitive effects of polyunsaturated fatty acids in children with attention deficit hyperactivity disorder symptoms: a randomised controlled trial. Prostaglandins Leukot Essent Fatty Acids 2008;78(4–5): 311–26.

201. Rucklidge JJ, Frampton CM, Gorman B, et al. Vitamin-mineral treatment of attention-deficit hyperactivity disorder in adults: double-blind randomised placebo-controlled trial. Br J Psychiatry 2014;204:306–15.

202. Rucklidge JJ, Johnstone J, Gorman B, et al. Moderators of treatment response in adults with ADHD treated with a vitamin-mineral supplement. Prog Neuropsychopharmacol Biol Psychiatry 2014;50:163–71.

203. Rucklidge JJ, Frampton CM, Gorman B, et al. Vitamin-mineral treatment of attention-deficit/hyperactivity disorder (ADHD) in adults: a one year naturalistic follow up of a randomized controlled trial. J Atten Disord, in press.

204. Nigg JT, Lewis K, Edinger T, et al. Meta-analysis of attention-deficit/hyperactivity disorder or attention-deficit/hyperactivity disorder symptoms, restriction diet, and synthetic food color additives. J Am Acad Child Adolesc Psychiatry 2012;51(1):86–97.

205. Sonuga-Barke EJ, Brandeis D, Cortese S, et al, European ADHD Guidelines Group. Nonpharmacological interventions for ADHD: systematic review and meta-analyses of randomized controlled trials of dietary and psychological treatments. Am J Psychiatry 2013;170(3):275–89.

206. Faraone SV, Biederman J, Spencer TJ, et al. Comparing the efficacy of medications for ADHD using meta-analysis. MedGenMed 2006;8(4):4.

207. Kaplan BJ, Simpson JS, Ferre RC, et al. Effective mood stabilization with a chelated mineral supplement: an open-label trial in bipolar disorder. J Clin Psychiatry 2001;62(12):936–44.
208. Popper CW. Do vitamins or minerals (apart from lithium) have mood-stabilizing effects? J Clin Psychiatry 2001;62(12):933–5.
209. Simmons M. Nutritional approach to bipolar disorder [letter]. J Clin Psychiatry 2003;64(3):338.
210. Rucklidge JJ. Successful treatment of OCD with a micronutrient formula following partial response to cognitive behavioral therapy (CBT): a case study. J Anxiety Disord 2009;23(6):836–40.
211. Frazier EA, Fristad M, Arnold LE. Multinutrient supplement as treatment: literature review and case report of a 12-year-old boy with bipolar disorder. J Child Adolesc Psychopharmacol 2009;19(4):453–60.
212. Frazier EA, Fristad MA, Arnold LE. Feasibility of a nutritional supplement as treatment for pediatric bipolar spectrum disorders. J Altern Complement Med 2012;18(7):678–85.
213. Frazier EA, Gracious B, Arnold LE, et al. Nutritional and safety outcomes from an open-label micronutrient intervention for pediatric bipolar spectrum disorders. J Child Adolesc Psychopharmacol 2013;23(8):558–67.
214. Rodway M, Vance A, Watters A, et al. Efficacy and cost of micronutrient treatment of childhood psychosis. BMJ Case Rep 2012;2012.
215. Gately D, Kaplan BJ. Database analysis of adults with bipolar disorder consuming a micronutrient formula. Clinical Medicine Psychiat 2009;4:3–16.
216. Kirsch I, Deacon BJ, Huedo-Medina TB, et al. Initial severity and antidepressant benefits: a meta-analysis of data submitted to the Food and Drug Administration. PLoS Med 2008;5(2):e45.
217. Turner EH, Matthews AM, Linardatos E, et al. Selective publication of antidepressant trials and its influence on apparent efficacy. N Engl J Med 2008;358(3):252–60.
218. Vöhringer PA, Ghaemi SN. Solving the antidepressant efficacy question: effect sizes in major depressive disorder. Clin Ther 2011;33(12):B49–61.
219. Findling RL, Kafantaris V, Pavuluri M, et al. Post-acute effectiveness of lithium in pediatric bipolar I disorder. J Child Adolesc Psychopharmacol 2013;23(2):80–90.
220. Akhondzadeh S, Gerbarg PL, Brown RP. Nutrients for prevention and treatment of mental health disorders. Psychiatr Clin North Am 2013;36(1):25–36.
221. Potter M, Moses A, Wozniak J. Alternative treatments in pediatric bipolar disorder. Child Adolesc Psychiatr Clin N Am 2009;18(2):483–514, xi.
222. Bogarapu S, Bishop JR, Krueger CD, et al. Complementary medicines in pediatric bipolar disorder. Minerva Pediatr 2008;60(1):103–14.
223. Rucklidge JJ, Johnstone J, Kaplan BJ. Nutrient supplementation approaches in the treatment of ADHD. Expert Rev Neurother 2009;9(4):461–76.
224. American Psychiatric Association. Diagnostic and statistical manual of mental disorders. 5th edition. Arlington (VA): American Psychiatric Publishing; 2013.
225. Adams JB, Holloway C. Pilot study of a moderate dose multivitamin/mineral supplement for children with autistic spectrum disorder. J Altern Complement Med 2004;10(6):1033–9.
226. Adams JB, Audhya T, McDonough-Means S, et al. Effect of a vitamin/mineral supplement on children and adults with autism. BMC Pediatr 2011;11:111.
227. Mehl-Madrona L, Leung B, Kennedy C, et al. Micronutrients versus standard medication management in autism: a naturalistic case-control study. J Child Adolesc Psychopharmacol 2010;20(2):95–103.

228. Blum K, Trachtenberg MC, Elliott CE, et al. Enkephalinase inhibition and precursor amino acid loading improves inpatient treatment of alcohol and polydrug abusers: double-blind placebo-controlled study of the nutritional adjunct SAAVE. Alcohol 1988;5(6):481–93.

229. Blum K, Trachtenberg MC, Ramsay JC. Improvement of inpatient treatment of the alcoholic as a function of neurotransmitter restoration: a pilot study. Int J Addict 1988;23(9):991–8.

230. Blum K, Trachtenberg MC. Neurogenetic deficits caused by alcoholism: restoration by SAAVE, a neuronutrient intervention adjunct. J Psychoactive Drugs 1988; 20(3):297–313.

231. Brown RJ, Blum K, Trachtenberg MC. Neurodynamics of relapse prevention: a neuronutrient approach to outpatient DUI offenders. J Psychoactive Drugs 1990;22(2):173–87.

232. Guenther RM. The role of nutritional therapy in alcoholism treatment. Int J Biosoc Res 1983;4(1):5–18.

233. Poulos CJ. What effects do corrective nutritional practices have on alcoholics? Orthomolecular Psychiatr 1981;10(1):61–4.

234. Blum K, Allison D, Trachtenberg MC, et al. Reduction of both drug hunger and withdrawal against advice rate of cocaine abusers in a 30-day inpatient program by the neuronutrient Tropamine. Curr Ther Res 1988;43(6):1204–14.

235. Grima NA, Pase MP, Macpherson H, et al. The effects of multivitamins on cognitive performance: a systematic review and meta-analysis. J Alzheimers Dis 2012;29(3):561–9.

236. Kesse-Guyot E, Fezeu L, Jeandel C, et al. French adults' cognitive performance after daily supplementation with antioxidant vitamins and minerals at nutritional doses: a post hoc analysis of the Supplementation in Vitamins and Mineral Antioxidants (SU.VI.MAX) trial. Am J Clin Nutr 2011;94(3):892–9.

237. Neri M, Andermarcher E, Pradel JM, et al. Influence of a double blind pharmacological trial on two domains of well-being in subjects with age associated memory impairment. Arch Gerontol Geriatr 1995;21(3):241–52.

238. Summers WK, Martin RL, Cunningham M, et al. Complex antioxidant blend improves memory in community-dwelling seniors. J Alzheimers Dis 2010;19(2): 429–39.

239. Wouters-Wesseling W, Wagenaar LW, Rozendaal M, et al. Effect of an enriched drink on cognitive function in frail elderly persons. J Gerontol A Biol Sci Med Sci 2005;60(2):265–70.

240. Cockle SM, Haller J, Kimber S, et al. The influence of multivitamins on cognitive function and mood in the elderly. Aging Ment Health 2000;4(4):339–53.

241. Kang JH, Cook NR, Manson JE, et al. Vitamin E, vitamin C, beta carotene, and cognitive function among women with or at risk of cardiovascular disease: The Women's Antioxidant and Cardiovascular Study. Circulation 2009;119(21): 2772–80.

242. Manders M, De Groot LC, Hoefnagels WH, et al. The effect of a nutrient dense drink on mental and physical function in institutionalized elderly people. J Nutr Health Aging 2009;13(9):760–7.

243. McNeill G, Avenell A, Campbell MK, et al. Effect of multivitamin and multimineral supplementation on cognitive function in men and women aged 65 years and over: a randomised controlled trial. Nutr J 2007;6:10.

244. Kang JH, Cook N, Manson J, et al. A trial of B vitamins and cognitive function among women at high risk of cardiovascular disease. Am J Clin Nutr 2008; 88(6):1602–10.

245. Alavi Naeini AM, Elmadfa I, Djazayery A, et al. The effect of antioxidant vitamins E and C on cognitive performance of the elderly with mild cognitive impairment in Isfahan, Iran: a double-blind, randomized, placebo-controlled trial. Eur J Nutr 2013. [Epub ahead of print].
246. Gariballa S, Forster S. Effects of dietary supplements on depressive symptoms in older patients: a randomised double-blind placebo-controlled trial. Clin Nutr 2007;26(5):545–51.
247. Grodstein F, O'Brien J, Kang JH, et al. Long-term multivitamin supplementation and cognitive function in men: a randomized trial. Ann Intern Med 2013;159(12): 806–14.
248. Smith A, Clark R, Nutt D, et al. Anti-oxidant vitamins and mental performance of the elderly. Hum Psychopharmacol 1999;14(7):459–71.
249. Wolters M, Hickstein M, Flintermann A, et al. Cognitive performance in relation to vitamin status in healthy elderly German women: the effect of 6-month multivitamin supplementation. Prev Med 2005;41(1):253–9.
250. Cardoso BR, Cominetti C, Cozzolino SM. Importance and management of micronutrient deficiencies in patients with Alzheimer's disease. Clin Interv Aging 2013;8:531–42.
251. Gillette-Guyonnet S, Secher M, Vellas B. Nutrition and neurodegeneration: epidemiological evidence and challenges for future research. Br J Clin Pharmacol 2013;75(3):738–55.
252. Smith PJ, Blumenthal JA. Diet and neurocognition: review of evidence and methodological considerations. Curr Aging Sci 2010;3(1):57–66.
253. Vassallo N, Scerri C. Mediterranean diet and dementia of the Alzheimer type. Curr Aging Sci 2013;6(2):150–62.
254. Carroll D, Ring C, Suter M, et al. The effects of an oral multivitamin combination with calcium, magnesium, and zinc on psychological well-being in healthy young male volunteers: a double-blind placebo-controlled trial. Psychopharmacology (Berl) 2000;150(2):220–5.
255. Kennedy DO, Veasey R, Watson A, et al. Effects of high-dose B vitamin complex with vitamin C and minerals on subjective mood and performance in healthy males. Psychopharmacology (Berl) 2010;211(1):55–68.
256. Kennedy DO, Veasey RC, Watson AW, et al. Vitamins and psychological functioning: a mobile phone assessment of the effects of a B vitamin complex, vitamin C and minerals on cognitive performance and subjective mood and energy. Hum Psychopharmacol 2011;26(4–5):338–47.
257. Scholey A, Bauer I, Neale C, et al. Acute effects of different multivitamin mineral preparations with and without guaraná on mood, cognitive performance and functional brain activation. Nutrients 2013;5(9):3589–604.
258. Kennedy DO, Haskell CF, Robertson B, et al. Improved cognitive performance and mental fatigue following a multi-vitamin and mineral supplement with added guarana (*Paullinia cupana*). Appetite 2008;50:506–13.
259. Willemsen MS, Petchot-Bacqué JP, Alleaume B, et al. A double-blind placebo-controlled study of the effects of an oral multivitamin combination with calcium and magnesium on psychological well-being and cardiovascular reactions to stress in healthy young male volunteers. Europ J Clin Research 1997;9:175–84.
260. Benton D. Micro-nutrient supplementation and the intelligence of children. Neurosci Biobehav Rev 2001;25(4):297–309.
261. Eilander A, Gera T, Sachdev HS, et al. Multiple micronutrient supplementation for improving cognitive performance in children: systematic review of randomized controlled trials. Am J Clin Nutr 2010;91(1):115–30.

262. Manger MS, McKenzie JE, Winichagoon P, et al. A micronutrient-fortified seasoning powder reduces morbidity and improves short-term cognitive function, but has no effect on anthropometric measures in primary school children in northeast Thailand: a randomized controlled trial. Am J Clin Nutr 2008; 87(6):1715–22.

263. Schoenthaler SJ, Amos SP, Eysenck HJ, et al. Controlled trial of vitamin-mineral supplementation: effects on intelligence and performance. Person Individ Diff 1991;12(4):351–62.

264. Vazir S, Nagalla B, Thangiah V, et al. Effect of micronutrient supplement on health and nutritional status of schoolchildren: mental function. Nutrition 2006; 22(Suppl 1):S26–32.

265. Wang Y, Yin S, Zhao X, et al. Study on the effect of micronutrients supplementation on health status of children. Wei Sheng Yan Jiu 2003;32(5):455–8 [in Chinese].

266. Carroll JB. Human cognitive abilities: a survey of factor-analytic studies. New York: Cambridge University Press; 1993.

267. Haskell CF, Scholey AB, Jackson PA, et al. Cognitive and mood effects in healthy children during 12 weeks' supplementation with multi-vitamin/minerals. Br J Nutr 2008;100(5):1086–96.

268. Long SJ, Benton D. Effects of vitamin and mineral supplementation on stress, mild psychiatric symptoms, and mood in nonclinical samples: a meta-analysis. Psychosom Med 2013;75(2):144–53.

269. Harris E, Kirk J, Rowsell R, et al. The effect of multivitamin supplementation on mood and stress in healthy older men. Hum Psychopharmacol 2011;26(8): 560–7.

270. Long SJ, Benton D. A double-blind trial of the effect of docosahexaenoic acid and vitamin and mineral supplementation on aggression, impulsivity, and stress. Hum Psychopharmacol 2013;28(3):238–47.

271. Schlebusch L, Bosch BA, Polglase G, et al. A double-blind, placebo-controlled, double-centre study of the effects of an oral multivitamin-mineral combination on stress. S Afr Med J 2000;90(12):1216–23.

272. Popovic IC. Neurotropic vitamin-mineral combination in the therapy of stress: results of a multi-centre study among general practitioners in Switzerland. Schweiz Zschr Ganzheitsmedizin [Swiss Journal of Integrative Medicine] 1993;3:140–3 [in German].

273. Selishchev GS, Petchot-Bacqué JP, Volkov AK, et al. An open non-comparative study on the efficacy of an oral multivitamin combination containing calcium and magnesium on persons permanently exposed to occupational stress - predisposing factors. J Clin Res 1998;1:303–15.

274. Haskell CF, Robertson B, Jones E, et al. Effects of a multi-vitamin/mineral supplement on cognitive function and fatigue during extended multi-tasking. Hum Psychopharmacol 2010;25(6):448–61.

275. Stough C, Scholey A, Lloyd J, et al. The effect of 90 day administration of a high dose vitamin B-complex on work stress. Hum Psychopharmacol 2011;26(7): 470–6.

276. Camfield DA, Wetherell MA, Scholey AB, et al. The effects of multivitamin supplementation on diurnal cortisol secretion and perceived stress. Nutrients 2013;5(11):4429–50.

277. Pipingas A, Camfield DA, Stough C, et al. The effects of multivitamin supplementation on mood and general well-being in healthy young adults. A laboratory and at-home mobile phone assessment. Appetite 2013;69:123–36.

278. Sarris J, Cox KH, Camfield DA, et al. Participant experiences from chronic administration of a multivitamin versus placebo on subjective health and well-being: a double-blind qualitative analysis of a randomised controlled trial. Nutr J 2012;11:110.

279. Heseker H, Kübler W, Pudel V, et al. Psychological disorders as early symptoms of a mild-to-moderate vitamin deficiency. Ann N Y Acad Sci 1992;669:352–7.

280. Li X, Huang WX, Lu JM, et al. Effects of a multivitamin/multimineral supplement on young males with physical overtraining: a placebo-controlled, randomized, double-blinded cross-over trial. Biomed Environ Sci 2013;26(7):599–604.

281. Rucklidge J, Johnstone J, Harrison R, et al. Micronutrients reduce stress and anxiety in adults with attention-deficit/hyperactivity disorder following a 7.1 earthquake. Psychiatry Res 2011;189(2):281–7.

282. Rucklidge JJ, Blampied NM. Post-earthquake psychological functioning in adults with attention-deficit/hyperactivity disorder: positive effects of micronutrients on resilience. NZ J Psychol 2011;40(4):51–7.

283. Rucklidge JJ, Andridge R, Gorman B, et al. Shaken but unstirred? Effects of micronutrients on stress and trauma after an earthquake: RCT evidence comparing formulas and doses. Hum Psychopharmacol 2012;27(5):440–54.

284. Rucklidge JJ, Blampied N, Gorman B, et al. Psychological functioning 1 year after a brief intervention using micronutrients to treat stress and anxiety related to the 2011 Christchurch earthquakes: a naturalistic follow-up. Hum Psychopharmacol 2014;29(3):230–43.

285. Simpson JS, Crawford SG, Goldstein ET, et al. Systematic review of safety and tolerability of a complex micronutrient formula used in mental health. BMC Psychiatry 2011;11:62.

286. Rucklidge JJ. Could yeast infections impair recovery from mental illness? A case study using micronutrients and olive leaf extract for the treatment of ADHD and depression. Adv Mind Body Med 2013;27(3):14–8.

287. Halliwell C. Dietary choline and vitamin/mineral supplement for recovery from early cortical injury [Master of Science thesis]. Department of Psychology and Neuroscience, Faculty of Arts and Sciences, University of Lethbridge, Lethbridge, Alberta, Canada; 2003. Available at: https://www.uleth.ca/dspace/handle/10133/222.

288. Halliwell C, Kolb B. Vitamin/mineral supplements enhance recovery from perinatal cortical lesions in rats [abstract]. Soc Neurosci Abs 2003;29:459.11 [Poster presented with title "Diet can stimulate functional recovery and cerebral plasticity after perinatal cortical injury in rats"].

289. Halliwell C, Comeau W, Gibb R, et al. Factors influencing frontal cortex development and recovery from early frontal injury. Dev Neurorehabil 2009;12(5):269–78.

290. Kolb B, Teskey GC, Gibb R. Factors influencing cerebral plasticity in the normal and injured brain. Front Hum Neurosci 2010;4:204.

291. Kolb B, Mychasiuk R, Muhammad A, et al. Brain plasticity in the developing brain. Prog Brain Res 2013;207:35–64.

292. Kolb B, Mychasiuk R, Muhammad A, et al. Experience and the developing prefrontal cortex. Proc Natl Acad Sci U S A 2012;109(Suppl 2):17186–93.

293. Wurtman RJ. A nutrient combination that can affect synapse formation. Nutrients 2014;6(4):1701–10.

294. Wurtman RJ. Non-nutritional uses of nutrients. Eur J Pharmacol 2011;668(Suppl 1):S10–5.

295. Morrison RD, Blobaum AL, Byers FW, et al. The role of aldehyde oxidase and xanthine oxidase in the biotransformation of a novel negative allosteric

modulator of metabotropic glutamate receptor subtype 5. Drug Metab Dispos 2012;40(9):1834–45.

296. Xu Q, Parks CG, DeRoo LA, et al. Multivitamin use and telomere length in women. Am J Clin Nutr 2009;89(6):1857–63.

297. Fortmann SP, Burda BU, Senger CA, et al. Vitamin, mineral, and multivitamin supplements for the primary prevention of cardiovascular disease and cancer: a systematic evidence review for the US Preventive Services Task Force. Rockville (MD): Agency for Healthcare Research and Quality (US); 2013. Report No: 14-05199-EF-1. U.S. Preventive Services Task Force Evidence Syntheses, formerly Systematic Evidence Reviews. Available at: http://www.ncbi.nlm.nih.gov/pubmedhealth/PMH0060787/.

298. Macpherson H, Pipingas A, Pase MP. Multivitamin-multimineral supplementation and mortality: a meta-analysis of randomized controlled trials. Am J Clin Nutr 2013;97(2):437–44.

299. Chang SM. Should meta-analyses trump observational studies? Am J Clin Nutr 2013;97(2):237–8.

300. Hemilä H. Vitamin supplements and mortality in older people. Am J Clin Nutr 2013;98(2):502.

301. Macpherson H, Pipingas A, Pase MP. Reply to H Hemilä. Am J Clin Nutr 2013; 98(2):502–3.

302. Lawson KA, Wright ME, Subar A, et al. Multivitamin use and risk of prostate cancer in the National Institutes of Health-AARP Diet and Health Study. J Natl Cancer Inst 2007;99(10):754–64.

303. Mursu J, Robien K, Harnack LJ, et al. Dietary supplements and mortality rate in older women: the Iowa Women's Health Study. Arch Intern Med 2011;171(18): 1625–33.

304. Omenn GS, Goodman GE, Thornquist MD, et al. Effects of a combination of beta carotene and vitamin A on lung cancer and cardiovascular disease. N Engl J Med 1996;334:1150–5.

305. Watkins ML, Erickson JD, Thun MJ, et al. Multivitamin use and mortality in a large prospective study. Am J Epidemiol 2000;152(2):149–62.

306. Bjelakovic G, Nikolova D, Gluud LL, et al. Antioxidant supplements for prevention of mortality in healthy participants and patients with various diseases. Cochrane Database Syst Rev 2008;(2):CD007176.

307. Druesne-Pecollo N, Latino-Martel P, Norat T, et al. Beta-carotene supplementation and cancer risk: a systematic review and metaanalysis of randomized controlled trials. Int J Cancer 2010;127(1):172–84.

308. Ristow M, Zarse K, Oberbach A, et al. Antioxidants prevent health-promoting effects of physical exercise in humans. Proc Natl Acad Sci U S A 2009;106:8665–70.

309. Roswall N, Larsen S, Friis S, et al. Micronutrient intake and risk of prostate cancer in a cohort of middle-aged, Danish men. Cancer Causes Control 2013;24(6): 1129–35.

310. Satia JA, Littman A, Slatore CG, et al. Long-term use of beta-carotene, retinol, lycopene, and lutein supplements and lung cancer risk: results from the VITamins And Lifestyle (VITAL) study. Am J Epidemiol 2009;169:815–28 [Erratum regarding dosing error in Am J Epidemiol 2009;169:1409].

311. Zhang SM, Cook NR, Albert CM, et al. Effect of combined folic acid, vitamin B6, and vitamin B12 on cancer risk in women: a randomized trial. JAMA 2008;300: 2012–21.

312. Comerford KB. Recent developments in multivitamin/mineral research. Adv Nutr 2013;4(6):644–56.

Index

Note: Page numbers of article titles are in **boldface** type.

A

Acceptance and commitment therapy (ACT), 492
ACT. *See* Acceptance and commitment therapy (ACT)
ADHD. *See* Attention-deficit/hyperactivity disorder (ADHD)
Affective disorders
    in children and adolescents
        music therapy and music medicine for, 538
Aggressive behaviors
    HUFAs and, 571–573
    music therapy and music medicine for
        effectiveness research related to, 542
Agricultural developments
    unfortunate dietary consequences of, 560–562
Antisocial behavior
    in youth and adults, 621–624
Anxiety disorders
    management of
        music therapy and music medicine in
            effectiveness research related to, 544–545
        NF in, 444–445, 450–451
        relaxation therapy in
            studies with youth and family, 515–516
Attention-deficit/hyperactivity disorder (ADHD)
    EEG power spectrum regulation in, 439
    HUFA abnormalities in, 563–566
    HUFA supplementation in youth with, 566–571
        meta-analyses and reviews of, 570–571
    management of
        broad-spectrum micronutrients in, 624–629
        music therapy and music medicine in
            effectiveness research related to, 542
        NF in, 470–474
            in comorbidity with substance use disorders, 446–447
        pharmacologic, 570
        SYM in, 508–510
        Tai Chi in
            studies with youth and family, 519–520
    TM for
        studies with youth and family, 510–511
Attention-deficit/hyperactivity disorder (ADHD)–type symptoms
    HUFA supplementation in youth with, 566–571

Child Adolesc Psychiatric Clin N Am 23 (2014) 673–685
http://dx.doi.org/10.1016/S1056-4993(14)00054-6
1056-4993/14/$ – see front matter © 2014 Elsevier Inc. All rights reserved.

childpsych.theclinics.com

Printed and bound by CPI Group (UK) Ltd, Croydon, CR0 4YY

03/10/2024

01040492-0008